SIGHT CORRECTION

Peculiar Bodies: Stories and Histories

CAROLYN DAY, CHRIS MOUNSEY, AND WENDY J. TURNER, EDITORS

SIGHT CORRECTION

Vision and Blindness in
Eighteenth-Century Britain

CHRIS MOUNSEY

UNIVERSITY OF VIRGINIA PRESS
Charlottesville & London

UNIVERSITY OF VIRGINIA PRESS
© 2019 by the Rector and Visitors of the University of Virginia
All rights reserved

ISBN 978-0-8139-4331-2 (cloth)
ISBN 978-0-8139-4332-9 (paper)
ISBN 978-0-8139-4333-6 (ebook)

First published 2019

1 3 5 7 9 8 6 4 2

Library of Congress Cataloging-in-Publication Data
is available for this title.

Cover art: Detail from *Recueil de planches, sur les sciences, les arts libéraux, et les arts méchaniques: avec leur explication*, vol. 2, part 2, plate XXIV, 1762. (Flory/iStock)

CONTENTS

ACKNOWLEDGMENTS   vii

PART I. Philosophy

1. Philosophy, Sight, and Blindnes   3
2. Blindness Is Not a "Disability": Before Compulsory Able-Bodiedness   16
3. Text as Theory: Understanding Sight and Blindness in the Eighteenth Century   39

PART II. Medicine

4. Unofficial Eye Care: William Read and Mary Cater   65
5. Official Eye Care: William Cheselden and Peter Kennedy   105
6. A Profession of Couching: John "Chevalier" Taylor   129
7. Free and Accessible Eye Care for All: John Taylor, Oculist of Hatton Garden   168

PART III. Lives

8. Thomas Gills of St. Edmunds-Bury and the Itinerant Giver   199
9. John Maxwell: The Beauty of Gardens   224
10. Priscilla Pointon Gets Married   250

NOTES   277
SELECTED BIBLIOGRAPHY   315
INDEX   325

ACKNOWLEDGMENTS

I would like first and foremost to thank Stan Booth, who has been my eyes over the years, from our first trips to York, to the conferences where most of the chapters were first read, to the preparation of the manuscript. You've always had faith in me. Thanks also to the Access to Work program, which has helped you be beside me when I needed you most.

Thanks also to my students, who have always listened to my ideas as they developed and told me when I was being stupid.

Thanks also to my family, John and Fernando, Barbara and Ben, who put up with me going on and on about blind people and cataract operations.

Last but not least, thanks to the anonymous readers who helped me turn this from a quarter of a million words to something, I hope, more manageable. Your wisdom is worth more than gold.

PART I

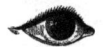

PHILOSOPHY

1

PHILOSOPHY, SIGHT, AND BLINDNESS

"Seeing" the Truth

The truth in eighteenth-century Enlightenment philosophy, argues Michel Foucault, can be understood in metaphors of sight and blindness: "What allows man to resume contact with childhood and rediscover the permanent birth of truth is this bright, distant, open naïvety of the gaze. Hence the two great mythical experiences on which the philosophy of the eighteenth century wished to found its beginning: the foreign spectator in an unknown country and the man-born-blind restored to the light."[1] In this quote, "the two great mythical experiences" of sight were, it is true, often used as rhetorical devices, but just as Oliver Goldsmith's *Chinese Letters*[2] can be met with the accounts of real travelers to Britain such as Karl Philipp Moritz,[3] so can metaphors of the restoration of sight to the blind be met with couching, the operation to remove a cataract from the eye, which became commonplace during the eighteenth century.[4]

This book explores the realities behind the metaphors of sight, as I live a life where blindness is no metaphor and find many visual metaphors for truth disappointingly vague. Do you see what I mean? Am I writing clearly? I do not know what it would be like to see again clearly. Nor what exactly is seeing. Did I ever see clearly? How would I know? Instead, I will explore blindness from an empirical standpoint, in a way not dissimilar to that of the eighteenth century. The first section of this book, therefore, begins with a discussion about blindness in terms of disability theory and argues that instead of working from a theoretical starting point, either the medical model of disability or the cultural model of disability, a historical study might better begin with the lives of historical people. Blindness and sight were, as now, lived experiences; that is, experiences lived by people who are as like ourselves as they are different from us, following the expectation of Variability,[5] that all people are "the same only different" from one another.

Variability, however, is by no means transhistorical, as it would expect blind people in the eighteenth century to be different from blind people in the twenty-first century in the way they were treated or understood, in the same way that we would expect that every person in each century had different experiences of and with their peculiar abilities. But Variability would nevertheless expect that someone who was blind in the eighteenth century would have similar difficulties in, say, accessing text, as blind people in the twenty-first century, although they would understand themselves in a different way and expect different solutions. Above all, Variability would not suggest that difference was binary and define disability against its absence in a term such as "compulsory able-bodiedness." Deaf people in the eighteenth century were as different from blind people as they were different from those who thought themselves normal. There never was a reference point of "normal" that defined those who were not. Variability would expect that every "normal" person was as different (Variable) as every other "normal" person.

Variability is a way of analyzing that enshrines uniqueness, has the patience to discover the peculiarities of each individual, and by so doing captures particular people rather than an "institutionalized representation of disabled people." As such it is a useless concept for those who are seeking "power relations" between groups who define themselves against an "other." But it is a good way to notice individuals in history.

What is different between individual variable people is our capability to live with the peculiar capacity of the body in which we live. Capability I understand as the mind's facility to accept differences in physical (or mental) capacity and live with it or deny it. Some can accept the physical constraints of visual impairment, some find it harder. Capability is experiential and nonjudgmental. It is not predictable and adds to the peculiarity of an individual. And it is another element to be added to capacity as a way of noticing people encountered in our own lives and in historical research. But if it is argued that I have set up yet another binary between capacity as body and capability as mind, it must be remembered that capacity and capability only become apparent in encounters with people (in our lives or in our research), and the three exist as a triplet.

What I want to maintain in the expectation of Variability is the immediacy of individual lived experience. I believe that the three elements capacity, capability, and encounter (which are meant only to illuminate the central word) can help to guide the analysis of historical experience and highlight the relationship between body, mind, and other people. However successful the method might be thought to be—and it is intended to be little more than a set of linked concepts from which to tell the story of a life—Rosemarie Garland-Thomson noted at the first Variabilities conference that it marked a move from objective study to subjective study of impaired people. As Variability develops, I hope that the increasing number of individual examples begs the question of why we need a unifying concept at all.

In 2011, Dwight Christopher Gabbard defined "disability studies" as "a uniquely interdisciplinary field operating in the humanities, social sciences, and legal studies as well as in public policy, education, health, and medicine."[6] While this is certainly so and must be celebrated, "disability studies" has always had a conflicted relationship with health and medicine as curative: as (re)making "normal." If anything, however, the hard line originally taken has begun to soften, while it remains true that "disability studies is not the same as, and frequently is at odds with, the medical, therapeutic, and rehabilitative sciences oriented toward treating disability. Indeed, the field was born in opposition to these traditional orientations [but] at present can be said to be in conversation with them."[7]

This book began as one of those conversations, and in the interplay between its three parts we shall find that, as in any good conversation, the entrenched positions of the medical model and the cultural models of "disability" are transformed.

In Lieu of a Medical Model of Disability

The second section of the book explores the way in which people with sight problems were understood from a medical perspective. It finds that by the end of the century, John Taylor had worked out a method of delivering properly financed and genuinely free eye care at the point of delivery for the poor blind, a goal not fully realized for other branches of medical care until the British National Health Service provision after the Second World War.

The road to John Taylor of Hatton Garden's utopia of eye health was not straight, and the story of getting there is peopled with characters who would be more at home in the dramatic than the operating theater. The section begins with the official baddy Sir William Read, who called himself "The Accomplish'd Oculist," and who became oculist in ordinary for William III, Queen Anne, and George I, but who struggled to make a living out of eye surgery and has been remembered only as a quack. We also meet a woman practitioner, Mary Cater, who refused to operate on eyes, preferring to use herbal preparations. Her preparations, though effective throughout her thirty-year career, were derided by Read and only advertised after his death. Next is the official hero, William Cheselden, behind whose mask we shall find was exposed a fast operator whose malpractice was openly attacked by the specialist eye doctor Peter Kennedy, and whose botched couching of the boy William Taylor, which was made famous by Condillac and Foucault as an example of the "blind made to see," left his patient always unable to tell his cat from his dog except by touch. Lastly before John Taylor of Hatton Garden, we meet a tortured and misunderstood showman, John "Chevalier" Taylor, who might be the prototype for the twentieth-century pianist-entertainer Liberace, complete with bejewelled buttons and pectoral cross, but who was also the best and most accomplished operator on eyes in Europe in the eighteenth century.

The problem, however, is not only how to present the complex story but how to discuss the development of ophthalmology without interpreting historical data from a twentieth-century perspective. If I were writing a history of ophthalmology in the eighteenth century, I would ignore England and concentrate on technical developments in France and the pioneering work of Antoine Maître-Jean, in *Traité des maladies de l'oeil* (Treatise on eye diseases, 1707), Pierre Brisseau in *Traité de la cataracte et du glaucoma* (Treatise on cataracts and glaucoma, 1709); Charles de Saint Yves in *Nouveau traité des maladies des yeux où l'on expose leur structure, leur usage, les causes de leurs maladies, leurs symptômes, les remèdes et les opérations de chirurgie qui conviennent le plus à leur guérison, avec de nouvelles découvertes sur la structure de l'oeil, qui prouvent l'organe immédiat de la vue* (New treatise of eye diseases, with description of eye structures and uses, the origins of their illnesses along with their symptoms, the most appropriate remedies and surgery treatments, including new discoveries concerning eye structure that prove the exact location of sight, 1722); and Francois Pourfour du Petit in *Lettre dans laquelle il est demonstre que la crystallin est fort près de l'uvee, et ou l'on rapporte de nouvelles preuves de l'operation de la cataracte* (Letter demonstrating that the lens is very close to the uvea, and in which evidence is reported on the operation for cataract, 1729). These publications laid out much of the development in the treatment of blindness in its various forms, and of them, Saint-Yves's *Treatise* might be called the European reference book on blindness. It was republished in French in Amsterdam (1736) and Leipzig (1767), and translated into German (Berlin, 1730), Dutch (1739), English (London, 1741 and 1744), and Italian (Venice, 1750, 1768, and 1781). The advances in France were perhaps no surprise as the French system of medical education was predicated upon specialism as the mark of a successful career. The opposite was the case in Britain, where general practice was the guiding principle.

The English word "empirick" in the seventeenth century was applied disparagingly to a medical practitioner who specialized in one type of cure. The *OED* tells us that the word was used "in direct or implied contrast to the approach of Galen, whose rational system formed the intellectual basis of Western medicine until the early modern period, and whose disparaging view of the rival empiric school has tended to invest the term with negative connotations in most medical contexts."[8] Francis Bacon recalled a conversation with Queen Elizabeth in which the disparagement of specialist medicine became a key to a point of politics:

> I call to mind, her Majesty was speaking of a Fellow that undertook to cure, or at least to ease my Brother of his Gout, and asked me how it went forwards? And I told her Majesty, that at first he received good by it, but after, in the course of his Cure, he found himself at a stay, or rather worse: The Queen said again, I will tell you, Bacon, the Errour of it; The manner of these Physitians, and especially these Empiricks, is, to continue one kind of medicine, which, at the first, is proper, being to draw out the ill humour; but after, they have not the discretion to change their medicine, but apply still drawing medicines, when they should rather intend to cure and corroborate the part.[9]

Although the OED suggests the use of the term, and presumably the disparagement of empirical medicine, was curtailed in "the early modern period," it can still be found in the middle of the eighteenth century even in the titles of books disparaging forms of medical practice.[10] And the separation between generalists and empiricks continued into the English history of medicine until the twentieth century in the use of the terms "Orthodoxy" and "the Quacks" in the most comprehensive history of eye care to date.

Robert Rutson James's *Studies in the History of Ophthalmology in England Prior to the year 1800* is the work of a former consulting ophthalmic eye surgeon to St. George's Hospital, London.[11] According to his obituary's report, Rutson James lacked "the temperament of a surgeon," and "his best work was done as secretary and editor of the Ophthalmological Society and editor of the *British Journal of Ophthalmology*," where his publications were described as "models of accuracy."[12] The chapters in *Studies in the History of Ophthalmology* Rutson James himself described as "abstractions" of papers published elsewhere, as "superficial" and "not ... exhaustive,"[13] which might be argued to be the result of his early retirement to Suffolk and occasional journeys to the British Museum for research. For example, in his very brief biography of Peter Kennedy, he notes the *Ophthalmographia; or a treatise of the eye, in two parts*,[14] but not the *Supplement to Kennedy's Ophthalmographia*,[15] which was published twenty-six years later, in which the specialist eye surgeon attacks the generalist William Cheselden for his botched operation on the boy.

Thus, where Rutson James's chapters on the eighteenth century, "the heyday of ophthalmic quackery," begins with a separation of "Orthodoxy" and "The Quacks" (whom I shall call sheep and goats as this book questions the use of the word "quack"), we must be careful in accepting his judgment. He claims, for example, that "Cheselden's operation of iridotomy is a landmark in our science."[16] But whether or not it might have been so in the twentieth century, Peter Kennedy's *Supplement* noted that the only time Cheselden performed the operation, it, too, was botched, such that Mrs. Crome of Deptford was barely able to distinguish a four-inch-long key.[17] Rutson James dismissed what he knew of Kennedy's work as "ophthalmologically speaking, worthless" but nevertheless called Kennedy "an honest man" since "In his remarks on any condition which he considers incurable he usually ends up 'as I look at it as an incurable disease, I leave it.'"[18]

But if Kennedy was an honest man and Rutson James had access to Kennedy's *Supplement*, what would he have thought of the iridotomy? Would he have accepted his honest man's judgment? Historical counterfactuals are never useful as they cannot be resolved. But then the question is nevertheless begged: just because the iridotomy has become "a landmark" of ophthalmology, should it be considered "a landmark" in its context when its use was thought to be negligible and its efficacy questionable? Mrs. Crome, Kennedy tells us, would not have been able to marry her husband had she been totally blind, but Kennedy tells us that Cheselden had spoiled her visual acuity by couching her as well as performing the iridotomy. In the event, although Cheselden continued to advertise his patented iris operation, he is not recorded ever to have performed it again.[19]

Likewise, when *Studies in the History of Ophthalmology* tackles John Taylor, oculist of Hatton Garden,[20] Rutson James claims that he made his fortune from quack remedies and that "No hospital was founded."[21] Nevertheless, he goes on to quote from the lyrics of the foundation anthem, which was set by the musician William Boyce, though Rutson James mistakenly claims the poem itself was by "a certain Mr. Boyce."[22] Would such a major musician set lyrics for the foundation of a hospital that never existed? Handel's *Messiah* is associated with the Foundling Hospital, and that was a large building, necessarily so as there were so many illegitimate children or children of paupers in London. But the first eye hospital had no need to be a larger building than the single dwelling at No. 6 Hatton Garden as there was little need for aftercare. And John Taylor, the son of the oculist of Hatton Garden, notes that he was brought up in another house in Highgate, leaving the Hatton Garden property vacant for patients if they needed to remain for a while to recover from their surgery; and William Taylor of Ightham, the boy who was born blind, is recorded to have stayed in John Taylor's house in Hatton Garden after his first eye was couched.

If our official hero was a bungler who made a chance innovation, and the founder of the first eye clinic a peddler of quack remedies, how, then, should they best be recorded in history? And how the other sheep and goats? The present state of "our science" employed by Rutson James is not an appropriate measure.

William Read may not have known what a "gutta serena" was, but he was able to couch a cataract and remove a spot from a lens. His newspaper advertisements for his practice can be found from 1696 until his death in 1715, and he named many of those whom he cured. Likewise, John "Chevalier" Taylor was outrageous, but he was also outrageously successful. Encomiums to his skill queue as long in his autobiography as the patients for his curing hand. He cannot have been a bungler. No matter how outrageous his manner and dress, so many thousands of people would not have offered him their eyes without hope of cure. But nor can we believe that either of these itinerant ophthalmic operators "cut and ran," as Roy Porter argued, suggesting that "it made better sense for the irregular doctor to be itinerant (mobility . . . gave the unscrupulous the advantage of being able to make himself scarce before his failures became obvious to all)."[23]

William Read's and John "Chevalier" Taylor's itineraries were advertised well in advance, and they also advertised (as the itineraries show) that they would return to visit their patients within two weeks of a procedure. Furthermore, William Read's address in Durham Yard on the River Thames side of the Strand was advertised weekly throughout his career, and when he was out on tour his wife remained at home, trained by him to perform any couching operations for those who called.

Nor can it be argued that the difference between Rutson James's sheep and goats was that the first were hospital-trained doctors whereas the second were apprentices like Lady Read. William Cheselden was also trained by apprenticeship to two doctors (Fern and Cowper) and passed his exams for the Company of Barbers and Surgeons on 29 January 1711 without taking a degree, which was not thought necessary for a surgeon. And it was he who trained John "Chevalier" Taylor, and the Chevalier who trained his son John Taylor, oculist of Hatton Garden. To be sure, no one knows who taught William Read how to couch a cataract, to treat a breast cancer, or to correct a harelip. However, his extensive travels throughout England took him regularly to Norwich, and it is not out of the question to argue that as a boy John "Chevalier" Taylor watched him operate in that town and determined in 1729 to make a "profession of Couching."

If anything differed in the practice of Rutson James's sheep and goats, it is their method of advertising their profession. Whereas the sheep were ensconced in hospitals with patient streams bringing their work to them, the goats were on the road searching for patients and therefore advertising their skills in newspapers. The sheep wrote textbooks presenting themselves down the generations of doctors as the founding fathers of a new profession, whereas the goats left only extravagant-sounding paeans to their own skill. But we must not simply dismiss the contribution of the goats to the history of medicine. If one is successfully to advertise something, it has to be readily comprehensible what is on offer, so it is best to advertise a single product. At the same time, it is true that if one is to become skilled at a medical procedure, it is best to perform it as many times as possible. Where hospital-bound doctors in England chose to be generalists, it must be argued that this was because they had to be so. A hospital doctor had to address each patient's individual condition as they came to the hospital. But an itinerant doctor could perform one procedure—couching, for example—as he journeyed throughout England (or Europe, as did John "Chevalier" Taylor) and become very skilled in that one specialism.

At the same time, it must also be remembered that hospitals were becoming large enough that doctors could begin to specialize in a particular procedure, and Rutson James tells us that "in 1727, John Freke was placed in charge of the eye patients at St Bartholomew's Hospital, and authorized to couch for cataract; a fee of 6s. 8d. was paid for each couching."[24] Furthermore, there is little doubt that William Cheselden was probably in his day the most competent cutter for the bladder stone. But Cheselden also presented himself in his textbooks as capable of operating on eyes as well as many other organs, and claimed successfully to have performed operations for which he was not skilled. Rutson James even confirms this fact when he tells us that John Ranby, another excellent cutter for the bladder stone, was elected in 1733 to couch cataracts at St. Thomas's Hospital (Cheselden's own hospital), although he was not "formally elected a member of staff."[25] After William Read, however, most itinerant practitioners learned to advertise one procedure and were de facto specialists. And specialism is perhaps the goats' greatest contribution to the history of medicine.

This is not to read the goats as the sole founders of medical specialism but rather to acknowledge their contribution against the torrent of abuse from which they have hitherto suffered in the history of medicine. This book is intended to give a "variable" account of the medical model of "disability," drawn from close attention to evidence and context, of the differing roles of the "sheep" and "goats" already presented (in part and partially) in Rutson James's *Studies in the History of Ophthalmology* and answer the question why he included George Coats's chapters on John "Chevalier" Taylor with his own on the rest of the goats. But it is also meant to tell the story of free at the point of access eye care which began at No. 6 Hatton Garden, where a poor patient could be couched "gratis" and did not have to pay the 6s. 8d. charged in the hospitals.

In Lieu of a Cultural Model of "Disability"

The third section of the book explores the problem at the heart of writing about individual impaired people from history: finding enough information about each and deciding what counts as a legitimate source for a biographical sketch.[26] However, the strength of the method is that neither a single account, nor the sum of the three lives explored here, adds up to "A History of the Blind in the Eighteenth Century." Just as now, the life as well as the experience of vision of each person with impaired sight is different. The question might be asked: Do those blind people who leave enough biographical traces of their lives in the form of texts lend themselves to this type of study and skew the conclusions in favor of the idea that blind people were able to fend for themselves? But the answer has to be agreed that no sample so small can be used to draw an overall conclusion that other blind people did, or did not, suffer from the problems associated with the cultural model of "disability": social obstacles that disabled them, or compulsory able-bodiedness. We can only work with the evidence we have. And this, I would argue, is the strength of a variable methodology. Applying an overarching theory will always produce similar conclusions whatever amount of evidence is found, and the cultural model of "disability" would predetermine that all three blind writers explored in this book would have been "disabled" by the obstacles society put in their way, which does not appear to have been the case for any of them. Thomas Gills was moderately successful at keeping his wife and daughter fed and housed, and after a horrid experience living in London, which he made the most of in a wonderfully funny poem, he was able to return to St. Edmunds-Bury and die in his hometown, which was his dearest wish while he was stuck "in the smoke." John Maxwell was the only beneficiary from a charity in the group, but that was a chance occurrence due to his living in the city of York, where the first charity for blind people was instituted. By the time his economic method was perfected, of writing short pieces "By John Maxwell, of York, being Blind" and with long subscription lists, he had become a freeman of the city and removed himself from charitable handouts. Maxwell's method of making money by publicizing his blindness was used by Joseph Spence, who gathered a similar list for Thomas Blacklock, which financed the rest of the Scottish poet's life. Priscilla Pointon perfected the subscription list method of publication with one of the longest subscription lists of the century, which allowed her to buy a house in the place of her choice and to marry the man she loved.

None of the three blind people whom this book explores might be thought of as exceptional people who "triumphed over their disabilities . . . [to] have lives of astonishing richness and diversity." But for me it is the very ordinariness of their lives that is to be celebrated and cherished, for ordinariness is not drab or boring; rather, it shows they had lives "the same only different" from ours. We are all Variable people.

Thus as we explore the altering capacity of Thomas Gills as his paralysis and blindness came and went, we notice that his capability was unaltered. He continued to encounter the world and through unshakeable faith in his god he accepted his continually changing self as a gift to work through, and a topic to write about. Likewise, he believed he was not intelligent, so wrote catechisms that describe encounters with children, with whom he believed he shared intellectual capacity, to teach them the sort of faith he held so they too could have the capability to face the world with fortitude.

John Maxwell's and Priscilla Pointon's capacity for business links them, even though it does not signify anything that might be called a trend in the business acumen of blind people in the eighteenth century. Their visual capacities were rather different, with Maxwell being totally blind, and Pointon severely visually impaired. Nevertheless, each found they could be successful according to their capacity. Maxwell found ways to encounter nearly eight hundred individual subscribers collected over five publications in a single city over a twenty-five-year period, and Pointon traveled throughout the Midlands of England in a two-year period, encountering her 1,600 subscribers by performing in theaters. It is a question that is probably unanswerable, but it is tempting to argue that since both Maxwell and Pointon became socially acceptable through their business success (Maxwell as a freeman of York, and Pointon in marrying her sweetheart after ten years' courting), there was a link between the two. This in turn might be argued to be an aspect of the cultural model of "disability," showing Maxwell and Pointon (and Gills) struggling but eventually winning out against a tide of feeling that demanded their compulsory ablebodiedness. But this is not the case. All three writers made capital out of their lack of sight, writing about it and using it as advertisement to sell their writing.

A Note on Eighteenth-Century Newspaper Advertisements

Much of the evidence for this book comes from newspaper advertisements which are now readily available in the databases founded on the British Library collections. But finding advertisements in newspapers is fraught with difficulties. About fifteen years ago I trawled through all the original copies of all the newspapers for 1706 in the Burney Collection. I was looking for news items and advertisements about one particular event, and it took me a year to turn all the pages and scan all the issues. How many advertisements I recorded, and how many I missed because of the sheer boredom of the task, I shall never know. I stopped the search and did not go on to 1707 when I was told about the new electronic Burney Collection, which would feature searchable digital copies of the newspapers. But when that came online, it quickly became apparent that it did not solve all the problems of accurate searching through huge bodies of information. Searching is quick, but since the OCRing can be so poor that the search facility probably brings forth fewer results than the visual searching I had done years before, and when I could still barely see, though of course the searches took seconds rather than years.[27] Given also that few copies of and no full runs of early newspapers survive, finding, say, a single advertisement for 1696 should not suggest that William Read placed only one advertisement that year. Even a haul of forty advertisements for 1705 might be no more than the tip of an iceberg of lost advertisements. However, I believe that the regular occurrences of certain forms of advertisements can suggest that whoever spent the three shillings to place the advertisement was aware that they were using the news media in particular ways, and it is on this evidence, read positively and negatively, rather than the total of advertisements understood as the sum total available of evidence on which I shall base my version of Read's life, and the lives of Mary Cater, John "Chevalier" Taylor, and John Taylor, oculist of Hatton Garden.

2

BLINDNESS IS NOT A "DISABILITY"

Before Compulsory Able-Bodiedness

The "Disabled" Body?

In the latter part of the twentieth century, we "disabled" people became the object of much heated debate. Either we were not people, or we were the objects of literary theory. In 1980 Peter Singer's *Practical Ethics*[1] killed us as part of a thought experiment, an experiment in which I was an eager participant during my first year as a philosophy undergraduate at Warwick University when the book was new. I was a sheep in wolf's clothing, a "reasonable"[2] murderer who believed with Singer that "killing a disabled infant is not morally equivalent to killing a person." Little did I think then that the fact I could read only with one eye covered was the sign of worse eye problems to come. If I had known what it was like to live without sight, how differently would I have reacted to the "arguments . . . in this [Singer's] book defending euthanasia in the case of the fetus or an infant with a severe disability . . . which presuppose that life is better without a disability than with one."[3] How easy it is to be taken in by the continuation of such sentences, which explains that this is "a prejudice held by people without disabilities." But this is because Singer's is a "reasonable" project, which he defines as one "to which philosophical reasoning can contribute." And philosophical reasoning is always at one remove from the practical issues that Singer analyzes. To be sure, on one level I can understand his point about human speciesism: Why do we believe it is ethical to experiment on or eat animals and not imbeciles, when faced with the possibility that "there are intellectually disabled humans who have less claim to be regarded as self-aware or autonomous than many nonhuman animals"?[4] But even then, when I first read the book, I could only appreciate and support the argument with its secondary goal, its aim "to elevate the status of animals rather than lower the status of humans." My own future euthanasia at the heart of the thought experiment passed me by in the reasonableness of the project.

Rereading the book now, I would suggest Singer's argument must be held up to scrutiny every time he moves out of the realms of the "reasonable" and enters the practical, to discuss "the most relevant issues [which] are those that confront us daily," or at least those issues that confront us, the impaired: "It is one thing to argue that people with disabilities who want to live their lives to the full should be given every possible assistance in doing so. It is another, and quite different thing to argue that if we are in a position to choose, for our next child, whether that child will begin life with or without a disability, it is mere prejudice or bias that leads us to choose to have a child without a disability."[5] It takes a while to come to terms with the knowledge that one has an impairment, but I know few impaired people who would think like this: I know deaf parents who do not want to have hearing children who would be excluded from the deaf society in which they have lived all their lives: I know parents who have never known sight who do not wish to have a perfectly sighted child as they do not regard being sighted as a benefit.

The inevitability of Singer's syllogistic vision of the world is summed up concisely by Alison Kafer, who writes: "If disability is conceptualized as a terrible unending tragedy, then any future that includes disability can only be a future to avoid. A better future, in other words, is one that excludes disability and disabled bodies; indeed, it is the very absence of disability that signals this better future."[6] Although Singer is never this direct about the mechanistic nature of his reasonable argument, he does present the idea that it is a truth universally acknowledged that all impaired people would accept a miracle cure without side effects that would make people in wheelchairs walk (and one supposes the blind to see and the deaf to hear and the intellectually impaired to think more reasonably), and he backs up his belief with the unsubstantiated claim that the fact that many impaired people fund-raise for medical research demonstrates they would prefer a life without impairment. To make this claim, Singer must silently argue for the medical model of impairment over the cultural model; thus he suggests: "Some disabled people might say that they make this choice only because society puts so many obstacles in the way of people with disabilities. They claim that it is social conditions that disable them, not their physical or intellectual condition."[7] But this is in the nature of Singer's argument: that though "permanent" impairments lie at the far end of the spectrum of the medical model of "disease, treatment, cure," a cure will be discovered at some time in the future, and it is with this in mind that we must make our decisions about ethics in the world today. Not content with the inevitability of the logic of his reasonable argument, Singer goes on to claim that the cultural model of impairments is the source of the lies impaired people tell themselves:

> This assertion takes the simple truth that social conditions make the lives of the disabled much more difficult than they need be, and twists it into a sweeping falsehood. To be able to walk, to see, to hear, to be relatively free from pain and discomfort, to communicate effectively—all these are, under virtually any social conditions, genuine benefits. To say this is not to deny that people lacking these benefits may triumph over their disabilities and have lives of astonishing richness and diversity. Nevertheless, we show no prejudice against people with disabilities if we prefer, whether for ourselves or for our children, not to be faced with hurdles so great that to surmount them is in itself a triumph.[8]

At this point, I suspect that any impaired reader might have gotten the feeling that Peter Singer has never talked at length with a person with an impaired body. Rosemarie Garland-Thomson reminded me of this in a paper given at the first Variabilities conference held at Emory University, in Atlanta, Georgia, in 2013, and she, too, came to a similar conclusion, describing Peter Singer "as a situated person limited in his own knowing by his isolation from disabled people."[9] Garland-Thomson approaches Singer through the experience of Harriet McBryde Johnson, an impaired woman who had met Princeton's ethicist, who asked him to help her adjust her seating posture and in so doing gently challenged his reasonable conclusion about euthanizing impaired infants.

Garland-Thomson reads McBryde Johnson's "Case for My Life" beginning with its narrative and language, and the subject position in which McBryde Johnson "relegates" Singer to the third-person singular "he," in order that "Singer's awkwardness and outsider status become apparent to us . . . [so that] . . . [w]e come to understand him not as the voice of objective truth." My response to Peter Singer has so far been less consciously rhetorical but no less empirical. By turning to my own experience of my impairment, I bring evidence from one body's experience of life to make claims about others (those who might class themselves as "any impaired readers" mentioned above, for example). And thus, if I may go on speaking for others about whom I know only through the suspicion that their experiences might be the same only different from mine, I can confront Singer with a more or less united "we."

We do not triumph over our impairments to have lives of "astonishing richness and diversity" but, rather, work in the ways we can, to reach the goals we want to. Some of those goals are similar to those of people who would not count themselves impaired; some are not. Thus, like many other university professors, I have published a number of academic books. But unlike most of my colleagues, and unlike all of my students, I have set myself the goal of reading a novel every day. I do not have the attractions of the television, cinema, or visual media to divert my attention, and it takes about six hours to read a book with high-speed reading. This is not a triumph; it's the application of readily available technology that many sighted people do not notice: the audible book has a variable speed of reading, and I have learned to listen carefully.

Some of the methods I use to reach my goals are similar to those of people who would not count themselves as impaired; some are not. Thus, I have written a book to help students research and write essays. However, as a teacher I tell my students to listen to their essays using text-to-voice software, and it has improved their writing. This is a technique I would not have thought of had my eyesight not become impaired. If it had remained good, I would still be telling my students to read over their work and then print it out and read it again, marking it with a red pencil.

But nor would this innovation have been possible if software engineers had believed they had triumphed when they produced the first monotonous and hardly comprehensible text-to-voice synthesizer. Instead they continue to improve the program and have gone on to create voices like Apple's "Alex," which is barely distinguishable from that of a human, and with which I am reading Peter Singer's book at the moment as well as this introduction as it progresses paragraph by paragraph.

But how academic is this "we" from which I justify what I say, and with which I identify myself as distinct from "they" who perhaps regard themselves as unimpaired against my impairment? It could be said that what has gone before are little more than the ramblings of someone who, unlike Singer, has spent time talking to impaired people, or at least thinking about himself and others the same only different from himself. Is it possible to develop an academic rigor from the "we" that I have used, and which Rosemarie Garland-Thomson implies informs her interpretation of the language of Harriet McBryde Johnson? I believe it is, and in this introduction, I will demonstrate a methodology using the multivalent language of Variability as an alternative to the binary logic that animates Peter Singer's Anglo-American philosophical approach to ethics, as well as to the "disability studies" emphasis on the cultural model of "disability" that Singer attacks.

With One Eye on the Language of "Disability"

While it might be odd to begin a book about the history of sight and blindness in the eighteenth century in the late twentieth century, I do so as this was the time that concern for academic rigor turned to language. The poststructuralists of France attacked the assumptions of the binary logics of Anglo-American reasonableness, and for a brief moment philosophy became the most important field in the academy.[10] Among others, Jacques Derrida claimed that there was no outside of the text from which to make objective statements about truth, and Michel Foucault claimed that language was historically specific in the way "truths" gained their positivity in every different discourse.

Derrida might answer Peter Singer's claim that the medical model for "disability" was true and the cultural model a "sweeping falsehood," with the argument that there was no place outside the language of either model to make a stable truth claim about the benefit of nondisability. Foucault, in turn, might suggest that a study of the historical a prioris of neither the medical nor the cultural discourses of the eighteenth century (for example) would demonstrate that either "was closest to a primary, or ultimate, destination, which would formulate most radically the general project of a science."[11] That is, neither medical nor cultural discourse had any more truth value than the other. If their conclusions are the same, the difference between Derrida's and Foucault's approaches is characterized by their relation to history, with Derrida working synchronically and Foucault diachronically. For Derrida, meaning is always contextual, although it might be the product of a nexus of contexts. For Foucault, meaning builds up over time in an archaeological layering and is animated by the *historical a priori,* defined as, "An *a priori* not of truths that might never be said, or really given to experience; but the *a priori* of a history that is given, since it is that of things actually said."[12] Variability, the methodology and terminology which I have developed over five previous publications, picks up on Derrida's suppleness of understanding of language without going as far as slippage, that is, it argues that though words are not fixed to meanings out of context, they are more adherent to ideas than Derrida will allow: language succeeds in its intended meaning more often than it fails both within and between contexts that make up a nexus. For this reason, the durability of contexts, Variability goes further than Foucault in working with historical discourse as an account of empirical facts ("things actually said") when they gesture to the human condition.[13] This is because Variability holds to the belief that the human condition is, in certain circumstances, comprehensible across historical periods and between people without the need for a historical a priori because human bodies recognize their sameness and difference from one another, and impairment of body, such as blindness, is one such circumstance.

Peter Singer's failure to comprehend the expectations of impaired people may be explained in terms of Variability: he does not write from the experience of having an impaired body and makes unfortunate assertions about those who do as he does not recognize they are the same only different from him, while at the same time he makes the assertion that animals are the same only different from him. Another example is the fact that Rosemarie Garland-Thomson and Harriet McBryde Johnson can understand what it is for others and each other to be impaired as they both live/d their lives with impairments. But if this is the background of Variability, its rigor comes from both Derrida and Foucault, in its comprehension of the complexity of contexts in which historical a prioris are uttered. I shall begin with the example of the word "disabled," including its academic adjuncts "disability studies" and "disability history."

A History of the Word "Disabled"?

A reader using up-to-date text-to-voice software, or who is sighted, will have noticed that up to now I have not used the word "disabled" in any of its grammatical forms except in quotes from other sources, or in scare quotes.[14] This is because in the eighteenth century, the word was used in different ways from those common nowadays. The *Oxford English Dictionary* meaning #2 for "disabled"—"having a physical or mental condition which limits activity, movement, sensation, etc."—is preceded by the note: "The word disabled came to be used as the standard term in this sense in the second half of the 20th cent., and it remains the most generally accepted term in both British and North American English today."[15]

This precludes "disability history" before 1950, though the usual dates given for its start are the American Civil War or the Great War, at which times there were increased numbers of impaired men. What is important for the present project is that a search in the Burney Collection of Seventeenth- and Eighteenth-Century Newspapers[16] records 1,163 uses of the word "disabled," the earliest being in 1711, and for the first quarter of the century, the word was exclusively used to describe ships that were not serviceable for battle: "disabled from service," a fact noticed in the *Oxford English Dictionary*, which gives disabled ships as meaning #1 for "disabled." The same transitivity is recorded in the first association of "disability" with a person, the Holy Roman Emperor Charles VI, who was described in 1735 as "being disabled to continue the Pensions he paid to a great Number of his faithful Spaniards."[17] Two years later the pilot of the man-of-war

Louisa, lost at Helvoetsluys, was sentenced "to be forever disabled to pilot any Ships, or follow the Employment of Pilot in England during his Life."[18]

The first use of the term in a medical context follows the same transitive form as these and appeared in 1747, in an advertisement for a Balsamick Electuary, a medicine which is claimed to cure men with "seminal weaknesses . . . [who] are . . . wholly disabled . . . from propagating their Species."[19] In 1753, the first person who used the word "disabled" self-referentially likewise used the word in the transitive form: "Christopher Brewer . . . [who had] a very dangerous Rupture . . . that quite disabled him from getting his Bread by his daily Labours as a Journeyman Tanner; which work he was obliged to quit."[20] Brewer's use of the word "disabled" was not only transitive but ends with his cure (which was the claim for the Balsamick Electuary), and the information comes to us in an advertisement for his cure by "Mr. Woodward, Surgeon, at the King's Arms, near Half-Moon Street Piccadilly."

This brief survey suggests that for the first half of the eighteenth century the word "disabled" was not used to describe an object or person that was irreparable or incurable but rather one currently not fit for service though amenable to repair or cure. Recent work in social history has suggested that the eighteenth century was the beginning of medicalization,[21] and this pattern of use of the word "disability" demonstrates the growing strength of the medical model of "disability" at this time. However, further unpacking of the complex uses of the word "disabled" in the latter half of the century not only demonstrates that the medical model was not implied by the transitive use of the word "disabled" but that the binary between the medical and cultural models of "disability" are ultimately rendered otiose as a means of analysis of impairment in this period.

In 1745, John Griffin, Mariner, published *Proposals for the relief and support of maimed, aged, and disabled seamen, in the merchants service of Great Britain*. His idea was to set up a hospital for merchant mariners along the lines of Les Invalides in Paris,[22] and the Chelsea Hospital in London, but once again, the description of those "disabled" seamen who might be thought worthy of such charity and the explanation of those who should be relieved is given in a transitive form, as "a poor Man, who loses his Limbs (which are his Estate) in the Service of the Government, and is thereby disabled from his Labour to get his Bread, should be provided for, and not suffer'd to beg or starve for want of those Limbs he lost in the service of his Country."[23]

Where Griffin explains the word "disabled" transitively in terms of unfitness to work, it must be expected he was aware he was playing on words. As a "Mariner," he was no doubt aware of the term "able seaman," which the *Oxford English Dictionary* defines as "a sailor capable of performing all duties; spec. a rank of sailor in the Royal Navy above ordinary seaman and below leading seaman,"[24] and dates as early as 1653. Furthermore, Griffin was doubtless aware that many impaired able seamen were not "disabled" from getting their bread.[25] Many ship's surgeons, for example, John Atkins, have written up cases of named officers and able seamen whom they treated with amputations and for gunshot wounds which might have rendered them "disabled" in the modern sense but did not stop them from getting their bread.[26] Atkins describes the amputation made of the right arm of Galfridus Walpole (brother of Sir Robert) while he was in charge of HMS *Lion*, a 60-gun fourth-rate ship of the line.[27] Captain Walpole continued to serve in the navy after the amputation, his last commission being on the HMS *Peregrine Galley* from 1716 to 1720.[28] Atkins also describes the successful treatment of able seaman Alexander Henderson, who lost an eye "struck out by a splinter."[29]

Griffin's hospital came to fruition in 1767, when the *London Evening Post* noted that "an Hospital for the reception of disabled seamen in the Royal Navy is to be built this summer in Sheerness."[30] But this establishment still did not herald a commonplace use of the word "disabled" as an adjective for "soldier" or "sailor" without a sense of the transitive, or of cure. Nearly fifty years later, in 1814, Jane Austen described Fanny Price's mother as being willing to give up her eldest daughter since she had "A large and still increasing family, an husband disabled for active service, but not the less equal to company and good liquor, and a very small income to supply their wants."[31] Here, Austen's brief glimpse into the life of a sailor "disabled for active service" applied to a man who was not at all "disabled" from enjoying the good things in life was written by a woman who had two admiral brothers and who was well aware of the navy and its expressions. Thus, it may be argued that since Fanny Price's father is described transitively as "disabled for active service," it is unlikely that other uses of the word "disabled" in the eighteenth century were uttered in the modern sense in which Singer uses it, that is, in a way which fulfils the medical model of "disability."

It might be fair to argue that the word "disabled" began to be used as an adjective to describe sailors transitively as being unable to work, in a dyad that played on the idea of the qualified ships' crew[32] being called "able seamen." At the same time, it must also be remembered that it was possible to hold the rating of "able seaman" even if one was missing a limb or an eye. Brian Lavery, writing of Nelson's navy (and it must be remembered that Nelson himself was missing a limb and an eye), notes:

> Some captains made a habit of keeping "description books" of the men under their command, for they might be useful in tracking them if they deserted. They often depict the seaman as a rather un-military figure. Captain Rotherham's book for the *Bellerophon,* begun just after the Battle of Trafalgar, shows a great deal of diversity. Some of the men would not have been recruited by any modern navy—John Millikan was an "amaciated thing"; Thomas Jewell had lost his right eye, and Henry McGee was blind in one; Michael Carvel was "not a good character but very strong"; James Robinson was a "stupid fellow," and John Sullivan was "very old looking." . . . Jack Allen, a Negro from Grenada, was the tallest at 5 feet 11 inches. Some were very short . . . John Cook, a watch motion maker from Cripplegate in London, was only 4 feet 11 inches and worked in the cramped conditions of the hold, where small stature might be an advantage.[33]

What could be argued to follow from the evidence that the facts of the various impairments were kept in order to track sailors lest they desert the ship, is that "Able-Seaman" was a rating based on experience, not a normative body. And it was not only the navy that was a safe place for those missing limbs, and being impaired did not always preclude the getting of bread. Three notable miniaturists were deaf: Richard Crosse (1742–1810), Sampson Towgood Roch (1759–1847), and Charles Shirreff (1750–1831), as was the more famous artist and founder of the Royal Academy Joshua Reynolds (1723–1792). Musicians John Stanley (1712–1786) and George Frideric Handel (1685–1759) were blind. Other people known for their lack of limbs are Peter Stuyvesant (ca. 1612–1672), who served as the last Dutch director-general of the colony of New Netherland; Gouverneur Morris (1752–1816), an American statesman and a Founding Father of the United States; and Samuel Foote (1720–1777), an actor and farceur.

But where the medical model of "disability" can be argued to be at odds with the evidence of the eighteenth-century uses of the word "disabled," a second conclusion is also suggested. In this period the existence of impaired sailors and others who continued to work on board ships and in other professions suggests that society did not demand compulsory able-bodiedness, nor does it appear to follow from these illustrations that in the eighteenth century "society put so many obstacles in the way of people with disabilities." At this point we might therefore move on from the medical model of "disability" to explore how heuristic it is to use a cultural model as a tool to analyze impairments in the eighteenth century.

A History of "Disability Studies"

All five editions of Lennard J. Davis's *Disability Studies Reader* begin with two important points that enshrine the cultural model of disability: first, that in order to "understand the disabled body, one must return to the concept of the norm, the normal body . . . because the 'problem' is not the person with disabilities; the problem is the way normalcy is constructed to create the 'problem' of the disabled person."[34] Second, Davis informs us that "the word 'normal' as 'constituting, conforming to, not deviating or different from, the common standard, regular, usual' only enters the English language around 1840."[35] Here, Davis's move, which locates "the normal . . . in a particular moment in history,"[36] is made in order to link "disability studies" to other critical theories through "late eighteenth- and nineteenth-century notions of nationality, race, gender, criminality, sexual orientation and so on."[37] In the form of a historical a priori and in the language of the new mathematics of statistics, Davis argues, nineteenth-century thinkers used the idea of *l'homme moyen* to create the category of "disabled" person as an outgroup by which the "normal" could define themselves. In turn the new discourses of "normality" fueled the eugenics debate and the medicalization which leads ultimately to Peter Singer's position on "disability": "We can see evolution, fingerprinting, and the attempt to control reproductive rights of the deaf as all pointing to a conception of the body as perfectible."[38]

It is the medical model of "disability" against which Davis argues, since medicine is predicated against the (re)making of some atemporal notion of "normal," and which his essay collection opposes with the cultural model of "disability." Thus, *The Disability Studies Reader* explains: "Disability studies, for the most part, shuns this unequal power transaction in favor of advocacy, investigation, inquiry, archeology, genealogy, dialectic, and deconstruction. The model of a sovereign subject revealing or reveling in that subjectivity is put into question."[39] I have nothing but satisfaction with the outcomes of this method of study, not least because of the recent political developments brought about through the sea change wrought in the understanding of "disability": the Americans with Disabilities Act and the Equality Act in the United Kingdom, which have begun to guarantee services for those like myself who need some help to lead our lives.

However, it must be remembered that Davis dated statistical thinking about the body to 1829, and the term "norm" to 1855. To explain how society functioned before this date, Davis's introduction in the current edition of *The Disability Studies Reader* gives a brief account of "a world in which the concept of normality does not exist" as a world in which the "ideal" body is regarded as divine and therefore unattainable on earth.[40] Davis describes it in terms of Pliny's account of Zeuxis painting Aphrodite using the body parts of a number of different women of Crotona to suggest that "all members of the population are below the ideal. No one young lady of Crotona can be the ideal. By definition, one can never have an ideal body. And there is no social pressure, we would imagine, that populations have bodies that conform to the ideal."[41] Davis's conditional mode, introduced by "we would imagine," is a reworking of the same sentence presented as an undeniable fact in the first edition of the same essay: "There is in such societies no demand that populations have bodies that conform to the ideal."[42] Likewise, in the same paragraph, the fifth-edition version removes the first-edition reference to a late eighteenth-century account of Pliny's story in François-Andre Vincent's painting *Zeuxis Choosing as*

Models the Most Beautiful Girls of the Town of Croton (1789, Museum de Louvre, Paris).[43]

The withdrawal from history before the nineteenth century in *The Disability Studies Reader* began in the second edition, which retained only three of the original six essays in the section called *Historical Perspectives*.[44] By the fifth edition, Davis's "Constructing Normalcy" essay, retitled "Introduction: Disability, Normality, and Power" and rewritten with amendments such as those demonstrated above, is no longer in the "Historical Perspectives" section, which contains only three essays, all of which explore aspects of disability after the nineteenth century. The three essays that disappeared after the first edition appear to have been intended to give a historical backdrop to "disability studies,"[45] and the present book is intended to refocus and recommence the debate on impaired bodies in history, or at least before the nineteenth century, using the language and methodology of Variability.

The need to readdress the historical is, I believe, due to the methodological problem that runs throughout Davis's own essay from the "Historical Perspectives" section of the first edition, and which may be the reason why the historical was gradually removed from the project. "Universalizing Marginality" begins with an impossible statement: "Without a sense of group solidarity and without a social category of disability, they [deaf people] were mainly seen as isolated deviations from a norm."[46] Deaf individuals before 1840 may or may not have felt a sense of group identity with other deaf people, but if, as Davis argues, the concept of "norm" did not come about until this date, deaf people cannot have been conceived of as "isolated deviations from a norm" in the eighteenth because there was no concept of "norm." Davis's essay is intended to give reasons why the idea of the "norm" came about in the early nineteenth century, so he asks, "If the concept of the norm or average enters European culture, or at least the European languages, only in the nineteenth century, one has to ask what is the cause of this conceptualization?,"[47] and gives us two arguments in explanation, the first in terms of the growth of reading and the rise of the novel in the eighteenth century, and the second in terms of deaf education and the philosophers who explored the senses "which help us to place deafness as an emergent, constructed category." Raymond

Williams's notion of the "emergent" is a useful idea from which to argue the existence of "a norm" before the statistical "norm" of the nineteenth century,[48] but as the present argument will suggest, the theoretical idea of the emergent does not fit with the empirical facts we find in eighteenth-century records.

Davis's argument about reading and novels is based on the idea of language as a sign system and makes the experience of deafness central to the experience of all eighteenth-century people. He suggests: "Because the eighteenth century was a period in which readers on a large scale first began to experience reality through texts, they may be said to have had a different relation to reality and to texts. Part of that difference has to do with the fact that in order to become readers people in the eighteenth century had to become deaf, at least culturally so. That is, to read requires muteness and attention to nonverbal signs."[49] This move is made in order to draw attention to the fact that while hearing readers were becoming silent in their attention to the printed word, deaf sign language was contested as a method of teaching deaf people to communicate by oralists who enforced the primacy of spoken language on their deaf pupils. The inequality in sign systems was due, Davis argues, to the eighteenth-century belief that although deaf people appeared to be the same as hearing people since they were capable of reading and writing, there was a "powerful view of deafness woven into eighteenth-century culture . . . [which understands] the deaf person as someone who reasons, feels, thinks, and uses language just as hearing people do, *only the language used is different from that of the linguistic majority.* The language is in fact the language of texts, of writing, of novels."[50]

The deconstructive logic of this double move that both links and separates deaf sign language from printed text is elegant and makes a literary theory of "disability studies," but it is not borne out by the newly available contextual evidence about the texts Davis cites. At the time Davis wrote his essay it was still believed that Daniel Defoe (who was then also thought of as the first English novelist) had written the *Life and Surprizing Adventures of Duncan Campbell*, the deaf prophet. The inaccuracy allowed Davis to conclude that John Wallis, the seventeenth-century oralist teacher of a profoundly deaf boy, Alexander Popham, "and by extension Defoe, acknowledge that the deaf have their own pre-existing language and that language is mediated for the hearing world through writing and textuality."[51]

However, as Jaap Maat argues, Popham's notebook dated 1662, which was discovered in 2008, suggests instead that teaching "semantics and grammar w[as] at least as important as the production of speech sounds in Wallis's method."[52] Leila Frances Monaghan goes further, arguing that Wallis believed that "deaf people who spoke without comprehending were no better than parrots."[53] His rival, William Holder, with whom Wallis engaged in a long-running pamphlet war, "also taught his pupils the manual alphabet, together with the written alphabet, but only after he had attempted to teach articulation."[54] Thus, it might be argued that there are no grounds for accepting from Wallis's method that he believed the deaf had a different language from the hearing since they had to be taught all the aspects of English, just as hearing people do, in order to communicate. Furthermore, Wallis's and Holder's opposing methodologies of teaching deaf pupils suggest that there was no single methodology from which to draw unifying conclusions. Moreover, in 1706, a paper was presented to the Royal Society explaining that deaf people could lip-read.[55] Together this evidence suggests that in the seventeenth and eighteenth centuries, language to the hearing was not believed to be so far removed from language to the deaf, even if the medium of comprehension was different for each, and in the case of Duncan Campbell, who communicated his prophecies by writing rather than sign language, the parallels between his language and English are paramount.

Nevertheless, Davis concludes that deaf people did have their own distinct language in the eighteenth century, and he quotes a "correspondent" to *Spectator* no. 474 of 3 September 1712 who believed Mr. Spectator would know of the whereabouts of Duncan Campbell since she had heard "you are a dumb man too." Rather than this, I would argue that "Dulcibella Thankley," the addresser (factual or fictional) of the letter to the *Spectator* searching for Duncan Campbell, is joining in the play of satire and disguise that lay behind the use of literary personae to protect political writers, and reminds readers that Mr. Spectator calls himself dumb in *Spectator* no. 1 of 1 March 1710: "I had not been long at the University, before I distinguished myself by a most profound Silence: For during the Space of eight

Years, excepting in the public Exercises on the College, I scarce uttered the Quantity of an hundred Words." This ploy was used by Whigs Addison and Steele at a time of Tory government, to pretend their new journal was merely copying what other people had said after their more direct political journal, the *Tatler,* had been shut down. Moreover, the letter from Mrs. Thankley and its reply, though giving the requested directions for finding Campbell: "at the *Golden-Lion,* opposite the *Half-Moon* Tavern in *Drury-Lane,*" is also given so an "Inspector . . . [may] enquire . . . into the Merit of this silent Sage and report accordingly," and is therefore likely to have been understood as a warning against Campbell at a time when he was thought to be a Jacobite.

Turning the tables, after the publication of Campbell's biography, which is now attributed to William Bond, Duncan Campbell again became the object of satire for turning Whig, supporting the Hanoverian succession, and selling his book printed on expensive paper at half a guinea before it was reduced to the usual book price of five shillings.[56] The Tory satirist Eliza Haywood attacked Campbell in *A Spy on the Conjurer,*[57] and again in *The Dumb Projector: Or, a Trip to Holland made by Mr. Duncan Campbell,*[58] both for making a fortune from his overpriced volume after he bought a house on the proceeds of the subscription,[59] and for being presented to King George the First.[60] More importantly for the present argument, Haywood gives a number of accounts of Campbell using sign language to communicate with hearing people, sometimes successfully, sometimes not. At a fish market in Rotterdam, we read:

> He cheapned at every Stall in his way, by shewing his Money and pointing.— His dumb signs were little intelligible in that Place; all the women gather'd about him.—Some ask'd if he had been among the Turks, and had his Tongue cut out, and he understanding what they said by their Motions, much better than they did his Meanings by his Signs, made a doleful Face, and gave 'em to understand he had been served as they said, and in a worse manner also; at that some laugh'd—some cry'd—some pity'd—some were ready to throw Stones.[61]

If the fishwives had not understood his signs, on the next page we are told: "He was another time very handsomely entertained by the Widow

Toms, she is a Woman of great Sense, has translated several Things from the *French* and other Languages.—She seemed very well pleas'd with Mr Campbell, and they were agreeable Companions."[62] While the intention of the first of these accounts of Campbell communicating with the fishwives is probably salacious, the fact that Haywood has no compunction about expressing the idea of the intercommunicability of languages, be they formal or informal, oral or sign, does not suggest that deaf people were either defined against "a norm" or were believed to have a preexisting language, or were able to communicate with each other through a shared deaf understanding of the world.

I draw attention to these details only to supply reasons why Davis's *Disability Studies Reader* may have stepped away from the historical aspect of "disability studies," which might be argued to be due to the change in the availability of information over the last twenty years, evidence which may better be accounted for in another way than fitting it into a theory that was still emergent. The recently available historical databases give up more and more empirical evidence, from which it can not only be expected that we will map out wider contexts and connections between contexts and from which we can draw new and different conclusions. Furthermore, we may adopt new methodologies that center on the accounts of experiences of unique individuals the details of whose lives are becoming more open to discovery.

Before returning to Davis's second argument about deaf education and philosophers who worked on deafness as a concept in the eighteenth century, it will be useful here to make a few comments on how this new possibility for research affects the ramifications of Davis's formulation of "disability studies" which have become so influential through the work of David T. Mitchell and Sharon Snyder.

Much of the work in literary analysis from a "disability studies" perspective, as the five editions of *The Disability Studies Reader* itself, has centered on the modern experience of "disability" and the cultural model of disability, based on a development of Davis's foundational methodology focused through the ideas of David T. Mitchell and Sharon L. Snyder, in *Narrative Prosthesis: Disability and the Dependencies of Discourse.*[63] Mitchell and Snyder argue that narratives proceed on the basis of something needing fixing, that there is some flaw in the natural order, which is usually thematized through a disabled character, and they choose Oedipus, Richard III, and Captain Ahab as examples of this in practice. Their book led to an understanding of "disability studies" as a binary ableist/nonableist discourse of compulsory able-bodiedness, which owes a debt to sexuality studies and the idea of compulsory heterosexuality, against which the Crip and the Queer are ranged. The approach has been very influential and is the basis of a number of projects, monographs, collections of essays, and other contributions that have come to define "disability studies" as a form of contemporary political activism as well as an academic discipline. The same can be said as we look to "disability studies" in the nineteenth century,[64] where the age of the American Civil War and the buildup to the Great War, with their myriads of war wounded, is read as the politics which grounded the idea of "Disabled Rights" that were made law in the late twentieth century. But this can say nothing about impaired bodies before 1840.

The reason for the paucity of "disability studies" in the early modern period is explained by Vin Nardizzi, who, tracing the abnormal subject as a prior development to the notion of the concept of normality, argues that in Shakespeare, the word "disabled" is connected with failures in masculinity, but since the term implies "self-diminishment [that] . . . is volitional because it is purely rhetorical; [Nardizzi concludes] disability is not yet 'the master trope of human disqualification' that disability theorists David T. Mitchell and Sharon L. Snyder argue it has come to be."[65]

Toward a Philosophy of Impaired Bodies

Returning to Davis's second line of argument about the education of deaf people in the "Universalizing Marginality" essay, we can readily come to a similar conclusion about altering the trajectory of study away from working with "the disabled" as a group, toward the uniqueness of each historical person. The illustration of the education of the deaf that Davis uses is Pierre Desloges, a deaf bookbinder and paper hanger from Paris who wrote a pamphlet, *Observations d'un sourd et muèt, sur un cours élémentaire d'éducation des sourds et muèts*, which attacks the new oral method of teaching deaf children recommended by l'Abbé Deschamps, a teacher of the deaf in Orléans, and recommends sign language.[66] For a start, I must point out that I downloaded the text of Desloges's book free of charge from the Bibliothèque National de France's excellent digital service Gallica,[67] and so have not had to rely on the available reprinted text or the translation by Harlan Lane[68] used in Davis's essay. Thus, although Davis argues that the editor's explanation of his function ("[I] corrected the young man's quite faulty spelling. I pruned some repetitions and softened a few words that could have given offense. Aside from these minor emendations, the essay is entirely the work of the deaf Desloges")[69] is "a mark of difference that separates him from normal readers," since his "words immediately contextualize the otherness of Desloges, who must be linguistically sanitized and standardized,"[70] we might pause at the translation that leads to this conclusion. The whole paragraph from which it comes reads: "Voici, dans l'exacte verité, tout ce que j'y ai mis du mien. J'ai rectifié l'orthographe de ce jeune home, laquelle est assez défectueuse. J'ai supprimé quelques répétitions & adouci termes qui auraient pu paroître ofensans. A ces légères corrections près, l'Ouvrage est en entier de notre Auteur sourd & muèt. Ce sont ses pensées, son stile & ses raisonemens."[71]

I have restored the first and last sentences, which read as though intended to minimize the interference of the editor, who introduces his interventions as: "This is the exact truth of what I put of myself into Desloges's text," and concludes, "These are his thoughts, his style and his reasoning." To be sure, as Davis suggests, any protestations of genuineness should be treated with caution at the onset of realist prose, but it must also be argued that it is impossible to describe what an editor says and does without bringing on this charge. Daniel Defoe claims to be much more invasive as the editor of the fictional text by Moll Flanders, such that he writes "the original of this Story is put into new Words, and the Stile of the famous Lady we here speak of is a little alter'd,"[72] but this is effected to hide her "real name" and the "Newgate" language of the original, both of which are further levels of the realist device. But once again this is part of the conscious fun and play of language that we encountered in the reading of the *Spectator* so that we might conclude that an eighteenth-century reader might well take Defoe's own advice and choose to believe it or not: "The World is so taken up of late with Novels and Romances, that it will be hard for a private History to be taken for Genuine, where the Names and the Circumstances of the Person are concealed, and on this Account we must be content to leave the Reader to pass his own Opinion upon the ensuing sheets, and take it just as he pleases."[73]

Thus, while the story of Duncan Campbell being the son of a Scottish man and a Lapp woman reads like fiction, the story of Pierre Desloges's mutism does not, and the eighteenth-century reader might agree with his editor: "Je senti que le principal intérèt de cet Ouvrage viendrait de son Auteur; que come c'étoit peut-être la première fois qu'un sourd & muèt avait mérité les honneurs de l'impression" (I believe that the principal interest of the work derives as much from its Author, as from the probability that this is the first time one deaf and dumb has merited the honor of publication).[74] The fact that Desloges's book is introduced as a text which "justifier en même temps la méthode de Mr. l'Abbé de l'Epée, laquelle est toute fondée sur l'usage des signes" (at the same time will justify the method of Mr. l'Abbé de l'Epée, which is all based on the use of signs) becomes the more interesting in relation to the uniqueness of the author himself, who describes the other effects of the illness which caused his deafness— the paralysis of his lips and the loss of his teeth—"c'est principalement à ces deux causes que j'atribue mon mutisme" (it is principally to these two causes that I attribute my muteness).[75]

Thus, we understand why Desloges praises and recommends the method of sign language he has learned from de l'Epée because it is the only way he can communicate—his spoken language is too "faible" (feeble). And this is why he attacks the new oral method of Mr. l'Abbé Deschamps as it is useless to him. True, the use of sign language requires a community with competence in signing (and Desloges notes the existence of his "compagnons sourds & muèts de naissance" [companions of deaf and dumb from birth][76] in Paris) as well as translators who have access to other languages so that the signers are not isolated from other language communities (such a one as the editor of Desloges's pamphlet), but *Observations* is a pamphlet about the experience of one particular impaired person who had access to the book trade (he was a bookbinder) and who was telling the tale of his life as a deaf man with paralyzed lips and no teeth: it is not the life of "a working man" to be taken as some representative of the working class in a Marxist sense.[77] Thus, when Desloges discusses the fact that sign language is the best method of communication for "mes compagnons sourds & muèts de naissance, qui ne savent ni lire, ni écrire, & qui n'ont jamais reçu d'autres leçons que celles du bon-sens & de la fréquentation de leurs semblables" (my companions, deaf and dumb from birth, who can neither read nor write, and who have had no other lessons than common sense and the attendance of their fellows),[78] he is drawing attention to their being illiterate in the language of the hearing because they were deaf from birth, not because they were ill-educated due to their poverty or had a language of their own that was completely distinct from French.

Recent work on Pierre Desloges by Anne Quartararo discovered more about his life:[79] that his father was a tax collector in the Loire region of Touraine, that he left home for Paris when he was nineteen to escape the usual misunderstanding of an impaired person by their family members, that he engaged in continued debate with Deschamps and another hearing teacher of the deaf who recommended oralism, Jacob-Rodriguez Pereire, whom he came closer to convincing of the need for sign language.

Quartararo also notes: "With the publication of his book, Desloges momentarily became the center of attention in several of the Parisian salons. He would eventually meet with the Marquis de Condorcet, who was interested in the philosophical arguments set forth in *Observations d'un sourd et muèt* and attended other social gatherings among the intellectual élite."[80] It was just such a link between Desloges and the *philosophes* of Paris before the Revolution that licensed Davis to makes the claim that "deafness as a phenomenon engaged the intellectual movement of the period in a way that blindness and other disabilities did not."[81] However, considering the philosophers to whom Davis refers—Denis Diderot, Thomas Reid, Etiènne Bonnot de Condillac, Jean-Jacques Rousseau, and John Locke—the claim is hard to sustain. Diderot wrote a *Lettre sur les aveugles* (*Letter on the Blind*) in 1749 and another *Sur les sourds et muèts* (Letter on the deaf and dumb) in 1751. Reid and Condillac both wrote on all five senses, respectively: *An Inquiry into the Human Mind* (1764) and *Traité des sensa-*

tions (*Treatise on the Senses*) (1754). Rousseau considered both blindness and deafness in his works on education, and Locke makes equal mention of deafness and blindness in his *Essay concerning Humane Understanding* (1690).

However, if we set this claim against another which is quite as hard to sustain—"The blind were historically regarded as objects of charity, if not venerated for their alleged 'second sight'"[82]—we can begin to understand what "Universalizing Marginality" was trying to do. Given that Duncan Campbell was as well known for his prophetical predictions as his deafness,[83] we must conclude that underlying Davis's argument is an attempt to add the suppression of deaf language as a historical a priori of the Enlightenment to Michel Foucault's use of the metaphors of sight, blindness, and the regaining of sight as a way of understanding the desire for truth in eighteenth-century Enlightenment philosophy. Thus where Foucault argues:

> What allows man to resume contact with childhood and rediscover the permanent birth of truth is this bright, distant, open naïvety of the gaze. Hence the two great mythical experiences on which the philosophy of the eighteenth century wished to found its beginning: the foreign spectator in an unknown country and the man-born-blind restored to the light.[84]

Davis asks us to remember that at the same time textuality is the forgetting of our quietness when we read:

> But precisely because sign language will never actually become a universal language, we must stop and consider how truly hegemonic and controlling a concept is the notion of writing and speech as a "hearing" phenomenon. The argument I have tried to make is that deafness of textuality is one of the best kept secrets of the Enlightenment and beyond. It is not so much that convention has ruled here, but that there has been an active suppression of the insights I have proposed in this essay.[85]

More than forgetting, Davis argues, it is the "active suppression" of deaf language that marks Enlightenment philosophy—we must "see" all truth during our "deaf" times reading philosophical texts. In this way, it is the suppression of deafness understood alongside the lionization of sight which makes "disability studies" so important. And this is a statement with which I most heartily agree. The history of impairments is only now beginning to be considered as worth knowing, and as a blind man I want to know about my forefathers and foremothers. But I cannot agree with the way Davis goes on: "After all, the body is political. . . . An able body is the body of a citizen; deformed, deafened, amputated, obese, female, perverse, crippled, maimed, blinded bodies do not make up the body politic. Utterances must all be able ones produced by conformed, ideal forms of humanity."[86] From what has been argued in this chapter about able seamen in the eighteenth century, it is not certain from the examples of Duncan Campbell and Pierre Desloges, as well as Galfridus Walpole and Fanny Price's father, whether Alexander Henderson would or would not have felt a compunction to return to work or to seek refuge in a hospital for "disabled" seamen after losing his eye, and John Atkins does not tell us what the able seaman did when his ship returned to port. Furthermore, though the narratives of Walpole and Henderson come to us from a doctor's hand, Atkins's *The navy surgeon; or, practical system of surgery* is a collection of memories of patching up and make-do-and-mend with sailors' bodies and not a plea for a navy of physically complete or model specimens of humanity. Nor even was impressment, which would take men of any physical condition up to the age of fifty-five years to serve in the navy.

The mechanics, economics, and personal accounts of eye surgery, its successes as well as its failures, will be the topic of the rest of this book. And as this book will argue for a close study concentrating on the unique, it suggests the sort of personal agency that was noted by Vin Nardizzi rather than any underlying conceptualization of "disability" underscoring all of its stories.

3

TEXT AS THEORY

Understanding Sight and Blindness in the Eighteenth Century

Defining Blindness

It is impossible to give a brief definition of blindness as it might have been understood in the eighteenth century, except that it appears it was not as a simple binary of "sight and no sight." As now, it was known that people's vision might be more or less blurred and that sight might be more or less absent. The trustees of the Dorothy Wilson Trust, which was the first private charity in England, set up in 1718 to give money to blind people, chose the three beneficiaries of their generosity based in part on their degree of blindness. Anne Gill was one of six nominees to be among the first three beneficiaries in 1718, when the charity began, but she was not awarded monies until 1736. The reason given for her not being accepted in the first instance was that she was not completely blind. How they judged I do not know, since there was no eighteenth-century version of the Snellen chart (see fig 1).

On this chart, invented in 1862 by the Dutch ophthalmologist Herman Snellen, the top line represents a visual acuity of 20/200, which is nowadays regarded as legal blindness. What this means is that a person standing 20 feet away from the chart who cannot read the top letter because it is too indistinct is deemed to have a visual acuity comparable with a person who has "normal" (20/20) visual acuity who is standing 200 feet away from the chart. Even if there were such a chart, or the decision of the Dorothy

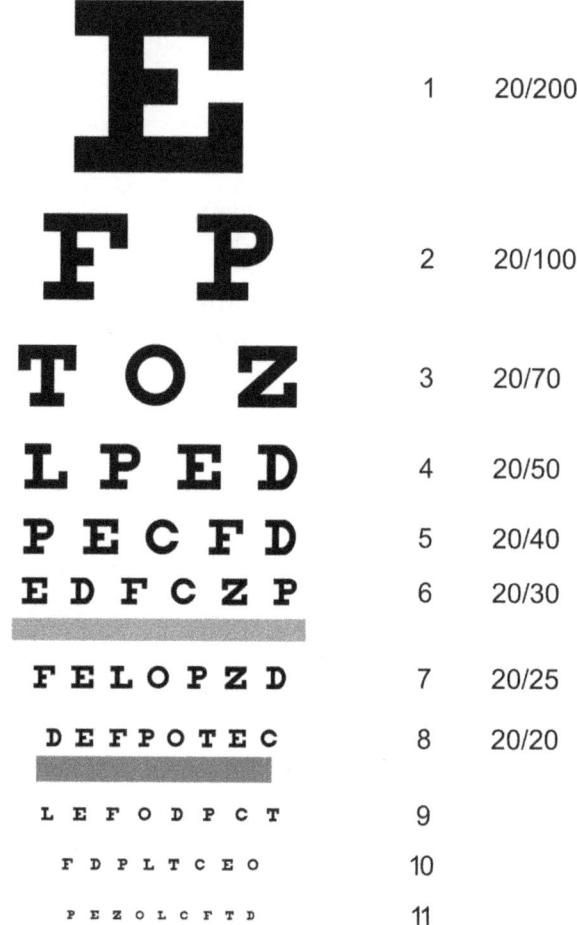

FIGURE 1. The Snellen chart, invented by Herman Snellen in 1862. (Jeff Dahl, CC BY-SA 3.0)

Wilson Trust made its decision about Anne Gill in some equivalent way, this would privilege the medical model of "disability" in the actions of a charity which was the first in England to favor the cultural model of "disability" in its payments of benefit for those who were blind. How we might understand blindness in the eighteenth century must then straddle what has become a divide in the twenty-first.

A methodology for the study of impaired people that addresses the problem of the medical model of "disability" and that works before the nineteenth-century onset date of the cultural model of "disability studies" will require some dexterous groundwork. If it is to center on the unique individual—and the personal experiences of impairment described in the previous chapter would suggest that a unifying account will not suffice—there needs to be a way of organizing a great number of particularities, as well as a way of filling in any gaps in the historical record. This is, in part, addressed by Variability, which begins from the expectation of sameness and difference between individuals in the phrase "the same only different." If I am "the same only different" from you, then you are not wholly "other" from me, and I can expect to find in our encounters that a great number of my particularities in terms of my capacities and capabilities are similar to yours, albeit you are within or outside my historical context. And this understanding suggests I do not have to repeat all of your particularities to make sense of you. Thus my description of you would center on our differences, and although this might appear to "other" you, it would, at the same time, be apparently to use myself as a theory to read you. But I am an individual, just like you, with particularities that are unique to me and inapplicable to you. I am not a theory; I am more like a text. I am not applicable in a number of different cases as a unifying principle. And this would suggest that anything I write about you is unique to me, is from my perspective and is only comprehensible by me. How could such a description be useful to anyone else but me?

For this reason, I propose the use of one literary or historical text to act in place of a theory for the purpose of interillumination of two or more texts. The methodology derives from the fact that texts and the detail of the historical record are becoming more and more accessible with the growth of the digital humanities. For example, Eliza Haywood, the author of two texts on Duncan Campbell, was little known when Lennard Davis wrote the essay discussed in the previous chapter. The ideas about sign language and political satire which Haywood's texts imparted added new perspectives on the life of the deaf prophet, and though the perspectives were biased to the Tory side, the reference to the *Spectator* counterbalanced them to the Whig. What emerged was neither a whole life of a deaf man nor a whole account of deafness in the early eighteenth century but more like a single tessera which adds to the mosaic of historical knowledge of deafness. A second tessera was added from the interplay between the unnamed editor's preface of Pierre Desloges's *Observations d'un sourd et muèt* and Daniel Defoe's preface to *Moll Flanders* from which we could derive information about the uniqueness of the author (real or fictional) from the debate about realism in fiction rather than move toward a theory to make a unifying statement about deafness.

Likewise, the account of the word "disabled" moved between a number of texts: newspaper advertisements, a novel, and a surgeon's manual, with each text acting as the theory with which to read the other. No "final" meaning of the word "disabled" in the eighteenth century emerged, but the different information streams informed one another, concentrating attention on certain particulars of the word and filling in the gaps of other streams. But nor was this a "final" account of even a single word because I—the manipulator of the texts in the nexus of contexts—am outside that context so can assert no stable objectivity.

Working with Text as Theory

It is the multiplication of textual examples, in effect the widening of the contexts informing the account—in this book, my account of blindness—which marks this methodology as a development from the theoretical. Michel Foucault's theoretical statement about couching a blind eye as a metaphor of the truth of the Enlightenment, which was discussed in the previous chapter, is derived from a single empirical source. As the *Stanford Encyclopedia of Philosophy* tells us: "Condillac was aware that [his claim that we do not need to learn to perceive depth] had been challenged by . . . empirical studies of recovered vision as were available at the time. In 1728, the English surgeon, William Chesselden [sic], had reported to the British Royal Society that subjects recovering from operations to remove cataracts that had blinded them since birth appeared to need to learn to associate what they saw with tactile experience before they could recognize shapes or objects."[1]

In fact, William Cheselden[2] had, according to the historical record, couched only one subject who had been born with cataracts, and on whom the 1728 report was based. But this was one of a number of similar operations noted in other philosophical sources as early as 1709 by George Berkeley in the addition made to the first edition of his *An Essay Towards a New Theory of Vision*:[3] "I am Inform'd that, soon after the First Edition of the Treatise, a Man somewhere near London was made to See, who had been Born Blind, and continued to for about Twenty Years. Such a one may be supposed a proper Judge to decide, how far some Tenets laid down in several Places of the forgoing Essay, are agreeable to Truth, and if any Curious Person hath the Opportunity of making proper Interrogatories to him thereon, I shou'd gladly see my Notions either amended or confirmed by Experience."

The operation had probably been carried out by William Read, the royal ophthalmologist, but we have no further record of it than Berkeley's hearsay. What is important is that this is a widening of the contextual record of people born blind and made to see. Following the idea of text as theory, if we begin with the many accounts of the experience of couching those born blind rather than with a theory based on a single case, we find a very different prospect for knowledge. The operation was not, as Foucault expressed it, a "great mythical experience" of the eighteenth century; it was a regular occurrence. I have, for example, found the names of seventeen children born blind who were treated throughout his career by John Taylor, of Hatton Garden.

> A few Days since, Master Smith, son of Captain Alexander Smith of Lombard Street, was restored to sight by Mr. Taylor, Oculist of Hatton Garden, after being deemed incurable.[4]

> A few Days since the Daughter of Mr Hargraft at the Blacksmith's Arms at Cuckhold's Point, Rotherhithe, was restored to Sight, by Mr John Taylor, Oculist of Hatton-Garden.[5]

> A few Days since the Daughter of Capt. Cuite, of Paradise-Row, Rotherhithe, who had laboured under a violent Inflammation, and loss of Sight for several weeks, was, by the Care of Mr. Taylor, Oculist of Hatton Garden, quite recovered.[6]

A few Days since a Child of Mrs. Price of Chichester Rents, Chancery-Lane, blind with the Gutta Serena, a Disease most Practitioners judged incurable, was nevertheless restored to perfect Sight by Mr Taylor, Oculist in Hatton-Garden.[7]

A few Days since a Son of Mr. Grant, Clerk to Mr. Knight, Proctor in Doctor's Commons, was restor'd to Sight by Mr Taylor, Oculist of Hatton-Garden.[8]

A few Days since a Son of Mr. Collup, Peruke-maker, in Fenchurch-street, was restored to Sight by Mr. Taylor, Oculist of Hatton-Garden.[9]

Three Weeks since arrived in Town a Son of Mr Lee, of Halifax, in Nova Scotia, after having been under the Care of an eminent Surgeon there, for an extraordinary Deprivation of Sight, and has already received much Relief, by the Assistance of Mr. Taylor, Oculist, whose house he is at in Hatton-Garden.[10]

A few Days since a Child of Mr. Bennet's, Engraver in Swan-yard, near the New Church in the Strand, was restored to Sight by Mr Taylor, Oculist of Hatton-Garden.[11]

A few Days ago a son of Mr. Roberts, painter, in Rochester Row, Tothill-fields, Westminster, was restored to sight by Mr. Taylor oculist, in Hatton Garden.[12]

A few Days ago a Child of Mr. Pinnick's at Mr. Walker's, Tin-Plate-Worker, near the Watch-house, High Holborn, was restored to Sight by Mr. Taylor, Oculist in Hatton Garden.[13]

A few Days ago the only son of Humphry Finnimore, Esq; at Dulwich, was restored to sight by Mr. Taylor, in Hatton-garden.[14]

In Justice to Mr. Taylor, Oculist in Hatton-Garden, and for the Benefit of those afflicted with Disorders in the Eyes, I make this public Acknowledgement for the great Blessings my Child has received, in being by his Judgment and Care, perfectly restored to Sight in both Eyes, after being blind some time. John Morgan, At the Ship, Little-Turnstile, Holborn, Nov. 5, 1774.[15]

A few Days ago a child of Mr. Hawxwell, grocer, in Church Lane, St Martin's-lane, was restored to sight by Mr Taylor, Oculist in Hatton-garden.[16]

A few Days a Son of Mr. Wright, Coal Merchant, in Wellclose-square, Goodman's Fields, was restored to Sight by Mr. Taylor, Oculist in Hatton-Garden.[17]

A few Days ago, a Son of Mr. Matthews, near the Asylum, St George's Fields, was restored to Sight on his Right Eye, by Mr. Taylor, Occulist, in Hatton-Garden.[18]

A few Days ago a Child of Francis Philips, in Bishop's Head Court, Gray's Inn Lane, was restored to Sight by Mr. Taylor, Oculist, in Hatton-Garden.[19]

A few Days ago a Child of Sarah Hunnins, blind in both Eyes, was recommended by Mr. Dale, Churchwarden of Christ-Church, Spital-Fields, to the Care of Mr. Taylor, Oculist in Hatton-Garden, and restored to perfect Sight.[20]

I cite each of these newspaper pieces because they give names to the people whose experience I believe should be central to any exploration of the various available facts. It will be noticed immediately that all but two of the pieces begin with the words "A few Days ago" or "A few Days since." The words introduce the pieces as news articles rather than advertisements, and they are placed typically under the main heading "London," with other news articles which are indented into separate paragraphs. In the *Public Advertiser* in which the Collup news article appeared, there are two other main news headings, "Deal," for shipping, and "Ireland." Advertisements take up more than three-quarters of the front page of this four-page daily; the second page is entirely news (mostly from London), as is a quarter of the third page. The rest of the third page and all the fourth page are advertisements, which cost three shillings to place and were separated from each other by lines or typeset in boxes.

Thus, readers of London's most popular newspaper would distinguish between a news article and an advertisement by the place and the way they appeared on the page. However, even if the articles about the cures of these children were presented as "news," they were attended with no great excitement. The occupation of the parent is usually given (two captains, two publicans, a clerk, a wig-maker, an engraver, a painter, a tin-plate worker, a grocer, two wives, and a lawyer—all middle-class people), and the address, perhaps so the child can be visited and the cure witnessed. But only John Morgan uses religious language to describe the cure as "the great Blessing my Child has received," and I wonder whether the news items raised any more curiosity than an eyebrow.

A second litany following the words "A few Days . . ." is "Mr. Taylor, oculist of Hatton Garden," the man responsible for the treatments, who was probably glad for the free advertisements for his work. Although children were not his sole patients, at a maximum of two recorded cures a year, we must understand that there were few interventions he could make, and his practice was more commonly with older people suffering from age-related cataracts. In his "Business as usual" advertisement,[21] which he placed twenty-seven times between 1757 and 1763, he notes the removal of foreign objects from eyes, for which he offers help. In this advertisement we also discover that he was available for only four hours a day, and there is evidence (in chapter 6) that he worked as an itinerant bleeder for Messenger Monsey, the physician at the Chelsea Hospital. Perhaps because of a lack of need or uptake of his services, near the end of his career John Taylor, oculist of Hatton Garden, also advertised his services to parents:

> The Small-Pox, Measles, and Colds from Birth, are often productive of very dangerous Disorders to the Eyes, but the latter Complaint is particularly fatal!—Mr. TAYLOR, Oculist, of Hatton-Garden, therefore, assures the Publick (and he speaks from the Experience of 30 Years Practice) that by his peculiar Method of Treatment, if called upon at the Commencement of the Disease, he can preserve the Eyes from every ill Consequence to which they are liable by those dangerous Disorders; preventing, by such a timely Assistance, either a Weakness of the Sight, a Defect therein, or a total Loss thereof. A Pamphlet of Cures gratis.[22]

The idea that a doctor should be called in the early stages of an illness to offer preventative care may appear to be a good one now, but reading the scare tactic of the "total Loss" of their child's sight if they have a cold, which "is particularly fatal!," suggests something of sharp practice: an attempt to ensure that anxious parents would pay for prophylactic care from John Taylor, oculist of Hatton Garden. If there was anything sensational about his medical interventions, it would appear to be something he had to secure for himself.

This analysis is text as theory: each advertisement adds another context, and the overall effect of the couching of cataracts is altered from a "great mythical experience" to the quotidian. Likewise, to give an account of blindness in the eighteenth century, a multiplication of contexts is necessary, and the ones I have chosen, which will give a variable rather than a "final" account, are Philosophical, Medical Intervention, Optical Correction, and the Religious.

Schematically, the philosophical tried to understand vision as one of the five senses that are foundational of empirical knowledge. The medical was interested in intervening in blindness by other means than optical correction, this largely being "eye-waters" and the treatment of cataracts. The optical explored the eye as a mechanism, how the image is focused on the retina and understood by the brain and how blurriness might be corrected with lenses. The religious centered on the miracles of Jesus, of which, according to Isaiah, curing blindness was one sign he was the Messiah.

Philosophical

How well Lockean philosophy was known in the general population is uncertain. Not so for medical interventions, which were advertised throughout the century in most newspapers, or the religious, which was always in eighteenth-century consciousness. What is certain is that the reality of the "blind man made to see," by which Foucault judged the project of the Enlightenment, has set many people thinking about blindness in its philosophical context in the eighteenth century. Marjolein Degenaar's *Molyneux's Problem* tells us that until William Cheselden's paper giving details of the cataract operation carried out in 1728, no philosopher "had posed the question as to whether a person born blind could really be given the power of sight."[23]

William Molyneux first suggested questioning the perception of a "blind man made to see" in a letter to John Locke of 2 March 1693 as a test of whether it was right to privilege the role of sight in the foundation of ideas in the first edition of the *Essay concerning Humane Understanding* (1690). Although he seemed at first to ignore what Molyneux called "a jocose problem," in the second edition of the *Essay* (1694), Locke made copious reference to Molyneux's "blind man made to see," finding himself in agreement with Molyneux's conclusions:

> Suppose a man born blind, and now adult, and taught by his touch to distinguish between a cube and a sphere of the same metal, and nighly of the same bigness, so as to tell, when he felt one and the other, which is the cube, which the sphere. Suppose then the cube and sphere placed on a table, and the blind man to be made to see: quaere, whether by his sight, before he touched them, he could now distinguish and tell which is the globe, which the cube? To which the acute and judicious proposer answers: Not. For though he has obtained the experience of how a globe, how a cube, affects his touch; yet he has not yet obtained the experience, that what affects his touch so or so, must affect his sight so or so; or that a protuberant angle in the cube, that pressed his hand unequally, shall appear to his eye as it does in the cube.[24]

Often called a "thought experiment," this aspect of Lockean empiricism was debated and is still debated by philosophers as though the curing of the blind man were some sort of miracle, or at least the details of the miraculous change from blindness to sight goes unnoticed, since Locke's agreement with Molyneux's conclusions has so great an importance to the way we understand the history of philosophy. The agreement quoted above is the underlying cause of Berkeley's rejection of Locke, which caused the shift from empirical materialism to empirical idealism in the English philosophical tradition. And here it should be remembered that George Berkeley's first publication, the year before the *Treatise Concerning the Principles of Human Knowledge* (1710), was *Towards a New Theory of Vision* (1709).

Laura Berchielli, writing in 2002, is one of a number of recent philosophers who has noticed that there is a basic problem in Locke's acceptance of Molyneux, and she rejects what she calls the "standard reading of Locke," which she characterizes thus: "The idea is that in Locke, only the sense of touch can receive ideas of three-dimensional figures, whereas sight always receives two. Therefore, when we believe we see a three-dimensional space or shape, what in fact happens is that we are making a judgement that moves from a visual to a tactile idea of figure."[25] Instead, Berchielli suggests that "Locke grants that it is possible for sight, under certain perceptual conditions, to receive ideas of three-dimensional figures,"[26] basing her argument on a reading of the first edition of the *Essay*. This approach is itself problematic as it is anachronistic in two senses: first, Locke did not know of Molyneux's "thought experiment" while he was writing the first edition of his *Essay;* and second, the theory of stereoscopic vision was not understood until the work on optics by Charles William Wells in 1792 and John Crisp in 1796.[27]

Nevertheless, the filiation of empiricism from Locke to Berkeley, and thus from materialism to idealism, was directly due to Molyneux's "thought experiment." As Désirée Park tells us, Locke suggests there is a real and material world outside us which is experienced by the senses. Countering this assertion, the Molyneux problem demonstrated the limitations of the sense organs: sight has to learn how to decode information brought to the "Presence Chamber" of the sensorium. Berkeley was more optimistic about human faculties, but this was easy for him because he did not have to suggest there is a world outside us that is being more or less accurately represented to the "presence chamber" of Locke's mind. For Berkeley, the fallible perspective of the viewer's sense data was the foundation of an idealist world. Thus, at the heart of Berkeley's rejection of Locke is the unsensed "substance," the mute material world, that Locke believed lay beneath the primary and secondary qualities of sense experience. Turning to Park's own, and very cogent explanation, we read:

> Locke argues . . . for the primacy of touch, as opposed to sight. Inevitably therefore, the agreement of sights and touches in a given case, for example seen and felt straight edges, brings us nearer to the presumed order of things. And further, whether Locke wishes it or not, he consequently is obliged to conclude that there is some uniquely "best" or "accurate" or

"true" perspective by which all others may be judged better or worse. From this vantage point, in principle at least, the revelations of the senses would indicate external objects as they are: that is, would give an accurate copy of them.

Substance Berkeley questions both as to its patently *ad hoc* role in shoring up primary qualities and, more especially, with regard to the plausibility of mindlessness entertaining any Lockean ideas at all. In the *Principles* it is in fact just this concept of substance that Berkeley dismisses as self-contradictory, as well as useless for Locke's purposes.

Berkeley's solution to the problem clearly must be in terms of coordinating various kinds of sensations, and this can be summarized as follows. If there is no real object distinct from the whole collection of its various appearances for any given observer, or mind, then not only is the primacy of touch rejected, but there is no reason whatever to suppose that any perspective of an object is uniquely privileged. . . . Rather the so-called true dimensions of the cube, so the argument runs, are the ones related to the present perceptual field and the viewer's present interest in it. For Berkeley then there are no unalterably pristine objects in the world, even in disguise. Apart from minds, there are only interpretations of experience which yield either expected or unexpected results, and reality is measured in these terms.[28]

It is therefore quite surprising that despite Berkeley's rejection of Locke's materialism in favor of idealism, Park argues, "In considering the Molyneux Problem both Locke and Berkeley, as well as Molyneux himself, arrived at the same correct conclusion,"[29] that is, the "blind man made to see" would not be able to recognize by sight the difference between a cube and a sphere which he had learned to recognize by touch. The problem in Park's conclusion, I would argue, is with the word "recognize."

Medical Intervention

Kate Tunstall's excellent *Blindness and Enlightenment*[30] draws us away from philosophical deliberations and reminds us that Berkeley speculated in the second edition of his *Essay Towards a New Theory of Vision,* whether the Molyneux problem would soon be answered empirically,[31] as it soon was by the physician William Cheselden.[32] In 1728 Cheselden performed a cataract operation on a boy of thirteen years old and reported, just as had Molyneux, Locke, and Berkeley, that, "When he [the boy who was blind and made to see] first saw, he was so far from making any judgment about Distances, that he thought all Objects whatever touch'd his Eyes, (as he express'd it) as what he felt, did his Skin; and thought no Objects so agreeable as those which were smooth and regular, tho' he could form no Judgment about their Shape."[33] The agreement between Locke and Berkeley on the Molyneux question now demonstrated by William Cheselden set in stone the shift in British empiricism from materialism to idealism, albeit unaccountable and counterintuitive, that empiricism should not hold as an inalienable truth the existence of a real world. Furthermore, Berkeleyian idealism was much more akin to Descartes's skeptical world of rational doubt than to Locke's materialism.

It therefore cannot be counted as odd that in the Francophone tradition philosophy latched onto Berkeleyian idealist empiricism, once again making a link, if somewhat ironically, through blindness. Kate Tunstall translates Denis Diderot's *Essai sur les Aveugles* (1749):

> The name Idealists is given to those philosophers who are conscious only of their existence and of the sequence of sensations they experience inside themselves, and therefore admit nothing else. It is an extravagant system which could only, it seems to me, have been born of the blind and which, to the shame of the human mind and philosophy, is the most difficult to refute, though the most absurd of all. It is set out with as much sincerity as clarity in three *Dialogues* by Doctor Berkeley, Bishop of Cloyne.[34]

Diderot continues with the argument that Berkeley and Condillac share the same philosophical idea:

> The author of the *Essay on Human Knowledge* [Condillac] should be invited to examine this work as it would give him the material for some useful, agreeable and subtle observations, in a word, for observations of the kind he does so well. It is well worth accusing him of idealism too, and this

claim is liable to excite him owing less to its singularity than to the difficulty of refuting it according to his own principles, which are exactly the same as Berkeley's. According to them both and according to reason, the terms essence, matter, substance, substrate etc. offer the mind no insights. Furthermore, as the author of the Essay judiciously observes, whether we raise ourselves into the heavens or descend into the abyss, we never go beyond ourselves and it is only our own thought that we perceive. Such is the conclusion of Berkeley's first dialogue and the very basis for his whole system.[35]

So dominant and powerful has been the belief that Berkeley's idealist argument was irrefutable, and that nothing existed but the philosopher's consciousness and the sequence of sensations they experience inside themselves, that, as Tunstall points out, "In the twentieth century, many French writers and philosophers—Bergson, Bataille, Merleau-Ponty, Foucault and Derrida—took a critical interest in the predominance of visual metaphors in Western thought and sought both to expose the assumptions such metaphors foster and to counter them by focusing instead on visual dysfunction, including blindness, and on the other senses, notably touch."[36]

David Hartley, a pupil of Nicholas Saunderson, gave just such a provoking example about the primacy of touch in *Observations on Man, his Frame, his Duty, and his Expectations* that appears to derive from observations of his teacher.[37] Having learned mathematics from a man who was completely blind, Hartley attempted to found a form of empiricism using touch rather than sight as the major sense. In order to do this, he gave an account of the difference between "a Person born Blind" and "a Person . . . born without feeling" in which the person born blind can know of a knife by touch, whereas a person born without feeling could be tricked by a picture of a knife into believing that knives can be indistinguishable from the flat surfaces on which they were placed.

Hartley's beguiling attack on the Molyneux problem is a counterfactual that can never be proven in fact, and thus may be regarded as being constructed with a lack of regard to the real example of sight used by Locke and Berkeley: the "blind man made to see" was not a myth, but nor was

Cheselden's boy the first person whose cataracts had been removed so he could see for the first time. Nevertheless, Locke's "blind man made to see" was unable to tell the sphere from the cube, although not for the reasons that made Locke reject vision as the primary sense and assert the primacy of touch, and which gave Berkeley his cue to reject materialism.

Optical Correction

The problem with the second edition of Locke's *Essay concerning Humane Understanding* is that it ceases to be empiricist when it takes on Molyneux's "thought experiment." In doing so, Locke becomes a rationalist and is therefore open to idealist criticism of his desire for a material world. But at the same time there is a problem with the second edition of Berkeley's *Essay Towards a New Theory of Vision* (1710), since as an idealist he ought not to have felt the need for empirical evidence like Cheselden's boy to make his point about there being nothing certain but thought. The problem with both Locke's and Berkeley's understanding of optics was that it was based upon a faulty assumption about the "blind man made to see."

If we carefully explore the additions Locke made to the first edition of the *Essay*, what we read is that the reason Locke agreed with Molyneux was because he came to know a man who had been cured of blindness while he was redrafting.[38] Locke mentions the relatively common operation of couching in both the first and second editions of his *Essay* in his arguments about innate ideas.

The mention of the "blind man made to see" in the first edition tells us:

> Few Children can be supposed to have those Idea's which they must begin to have sometime or other; and then they will also begin to assent to that Proposition, and make very little question of it ever after. But such assent upon learning, no more proves the Ideas to be innate, than it does, That one born blind (with Cataracts which will be couched to morrow) had the Ideas of the Sun, or Light, or Saffron, or Yellow; because when his Sight is cleared, he will certainly assent to this Proposition, That the Sun is lucid, or that Saffron is yellow: And therefore if such an assent upon hearing cannot

prove the Ideas innate, it can much less the Propositions made up of those Ideas. If they have any innate Ideas, I would be glad to be told, what, and how many they are.[39]

The paragraph is based on the possibility of couching a cataract to "clear" the vision of the "one born blind," but Locke here had no experience of couching, so the operation is put into the future. By so doing, his paragraph ends up with a rhetorical rather than a conclusive statement. A new paragraph added to the second edition tells a different story:

> Suppose a Child had the use of his Eyes till he knows and distinguishes Colours; but then Cataracts shut the Windows, and he is Forty or Fifty Years perfectly in the Dark; and in that Time perfectly loses all Memory of the *Ideas* of Colour he once had. This was the Case of a Blind Man I once talked with, who lost his Sight by the Small-Pox, when he was a Child, and had no more Notion of Colours, than one born Blind. I ask whether any one can say this Man had then any *Ideas* of Colours in his Mind, any more than one born Blind? And I think no Body will say, that either of them had in his Mind any *Idea* of Colours at all. His Cataracts are couch'd, and then he has the *Ideas* (which he remembers not) of Colours, *de novo*, by his restor'd Sight, convey'd to his Mind, and that without any Consciousness of a former Acquaintance, being thus in the Memory, are said to be in the Mind.... The use I make of this is, that whatever *Idea* being not actually in View, is in the Mind, is there only by being in the Memory; and if it be not in the Memory, it is not in the Mind; and if it be in the Memory, it cannot by the Memory be brought into actual View, without a Perception that it comes out of the Memory, which is this, that it had been known before, and is now remembred [sic].[40]

Here Locke is preempting the Molyneux problem by adding an explanation of the function of memory, in a way that explains why the man who has ideas of the sphere and cube by touch will not know them at first sight: because the ideas in his Mind of the sphere and cube which got there by touch have no conscious acquaintance with the new perceptions, and must be learned *de novo* as here with color.

This ought not to be the case in empiricism, for as Locke argues in a paragraph "*Of simple* Ideas *of diverse Senses*" which appears in both editions of the *Essay:* "The *Ideas* we get by more than one Sense, are of *Space, or Extension, Figure, Rest,* and *Motion:* For these make perceivable impressions, both on Eyes and Touch: and we can receive and convey into our Minds the *Ideas* of the Extension, Figure, Motion and Rest of Bodies, both by seeing and feeling."[41] Since Ideas of figure can be gained by touch AND sight, even though touch alone is the sense by which figure is learned, which is the jocose problem, this paragraph would suggest that the sphere and cube should be known at first sight, whereas the added paragraph quoted above suggests John Locke knew they could not be distinguished by a "blind man made to see."

But what the added paragraph also tells us is that Locke has learned this not from Molyneux's thought experiment, but from the experience of "a Blind Man I once talked with" who has been couched. And it is by "experience" that Locke's empiricism tells us by which we learn things: "Let us then suppose the Mind to be, as we say, white Paper, void of all Characters, without any Ideas; How comes it to be furnished? Whence comes it by that vast store, which the busie and boundless Fancy of Man has painted on it, with an almost endless variety? Whence has it all the materials of Reason and Knowledge? To this I answer, in one word, From Experience: in that, all our Knowledge is founded; and from that it ultimately derives it self."[42] The only way he could know that "one born blind and made to see" could not tell the sphere from the cube would be by asking his friend, or by being there at the unbinding of his eyes after the operation.[43] And if this were so, then he could have shown the man a cube and a sphere, and then he would have known by empirical evidence, by experience, that Molyneux was right.

Or at least he would have believed that Molyneux was right because the couched man would not have been able to recognize the difference between the two shapes. Cheselden's account of his boy's failure to recognize objects is rather charming: "When he first saw . . . he knew not the Shape of any Thing, nor any one Thing from another, however different in Shape, or Magnitude; . . . One Particular only (though it may appear trifling) I will relate; Having often forgot which was the Cat and which the Dog, he was asham'd to ask; but catching the Cat (which he knew by feeling) he was observ'd to look at her stedfastly, and then setting her down,

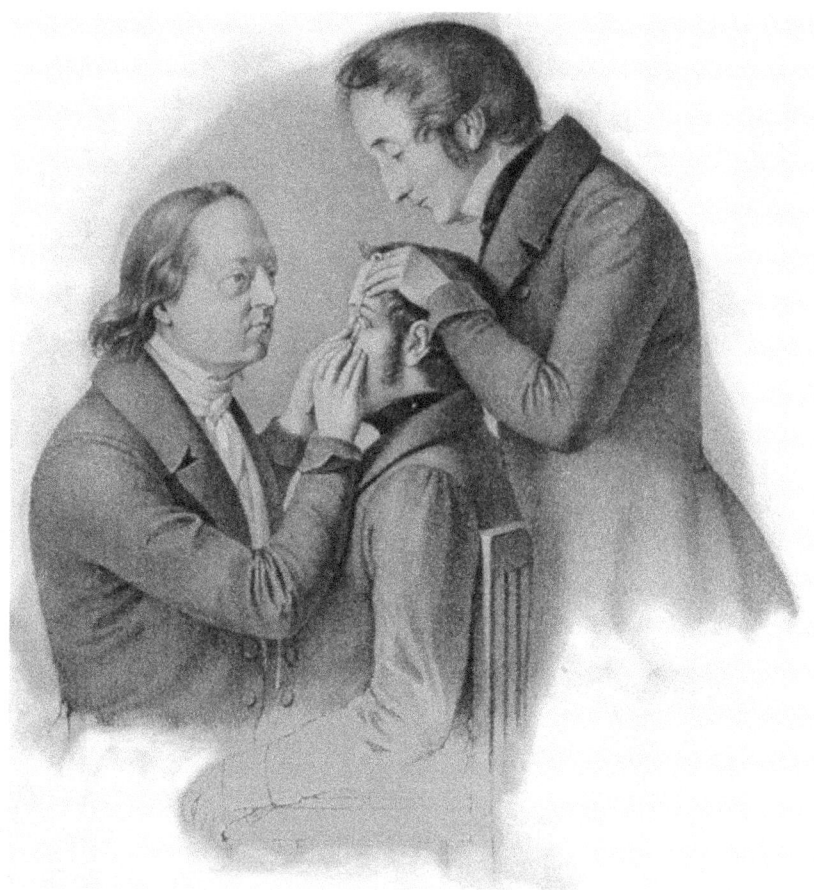

FIGURE 2. The couching operation depicted in *Operation for Cataract*. (Wellcome Collection, CC BY)

said, So Puss! I shall know you another Time."[44] However, as mentioned above, both Locke's and Berkeley's (and also Cheselden's) understanding of optics was faulty and it is merely an assumption that a "blind man made to see" by the process of couching could not, in perfect circumstances, discern objects directly the bandages are removed after recovery from the operation.

Couching is still a common practice in many parts of the world (see fig. 2). The clouded lens is cut out and pushed back into the aqueous humor, where it rests out of the way of the retina. The operation avoids damaging the iris, so the pupil continues to function nearly normally. If it is well done, there will be a minimum of corneal scarring, which would form a lenticular cataract that would itself reduce vision. Nevertheless, the practice was regarded as unsafe and ineffective until a 1995 study by Girard[45] suggested that a modified form of couching is effective and cheap.

But the operation of couching does not bring with it an instant recognition of objects newly perceived for the first time. William Taylor of Ightham, who was born with cataracts, was operated on by John Taylor, oculist of Hatton Garden, on 9 November 1751. After the operation he was asked by some of the company of sixteen who were present "*What he saw?* [and he] Answer'd in a kind of transport, and Wonder, at the strange Shapes, Forms and Colours of many Things, so incomprehensible about him, that *He beheld the Room full of Lights, and Moons.*"[46] However, this does not simply give the argument to Berkeley. Just because objects are first perceived upside down, or distance is unrecognized after a couching operation, and when consciousness has not made the reversal of the image it does in young sighted children, does not mean there is no substance or material world. Something is being perceived by William Taylor; it is just not comprehended or consonant with the previously existing plenum of the blind boy's experience.

Furthermore, William Taylor of Ightham would not see properly until his sight was corrected after the operation: Couched patients need to wear glasses if they are to see "clearly." Typically, a couched patient without refractive correction has eyesight of the order of 20/200, that is, they are what we would now call legally blind. We might therefore conclude that Cheselden is being absolutely truthful about his boy's failure to recognize the difference between the dog and the cat. Likewise, and probably to Locke's chagrin, when he met the man who had been couched, he came up against empirical evidence that a "blind man made to see" could not tell the difference between a sphere and a cube of the same color and the same size at a distance of about ten feet.

This is all well and good, but we need a further reason why Molyneux and Locke as materialists believed this was a question of tabula rasa and the brain's presence chamber, and failure to recognize a new sensation encountered for the first time, rather than a question of accommodation to the new sense and poor visual acuity. At the same time we also need a reason why Berkeley the idealist called for empirical evidence at the end of the second edition of his book on vision when he knew that he could rely on the failure of discernment between the two shapes as the cure of a person born blind and made to see had already been advertised as having been performed many times before 1710 by the queen's oculist, William Read. And the reason is that all three philosophers' understanding of optics suggested to them that the focus of the image upon the retina was a function of pupil diameter and the qualities of the vitreous humor, and not of the changing shape of the lens.

It was not until 1 May 1794, when David Hosack, an American physician, read a paper before the Royal Society called "Observations upon vision," that this version of optics was challenged.[47] Hosack began with the version that Molyneux, Locke, and Berkeley would have known: "By what power is the eye enabled to view objects distinctly at different distances? As the pupil is enlarged or diminished according to the greater or less quantity of light, and in a certain degree to the distance of the object, it would readily occur that these different changes of the pupil would account for the phenomena in question. Accordingly anatomists and philosophers, who have written upon this subject have generally had recourse to this explanation."[48] Hosack goes on to note the observations from his experiments: the pupil did not continue to contract when an object was brought very close, but dilated, and that the pupil contracted in bright sunlight when it ought to have dilated to see the distant sun in focus. He is therefore certain that it is not the iris alone that changes the focal length of the image to produce an image on the retina: "Were it from the contraction and dilation of the iris alone that we see objects at different distances, I naturally concluded it should operate regularly to produce its effects; but if to view an object at a few yards distance it be enlarged to the utmost extent, surely it must of itself be insufficient to view one at the distance of several miles; for example the heavenly bodies."[49] To be sure, Hosack's new proposal that there are transparent muscle filaments in the lens which change its focal length is somewhat wide of the mark, but he also argues that the whole eye shape can be altered by the six layers of muscles that surround it, which is still believed to be true. But this argument dates from a century after Molyneux, Locke, and Berkeley. For these philosophers, a couched patient with an undamaged iris and cornea ought to have been able to see in focus.

Marjolein Degenaar has also noted the reduction of visual acuity in couched patients, although as she points out, "this fact was missed by all the eighteenth-century commentators on Cheselden's report."[50] She also notes that "A cataract operation makes the patient far sighted [long-sited], and if good eyesight is to be restored there is need of optical correction, in the form of a lens or a glass."[51] As she points out, "The need for optical correction was already perceived by Benito Daza de Valves in 1623 in his *Uso de los antojos*, one of the first books about spectacles, [in which] he recommended the wearing of glasses by patients who had had a cataract operation."

This places knowledge of optical correction at least a hundred years too late. The 1519 English version of the comic tales of the German trickster Till Eulenspiegel, who was known as Howleglasse, notes that when asked by the bishop of Taer "what he was, . . . Howleglas [sic] answered I am a Spectacle maker cum out of Grabant."[52] The Worshipful Company of Spectacle Makers, which presumably was set up to regulate the poor practices of spectacle makers such as Howleglasse, dates from 1629. Likewise, in 1696 we find "The first True Spectacles" advertised by John Yarwell, "at the *Archimedes* and *Three Prospects, St Paul's Churchyard* and *Ludgate Street.*" What is more important, the same advertisement informs us that Yarwell made "other sorts of Concave and Convex glasses," suggesting that both farsightedness and nearsightedness could be corrected.[53] Nevertheless, the connection between couching and the use of lenses was not made until 1737, when William Porterfield presented a paper to the Royal College of Physicians of Edinburgh: "A Man having a Cataract in both Eyes, which intirely deprived him of Sight, committed himself to an Oculist, who finding them ripe, performed the Operation, and couched the Cataracts with all the Success that could be desired; but after they were couched, he could not distinctly see Objects, even at an Ordinary Distance without the help of a Convex Lens; which is what every Body has observed to be necessary to all those who have had a Cataract couched."[54]

The weasel words "which is what everybody has observed" read to me something like an in-joke—it is a fact that readers (or at least professional ophthalmologists) of the time would have known so well that they did not bother to explain it elsewhere. But for how long would this in-joke have been known, and would John Locke have known? Would his friend who had been couched, from whom Locke learned by empirical experience that Molyneux was correct, have had a pair of "couching spectacles"[55] ready beside him when his eyes were unbound? If he had, would they have been ground to the precise lens that would have allowed him to perceive the difference between a cube and a sphere? Edward Scarlett, the royal optician, is known to have ground graded lenses for different visual acuities.[56]

I would argue that following the contemporary belief in the optical characteristics of the eye, and the state of knowledge of optical correction, even if Locke expected reduction in visual acuity of a postoperative cataract patient if the iris remained intact, the overlaying contexts of information about sight occluded his thinking through the idea that new visual sense experience would not simply be included into the plenum of experience of a blind person to allow for something so subtle as "recognition" of something known previously by touch. Therefore, we must be careful when reading Michael Bruno and Eric Mandelbaum's suggestion that, "given Locke's views about primary qualities and common sensibles, it seems that he should have said that the blind person would be able to call up and deploy the tactually acquired idea when first visually presented with the sphere and the cube and thereby be able to tell which is which."[57]

And answer: it might be possible only if the person's sight were corrected perfectly. But as we now can conclude, Locke was truthful to his method and believed the empirical over the rational, and trusted the experience of the couched man with whom he had spoken. He put faith in his "blind man made to see" rather than the "thought experiment," which led to Berkeley's move to idealism. And for this reason I would agree with Désirée Park's conclusion "that the Molyneux Problem served to drive a wedge between the epistemological theories of Locke and Berkeley, a result which in turn makes somewhat doubtful the commonly accepted line of the empirical succession."[58]

Philosophically, then, we must conclude that in the eighteenth century the capacities and capabilities of sight remained indeterminately known and unknowable but in encounters with the sighted and the blind. It was not and could not be a metaphor for truth as its own truth was not understood. And yet sight and the restoration of sight did signify another route to truth.

Religious

If I have ignored the religious in this analysis, let me end with a miracle which might also have affected Locke's understanding of his "blind man made to see." In Mark 6:22–26 we read:

> And he cometh to Bethesda, and they bring a blind man to him, and besought him to touch him.
> And he took the blind man by the hand, and led him out of the town; and when he had spit on his eyes, and put his hand on him, he asked him if he saw ought.
> And he looked up, and said, I see men as trees walking.
> After that, he put his hands again upon the eyes, and made him look up: and he was restored, and saw every man clearly.

In Matthew Poole and Samuel Clarke's annotated Bible, this incident is glossed thus: "Christ was wont to heal at once, here he healeth by degrees; so as the Healing of this Blind Man, was a true pattern of his Healing spiritual Blindness, which usually is done gradually, but perfected at last as this bodily Cure was."[59] If Locke knew the passage from Mark, and it is difficult to believe he did not, then he had a revealed version of what he discovered empirically: that a "blind man made to see" did not begin to see in focus immediately. But where Locke avoided going into metaphors about blindness, we like sheep have followed Berkeley into the realms of thought experiments and spiritual blindness.

Conclusions

If this is the hinterland of the understanding of sight and blindness in the eighteenth century, we shall find that little of it appears at the surface of medical practice on eyes and in the personal experience of blindness. For this reason I shall now leave the problems inherent in the technical understanding of sight and blindness as a backdrop to the arguments made in the rest of the book, only to reiterate that the chapters on medical intervention and the chapters on the personal experience of blindness, as has been argued here, were very unlike either of the theoretical medical and cultural models of "disability" used in modern "disability studies" and probably because the very philosophical problems explored here have continued into modern philosophy.

PART II

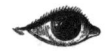

MEDICINE

4

UNOFFICIAL EYE CARE

William Read and Mary Cater

It was demonstrated in the introduction how difficult it is to be sure who are the luminaries and who the villains of the history of medical practice at a time when it was not only protectionist, but also when there was uncertainty about the relative status of medicine and surgery. The Royal College of Physicians, who required a degree for entry into their society, laid the charge of "quack" or "empirick" or "mountebank"[1] on any practitioner (be they trained or not) who stood on a bench (real or metaphorical) before a crowd to advertise a specific skill or a new medicine as they searched through the nation to find the individuals whom they could help. The physicians were equally dismissive of surgeons, whose training was by apprenticeship and required no degree, and the surgeons in their turn had little time for physicians. A third type of practitioner, whose success derived from cures known from time immemorial, appears to have been ignored by both branches of the profession. What was common to all was the fact that some patients were helped by the remedies offered, a fact widely advertised in the newspapers, which were becoming an important factor in British economic life, and in medical textbooks, which might be argued to have been intended to raise the status of the medical practice into a profession. Physicians, surgeons, and other medical practitioners all had to make a living, and treatments for conditions like blindness were equally important for patients who needed to see to work. But who could be trusted?

William Read, Experienced and Approved Oculist

Emilie Savage-Smith omits William Read's newspaper advertisements from the list of sources for her *ODNB* entry,[2] and thus it is remarkable that she can be as positive as to claim that "It is difficult to assess the validity of Read's claims ... to have performed many cures." It is less remarkable that Thomas Seccombe's account of Read in the original *DNB* dismissed him outright as an "empiric, [who] was originally a tailor, and became progressively a mountebank and an itinerant quack."[3] Seccombe based his assessment on three sources: a handbill listing Read's cures dating from 1696 called "Post nubila Phoebus, nihil absque Deo" (After the clouds, the sun, Nothing without God); his advertising having been satirized in the *Spectator* no. 547; and Jonathan Swift's letter to Stella of 11 April 1711 in which Swift reports that Read "has been a mountebank, and is the queen's oculist. He makes admirable punch, and treats you in golden vessels." On the evidence of the handbill, Seccombe attacks Read for offering too many cures for "Blindness, Cancers, Wens, Hare-lips, or Wry-necks" to be believed. On the other hand, it is implied that the substance of the attack by the authors of so august an organ as the *Spectator* must be believed, since it is an impeccable source, as is Jonathan Swift, who satirizes Read for using his wealth for social climbing and trying to gain legitimacy by association.

What makes Emilie Savage-Smith pause in accepting Seccombe's judgement is the sheer number of Read's reported cures and his knighthood granted for helping soldiers and sailors blinded in action, which leads her to the conclusion that "In London Read appears to have been considered by some to be skillful." And this despite her additional accusation against him that "The first part of the book [Read's *A short but exact account of all the diseases incident to the eyes*] is an unacknowledged reprint (with a few spelling changes) of the *Breviary of the Eyes*, written by Richard Banister in 1621." I cannot locate a copy of Banister's *Breviary of the Eyes*, which appears in the British Library catalogue as "Jacques Gillemeau, *A treatise of one hundred and thirteene diseases of the eyes, and eye-liddes. The second time published, with some profitable additions of certaine principles and experiments, by Richard Banister, Dr. in Chirurgery, Oculist, and Practitioner in*

Physick, Imprinted at London: by Felix Kyngston, for Thomas Man, dwelling in Pater-noster-row, at the signe of the Talbot, 1622."[4] The apparent plagiarism by Read was first noticed by Arnold Sorsby (1900–1980), an ophthalmologist, and was reported in Rutson James.[5] In fact, it must be argued that it was Banister who was the plagiarist. When Read published his only book, *A short but exact account of all the diseases incident to the eyes,* in 1710, it was also called a "Second edition,"[6] but only the third part, which makes up the final thirty-nine pages and is separately numbered and given a separate title, *Practical observations upon some extraordinary diseases of the eyes,* is introduced in the contents as "by Sir *William Read.*"

It might therefore be argued that Savage-Smith's ultimate dismissal of Read is overly harsh when she claims that "available evidence suggests that Sir William was a more effective self-promoter and plagiarist than he was an oculist." Furthermore, Swift's comment to Stella that guests at the Reads' were entertained from "golden vessels" suggests that a very great number of people in London (and around England) considered him to be skillful enough to pay him to couch their cataracts. He certainly did not make the money to buy his "golden vessels" from his service to the Crown that began as early as William III's reign, since it was advertised "gratis." The knighthood cannot have hindered his career and was awarded in July 1705 after his services to soldiers wounded in the battles of the Wars of Spanish Succession, a role he had also undertaken in the Nine Years' War for William III. But it must be asked whether Read would have been awarded so high a rank if he had been a bungler or made little or no improvement in the eyesight of the soldiers and sailors he treated.

There is no doubt that Read, as Savage-Smith claims, "flamboyantly advertised his medical and surgical skill," but if we explore the newspaper advertisements that document his working life in nearly daily detail, we get a very different sense of his achievement from that based on the small collection of cures listed in "Post nubila Phoebus, nihil absque Deo": the sheer weight of numbers of cures documented and his account of his meticulous business practice render us more able to judge how many cures might be thought bogus and how many real. Furthermore, the context of his advertising practice suggests that the satire of the *Spectator* no. 547 in November 1712 probably had a different cause than a swipe at Read's surgical skill.

Seccombe noted in his *DNB* article that Read advertised in the *Tatler*, but he does not tell us that these eighteen advertisements were placed throughout the life of that Whiggish magazine between November 1709 and January 1711, when it folded. Thereafter, Read continued to advertise in Addison and Steele's *Spectator*, stopping only when the eye surgeon began an extended tour of England. Read's name may well have been lampooned in the *Spectator* in November 1712 because he did not take up his advertisements with them on his return to London, choosing instead to advertise in Abel Roper's Tory *Post Boy*, or perhaps he was satirized simply because his move to the new source of advertisements indicated he had changed sides politically.

The confusion over Read's political change of sides may also account for Jonathan Swift's letter to Stella. Whereas Seccombe and Savage-Smith believe it to be unbiased, we must remember that the letter was written in April 1711, when it was not well-known that Read had become a Tory and was now of Swift's party: Read's first of a series of regular advertisements with the Tory *Post Boy* did not appear until the following month.[7] Furthermore, Swift's arch rival, the Whig writer "Mr. Observator," used Sir William Read as a metaphor to attack Swift as writer of the Tory newspaper the *Examiner* on the very day Swift sent the letter to Stella about Read's "golden vessels":

> OBS. I perceive you are acquainted with Sir *W. Read* her Majesty's principal Oculist, who cures People that are born blind, and has restor'd I don't know how many hundreds of Seamen and Pilots to their sight, so that they can see how to haul Ropes, and manage Rudder and other Tackling of the Ships, so as to prevent their stranding, and running soul upon Rocks and Shelves.
>
> COUNTRYM. Well, and what of it Master?
>
> OBS. Why you must speak to Sir *William, Roger*, and tell him that he ought to lend the *Examiner*, his brother *Abel*, and Dr. *Sacheverel* the three blind leaders of the Blind, a Cast of his Office; and since he can cure those who are born blind, 'twill be for him to help those who have only artificial Mists, Pins, and Cobwebs cast before their eyes.[8]

Swift cannot but have thought Read another Whig and a target for his pen, albeit in a letter to his friend.

The run of all of Read's available newspaper advertisements (including those in the *Tatler*) gives us a grounding for an account of the life of a man struggling with the beginnings of a new specialist practice and finally succeeding to make a profitable career as a surgeon at a time when the popular conception of medical intervention in eye conditions was changing from, to use Swift's term, the "mountebank" to the professional, which change we can understand again from Swift's letter to Stella when he follows the word "mountebank" with "and is the queen's oculist." Swift's words, I would argue, are not merely ironic but demonstrate his surprise, a genuine surprise in 1711, that an eye surgeon could be socially acceptable, an idea which would only begin to become concrete after 1745, when John Ranby and William Cheselden led the separation of the Company of Barbers and Surgeons in order to set up surgery as a profession. In effect, William Read was, like all other surgeons in Swift's mind, a Barber: he shaved your face, he cut your hair, he bled you when you were ill and sewed up your wounds on the battlefield. It is perhaps no surprise that John Ranby, the first Master of the new Company of Surgeons, and the source of Cheselden's influence with the Crown in bringing about its separation from the barbers, was sergeant-surgeon to George II and treated the Duke of Cumberland on the battlefield of Dettingen in May 1743 for a gunshot wound. Emilie Savage-Smith draws our attention to these practical aspects of barber/surgery, I believe unintentionally, when she describes Read's own contribution to *A short but exact account of all the diseases incident to the eyes* as a "discourse promoting his manual dexterity." It was his very "manual dexterity" that he was trying to sell, and which he advertised to found his career as a privately financed eye surgeon.

In order to do this, as this chapter will demonstrate, Read was very different from an orthodox surgeon who would tackle a myriad of surgical procedures, since he styled himself an oculist. The difference was that the orthodox surgeon (who would rarely operate on eyes) waited in his hospital until patients came to him, or called him out to their homes, whereas Read spent a good deal of his time touring the country looking for patients. In effect he was a field surgeon like John Ranby, performing procedures where they were needed. A second difference was that Read was far better than most orthodox surgeons at operating on eyes. By traveling around the country, he encountered more cataracted eyes, cancers, wens, harelips, and wry-necks and performed many more operations than a hospital-bound surgeon, so he gained more specialist practice than the orthodox. Since he toured extensively in East Anglia, he most probably set John "Chevalier" Taylor on his life's course to his "profession of Couching" in 1727, and as we shall find in chapter 5, it was John "Chevalier" Taylor who helped surgery take the next step forward toward the idea that specialism in a single operation could be a profession.

William Read's Self-Presentation

Much of his reputation for being a quack is based on "Sir William Read's Advertisement," as Rutson James calls "Post nubila Phoebus, nihil absque Deo," a handbill which describes multiple cures performed around England between 1687 and 1694. It is reproduced in *Studies in Ophthalmology*, along with a transcription that is given without comment as though its words alone are enough to damn Read. However, for a start it was not "Sir" William Read's advertisement, as he was not knighted until some ten years after the latest-mentioned procedure, an amputation of the leg of Mrs. Anne Crook on 14 July 1694, performed before the Duke of Northumberland, "without the loss of an Ounce of Blood after the Styptick-Water was applied."[9] The handbill gathers together information of Read's early cures before he turned to newspaper advertisements and is aimed at an illiterate audience since it is surmounted by five woodcut illustrations. The continuous mention of Read's "Styptick-Water" is without doubt product placement, and the account of his testimonial for numerous cures in Oxford from the vice chancellor of the university might be described as "flamboyant." But the handbill needs to be read in context.

If we explore the self-presentation of "orthodox" medical practitioners in London in the 1690s, we discover that even they encountered difficulties in getting their names known as practitioners. The example of Edward Hannes gives more than a suggestion that attacks on Read may have been (and continue to be) politically inspired rather than having anything to do with his skill as a surgeon. Queen Anne's physician, Edward Hannes, was also lowborn: his father was an herb seller at Bloomsbury Market. He was nevertheless educated at Westminster and Oxford, and came back to London in 1699 to set up as a doctor, whence J. H. Curthoys in the *ODNB* records:

> Not licensed with, even actively rejected by, the Royal College of Physicians, he found that, even for a man relying on his Oxford degrees, it was difficult to compete with established practitioners like John Radcliffe. In some desperation, and in order to make his name known in the city, he reportedly sent his footman out on to the streets of London to stop every carriage and make enquiries for the doctor. The servant continued the campaign into the coffee houses and, at Garraway's, encountered Dr Radcliffe who, in response to the servant's enquiry after the whereabouts of a nobleman who allegedly had called for Hannes, quipped that it was not the lords who needed Hannes but "the doctor wants those lords".[10] Eventually the strategy paid off; his practice grew, and he was appointed principal physician at court.

If this is a suggestion that Hannes advertised his profession more subtly than Read, it must be noted that John Radcliffe was not above advertising his own Cordial Tincture in public newspapers when his own career was at a low ebb.[11] Curthoys's account of Hannes's life itself also politicizes Hannes's role, noting that he attended the deathbed of William, Duke of Gloucester, in 1700, "whose death effectively ended the Stuart succession." Furthermore, Curthoys informs us that John Radcliffe believed that Hannes had misdiagnosed the duke's illness and that it was not smallpox but a heat rash brought on by excessive dancing. Again, Curthoys tells us that on Hannes's knighthood in 1705, "[Thomas] Hearne, rather acidly, drew attention to the liberality of the queen in her distribution of honours at this time." What Curthoys does not tell us is that John Radcliffe was "a confirmed Jacobite and violent tory,"[12] who had been dismissed from William III's Whiggish court in 1699 and who would not be welcome to serve the king's sister-in-law before her conversion to Toryism in 1706. Another high Tory, Thomas Hearne, derided Whigs as "Pharisaical People."[13] Thus, it would be scarcely credible if Hearne had welcomed the knighthoods of Hannes, as the queen's physician,[14] and William Read, as the queen's oculist,[15] which took place within two days of one another in July 1705 while she and presumably they were still Whigs.[16]

But in the context of William Read's gaining a knighthood, we should understand the handbill "Post nubila Phoebus, nihil absque Deo" as Read's first and failed attempt to draw attention to himself in London as a practitioner with an even less orthodox training than Hannes. Whereas Hannes could rely on his degrees from Oxford, Read had to rely on cures performed in that town and "a Testimonial from the Vice-Chancellor for several considerable cures he hath performed in the aforesaid University of Oxford." And whereas Hannes turned to the aristocracy to get his career going, Read's handbill is aimed at the general populous. He is listing the procedures he can perform and naming the names of those he has cured while touring the country as evidence of his ability. But a single handbill could never be effective in spreading his name and skill across a whole nation. Whereas Hannes's name spread through the relatively small number of Whig aristocrats eventually to be knighted as the queen's physician through their recommendation, Read had to turn to the medium of newspaper advertising to reach his target market and publicize a multitude of cures (sometimes repeating himself) eventually to become renowned enough to be knighted as the queen's oculist.

Another context from which to explore "Post nubila Phoebus, nihil absque Deo" is the milieu in which it suggests that William Read moved. In want of publishers' details, the subscription of the handbill informs the reader: "He [William Read] is to be spoken with at Mr. Agutters a musical-instrument-maker, at the sign of the Crown, over-against the York-Buildings in the Strand, from 8 in the morning till 6 in the evening, where you will see a bill of operations hang at the door."

Ralph Agutter was the most important English violin maker of this period,[17] and the premises in which he worked were newly built. George Villiers, 2nd Duke of Buckingham, sold the land on which the York Buildings had stood[18] to developers for £30,000 in 1672. He made it a condition of the sale that his name and full title should be commemorated by George Street, Villiers Street, Duke Street, and Buckingham Street, but to this day, the name "York Buildings" is associated with the area. If not fashionable, the development was made up of solid owner-occupier shops, and the lithograph of Hungerford Market by Thomas Hosmer Shepherd made early in the nineteenth century demonstrates that it still comprised wide streets and profitable businesses.

Read is associated with two other addresses in London during his career.[19] He names a house in Bartholomew Close in advertisements placed from 1696 until 1704, where his neighbors were the booksellers William Downing[20] and William Rawlins,[21] the printer J. Darby,[22] the upholsterer Augustin Crow,[23] and, of course, St. Bartholomew's Hospital. In February 1704 he moved back to the Strand to Durham Yard, which was another new development similar to where he began at Ralph Agutter's, and remained there until the end of his life. This time, the 5th Earl of Pembroke sold the land of Durham House,[24] which had acted as quarters for Parliamentarian soldiers during the civil war, to developers in 1682, whence "A few moderate-sized houses were erected on the south side of Durham Yard with gardens to the river." The account of Durham Yard continues: "From the first there were wharves on the river front used for commercial purposes, and soon the greater part of the site was covered with courts of little houses occupied by small traders and artisans. By the middle of the eighteenth century Durham Yard had become a slum, and by the time the Adam brothers took it over [to build the Adelphi Building in 1768] practically all the buildings were in ruins."[25] However, while William Read lived there (until 1715), it was in its brief ascendency, and his neighbors were the goldsmith William Walker,[26] a dealer in lace, Mr. Bird,[27] the Grecian Coffee House, probably in an early incarnation,[28] and a flourishing haberdasher's shop.[29]

It is not certain whether Read owned any of the addresses he called "his house." In the first newspaper advertisement he placed that I can locate, which dates from 1696, the year after "Post nubila Phoebus, nihil absque Deo," he mentions "his House over against St. *Mary's* Church in St. *Edmundsbury* in *Suffolk*,"[30] as well as William Downing's in Bartholomew Close as destinations for letters to be sent to him. The second advertisement records "his Abode at his House in *Great St. Bartholomew Close, near West Smithfield, London*," suggesting this was where he resided permanently and that the St. Edmunds-Bury house was a temporary home while Read was on tour in 1696. But what is important here is the constant reminder of his address in advertisements, which suggests that Read was not wholly itinerant and, furthermore, gave former patients a place of recourse should any of Read's procedures fail.

Thus I would argue that when we read an address, we are looking at a place of business, a mark of social status and a guarantee of professional quality. William Read placed more than two hundred advertisements giving his address throughout his working life from 1696 to 1715, and he quickly learned how to manipulate the news media not just as a reminder that, and of where, he was carrying on his business, but to keep his name and association with eye surgery familiar to readers. And he was good at manipulating the press: many of his advertisements are printed just above or just below the newspaper title "Advertisements," and he used a number of other eye-catching devices such as pointing fingers and repeats. It is particularly telling that when the *Spectator* lampooned him, it was his advertising style that they mocked: something which had formerly brought in a regular income from Read to the *Tatler*.

What we find in his advertisements is certainly his own idea of himself, and it can also be argued that outside the historical contexts employed by Seccombe and Savage-Smith there is a concept of "medical truth" from which it might be argued that William Read was a quack rather than a doctor because he was not properly trained or did not know his subject: Robert Rutson James's book claims just this. Looking no further than the first example in Read's "Practical Observations *relating to some extraordinary Cures, of the Diseases of the Eyes*," Rutson James addresses his own "professional Brethren,"[31] giving details of the treatment Read administered to Jeremiah Puttiford of Watford for the "*Gutta Serena* joyn'd with a *Glaucoma* . . . [caused by] . . . a violent contusion to the head and right eye."[32] But access to "medical truth" cannot be accepted blindly, and must itself be contextualized against the evidence given and to the results of the treatment rather than against a mythical reality of the correct cure for the diseased body to which Rutson James and his mid-twentieth-century "professional Brethren" appear to have believed they had direct access. Rutson James writes up the Puttiford case thus: "The Faculty put his blindness down to a total obstruction of the optic nerves. Read treated him with cephalics and cordial stomachics. This treatment having produced some slight improvements in the man's condition, and Read having made up his mind that the case was one of glaucoma, he proceeded to treat this with mallows, violets, eyebright, celandine and fennel, together with depletion: he then performed a couching operation and the man received full sight."[33]

Read's own write-up of Puttiford's situation demonstrates a typical contemporary understanding of the failure of nerves as an impediment in "the Natural course of the [Animal] Spirits of Sight to the Eye," caused by "*Amaurosis* or Obstruction of the Optick Nerves, . . . or *Symptosis* or *Depressing* of the same Nerves . . . [or] *Aporrexis* or breaking a sunder of that Nerve."[34] Read decides that Puttiford has an obstructed optic nerve, known as a *gutta serena*, by either of the first two causes rather than a broken nerve, and prescribes snuffs, deciding that "by their strengthening and subtilising quality, [they] were most proper to attenuate, dissolve and disperse those gross and vicid Humours, which had hitherto obstructed the natural Course of the Animal Spirits (commonly called the Spirits of Sight in those parts) through the Optick Nerves, and consequently their conveyance to the substance of the Eye."[35] He also regulates Puttiford's digestion to make him strong enough to help his body cure the nerve by itself. When this treatment brought his "patient to have some glimpses of Sight,"[36] Read looked again at Puttiford's eye, which was opaque, and decided that it was not a cataract of the lens ("the Crystalline Humour")[37] but a "Glaucoma," by which he meant an opaqueness further back in the eye. It was this which he treated with the herbs Rutson James mentions along with more snuff "intended only as Preparatives, to facilitate the Manual Operation."[38] But the procedure was not, as Rutson James records, a couching operation; rather it was a manipulation with "a Couch Needle, adapted properly to the removing of such like coagulated vicious Humours (which by Consent of all Artists in this kind, prove more difficult in the Operation than ordinary *Cataracts*) in which I succeeded so well, that in a short time the Patient recovered his full Sight."[39]

I have no medical knowledge and do not pretend to understand what Read did to restore Puttiford's sight. However, his procedures were all logical, considered, and followed contemporary thought and practice. On the other hand, even a layman can comprehend that he used medical terms such as "glaucoma" (a disease of the eye, characterized by increased tension of the globe and gradual impairment or loss of vision) in a way which would appear idiosyncratic to a twentieth-century doctor. But in the eighteenth century Samuel Sharp, whom Rutson James treats as an "orthodox" surgeon,[40] argued in his *A treatise on the operations of surgery, with a description and representation of the instruments used in performing them,* that "we must understand the Words *Cataract* and *Glaucoma* as synonymous Terms, since they are in fact one Disease."[41] If anything is to be learned from this intervention by Read, it is, as Emilie Savage-Smith tells us, no more than "a discourse promoting his manual dexterity" in his removal of the diffuse opaqueness in Puttiford's eye. But what is more important is that after treatment by Read, Jeremiah Puttiford was able to see again, and all who wanted to visit him to testify to the cure knew that he lived in "the Parish of *Watford* in *Hartfordshire.*"[42] And furthermore, if Puttiford's cure failed, or the account was a lie, he knew where to find William Read from the newspaper advertisements placed after the date that Read's *A short but exact account of all the diseases incident to the eyes* was first published.

These advertisements, through which Read presents himself to us now, and presented himself to his audience in the eighteenth century, can be classified in several forms, although many advertisements are also a combination of the following types:

- Named cures
- Curing the poor/queen's oculist
- Affidavits for cures
- Tour itineraries
- Warnings against imitators
- Product placement/other operations

Named Cures

Named cures make up the majority of the column inches. As with the handbill, they provide readers with the name and address of the person cured, which suggests that the doubting reader might go and find the named individual and ask for confirmation of what William Read had done. For example, from Read's first surviving advertisement, we read that "a Child of Sir William Luckyns Barronet, of Messing-hall near Kelvedon in Essex" and "Likewise Mrs Baily New-street in Ipswich, Suffolk" were cured with "Cephalic Restorative Medicaments to the Optick Nerves, which he [Read] hath lately found out."[43] And as we would expect, at the bottom of the advertisement Read gave his own two addresses (mentioned above) presumably because he was soon to be on his way back to London.

As a first advertisement, this was something of a coup. Sir William Luckyns's son (perhaps the child of the cure), another William Luckyns, inherited the estates of his great-uncle, Sir Samuel Grimston, whose name he assumed. These estates included Gorhambury, formerly the seat of the Bacon family, and carried an important Whig electoral interest at St. Albans. Luckyns was no politician and became the victim of a lampoon by Sarah Churchill, who was provoked by his refusal to support her grandson, John Spencer, and thus Sir William Luckyns was ousted from his seat between 1722 and 1725.[44] Nevertheless, in 1696, the name of the Luckyns family was unlikely to have been used lightly. It cannot be argued that they were country bumpkins who had no access to London doctors as might be the case with "Mrs Baily New-street in Ipswich, Suffolk," and we should be inclined to believe Read's claim that "Sir *Wm. Luckyns,* notwithstanding he paid honourably for the cure, desired it may might [sic] be put in print for the public good, as well as for the credit of the Oculist: If any person have occasion to make use of him."

We might be a little wary when we read of a similar demand after a "generous reward" for the cure of Sir Cecil Bishopp of a cataract eight years later, that "this might be printed for the public good of others in the like Condition."[45] But this time Read combined the demand with the fact that the procedure was observed by "Dr. Tyson and Mr. Bernard (Surgeon in chief to her Majesty) &c." Dr. Edward Tyson was a member of the Royal College of Physicians, with degrees from Oxford and Cambridge Universities, who had a particular interest in comparative anatomy. His major contribution to knowledge was the idea that the porpoise was a link between fish and land animals and the chimpanzee a link between monkeys and humans. The reason for his attendance at Read's procedure on Cecil

Bishopp can only be surmised, but it might have been due to his interest in the anatomy of the eye, or to find out how steady Read's hand was in action. On the other hand, Charles Bernard was appointed sergeant-surgeon to Queen Anne on her accession in 1702. He was an apprenticed surgeon and admitted a freeman of the Company of Barbers and Surgeons in 1677. Appointed assistant surgeon at St. Bartholomew's Hospital in 1683, he was full surgeon in 1686 and was lithotomist from 1693 to 1705. What makes him a useful witness to Read's couching operation was the fact that he was known as a conservative in operations and for saving Bishop Benjamin Hoadly's leg when other surgeons called for amputation.[46] As such, Bernard would appear to be a surgeon keen to learn new techniques for saving a part of the body, and in this case, the eye. If nothing else, the attendance of both a physician and a surgeon suggests that eye operations were not common in the hospitals, had traditionally been left to itinerant surgeons, much as today when opticians not only test visual acuity but also look for the first signs of glaucoma and cataract.

Other techniques Read employed in naming patients might easily suggest some chicanery, such as the repetition of the names of those cured, which practice would suggest he was not telling a lie but nor entirely to be trusted. For example, Read advertised his place of business in August 1702 "for one Month at Mr Pain's, Goldsmith, at the Raven over against Exeter Exchange, in the Strand, London."[47] The Exeter Exchange was on the north side of the Strand, opposite what is now the Savoy Hotel, and the Worshipful Company of Goldsmiths record one Edmond Payne (or Paine) at this address in 1702.[48] In December of the same year, Read advertises the successful couching of "Mrs. Payne, (Wife of Mr. Payne, Goldsmith, over against Exeter Exchange)."[49] It is not out of the question to argue that this is the wife of the same Goldsmith, although the Goldsmiths' Company register notes a "Payne,—" with an unknown first name at "Exeter Exchange—1702," and Read himself gives his address in the advertisement of December 1702 as "the Raven over-against Exeter Exchange," and no longer at Mr. Pain's, Goldsmith. The apparent repetition of the named cure comes three years later, when Read advertised the cure of "Mrs. Paine, Wife of Mr. Paine, Goldsmith, next Door to the Fountain Tavern in the Strand."[50] The Fountain Tavern, where the Kit Kat Club met, was opposite the Exeter Exchange, and this Mr. Paine is duly recorded by the Company of Goldsmiths. With no first names available, we might be victims of an expansion of the available evidence, but there may well have been two separate goldsmiths working close to each other, who were or were not related to each other, as it is a trade which runs in families, and thus there may well have been a Mrs. Pain and a Mrs. Payne, both wives of goldsmiths, and both in need of cataract operations. Examining the advertisements for each cure, we find them also to have similarities and differences, like their husbands' names. After the couching of Mrs. Payne in December 1702, Read recorded that she could "now see so perfectly well as to thread the finest needle, and read the smallest Print, tho' stone-blind before, as any Person may be satisfied of at the said Mrs. Payne's House." After the cure of Mrs. Paine in February 1705, Read used similar terms, claiming that he had "restored her to her perfect Sight of both Eyes, so as to see to thread a fine Needle, as any Person may be satisfied upon enquiring of Mr. Edmond Paine, who inserts this for the public Good." It would be so easy to dismiss the advertisements as Read repeating himself. Who would remember the names of those he claimed he cured after three years? And if they visited a goldsmith called Mr. Paine/Payne somewhere at the Fleet Street end of the Strand, his wife would attest to the cure, albeit that it was recent or three years old. However, I am inclined to believe Read because of a significant difference in the detail of the account of the cure in the second advertisement. Where we read: "Mrs. Paine, ... who was blind of both Eyes with Cataracts, and also Obstructions in the Optick Nerves, which did in some measure hinder the present Success after the Operation, notwithstanding she was Couched with all imaginable Care and Dexterity, by Dr. William Read, Her Majesty's Oculist, in Durham-yard in the Strand, London, who has since, by his great Skill and Care, supplied the said Mrs. Paine with those Medicines which have restored her to her perfect Sight in both Eyes."

From this detailed information, given soon after Read moved into his permanent residence in Durham Yard at the other end of the Strand, it might be argued that a not completely satisfied customer had returned to him for further care. There was but one Mrs. Paine/Payne, she had been couched in December 1702, her sight had become worse again, and in

March 1705 she reapplied to Read for assistance, whence he gave her medicines or repeated the couching, which cleared it again. This argument reduces the number of goldsmiths of the name Paine working in the Strand in the first five years of the eighteenth century, and it also evidences the possibility that patients did return to Read for further treatments, which I suggested above would be a necessary result of giving his address. The naming of the names of his patients was a strong incentive to good practice as patients could and did witness their own cures.

Curing the Poor/Queen's Oculist

As nowadays, performing cures however miraculous and however lucrative did not curry royal favor, though the title "queen's oculist," and the subsequent knighthood must have helped Read's business and looked good in his advertisements. Until the present survey of William Read, Jonathan Swift's tart comment about his rise from mountebank to queen's oculist has been treated as a mark of Read's quackery, but the evidence of his newspaper advertisements suggests the title was gained by hard work, examination, and giving his services gratis to the poor.

William Read's status and titles are as variable as the spellings of the name Paine, and in his first extant advertisement, he referred to himself as "an experienced and approved oculist."[51] Two years later, in 1698, in his second extant advertisement, he called himself "sworn Servant in Ordinary to His present Majesty,"[52] an association with William III repeated in two more advertisements in May and June of the same year.[53] Both also give his address as *"Great St. Bartholomew Close,* near *West-Smithfield, London"* and explain that "he Couches the Poor of Cataracts *gratis.*" In August 1698, Read changed his title to "his Majesty's Oculist" and claimed to have been "sent for to France, to Couch a Person of Quality."[54] Whether or not this was an official position, with or without a stipend, is hard to determine as in October 1698 Read's title was recorded as "His Majesty's Oculist in Chief, and Operator of Eyes in Ordinary," which sounds so grandiose it is unlikely to be more than a boast. But nor does the evidence suggest it was entirely out of order. Three years later, in 1701 (and in the interim, advertisements suggest Read had been on tour throughout England), Read began to advertise in the official *London Gazette,* in which it is unlikely that he could use pretended titles, and where he called himself "an Experienced and Approved Oculist, and in that Quality sworn Servant in Ordinary to His Majesty."[55] Whatever Read's actual title at this time, it is also important to note that his work was more directed toward "Persons of Quality" as only the two advertisements of June 1698 mentioned free cures for the poor.

A number of advertisements for cures placed after the death of William III suggest more of Read's patients might have been poor, such as that in November 1702 for James Silvester and John Collins, both couched "at Alderman Saunders's in Guilford" and "Mrs. Hilton at Esquire Blooms near Guilford."[56] Others suggest they were placed by and thus paid for by the person cured, such as that in July 1703 for John Blowes, who records his advertisement is "to be made known for the public Good of others."[57] The suggestion of the poverty of Silvester, Collins, and Hilton comes not only from the fact they were couched in the houses of the wealthy but also because Read's title is given in that advertisement as "the Approved and Experienced Occulist," which Read had used before, while the Blowes advertisement calls him "the Famous Occulist," a title Read does not use elsewhere, suggesting that Read placed the first advertisement and Blowes the second. It must also be noted that in each advertisement, which were both placed after the death of William III on 8 March 1702, Read is no longer styled oculist in ordinary to His Majesty.[58]

Rutson James, who does not note Read's title from William III, dates Read's entitlement to call himself "Oculist to Queen Anne" from 30 July 1705, though he does not find any record of it in the state papers.[59] Read's first newspaper advertisement calling himself "Sworn Oculist in Ordinary to Her Majesty" actually appeared a year earlier in the *London Gazette* on 24 July 1704.[60] The group of advertisements published up to this date suggest that the title was granted to him only after a public expression of his willingness to offer his services gratis to the poor and a demonstration of his skill by an appointed examiner, despite his having held the title for William III.

Two numbers of the *Daily Courant* of 17 January and 7 February 1704 list "People lately couch'd and brought to perfect Sight in London in 1703 by Dr. *William Read* the Approved Occulist," including "Mrs. Payn" and "John Blows," adding "he has cured above a hundred poor People *gratis* within this 18 Months, some of Cataracts, Albugo's, and Defluxion of Humours."[61] The *Post Man* of 10–12 February 1704 announces Read's move to his Durham Yard house, where the advertisement claims, "He gives advice to the Poor gratis in all Distempers incident to the Eyes, and has restored some hundreds to perfect Sight for Charity, that were recommended to him by the Ministers and Churchwardens of several Parishes in the Country, as well as in the City, since Christmas last; and will freely continue his kindness to the Poor."[62] Two weeks later, on 6 March and again on 11 March 1704, Read performed a number of couching operations before Sir Edmond King "to his great Satisfaction" at his new house in Durham Yard.[63] Edmond King, who was physician to Charles II and attended him in his last illness, had been an associate of the anatomist Robert Lower and Christopher Wren when they attempted blood transfusions between sheep and calves and a sheep and an Oxford student. However outlandish his experiments might appear nowadays, King was apparently happy with Read's technique, as he presented him with a set of gold couching needles. The advertisement was repeated at least twice more, in which Read called himself "principle Oculist and Operator of the Eyes to his late Majesty King William III,"[64] a title he had not used for over two years, suggesting he was hoping for an appointment from the queen. Further advertisements appeared in March and April 1704 numbering the poor he had cured, with one listing the operations in detail: "he has Couched and brought to perfect Sight since Christmas last 95; of Deflexions and Humours of the Eyes and Eye-lids, Clouds Specks, Ungula's and Albugo's 240; of the Fistula Lachrymalis 14; of Obstructions to the Optick Nerves, Dimness of Sight and Atoms flying before the Eyes 48; . . . and as many Persons of Name, having Couched in all since the time above mentioned 166, with so good Effect and Success, as not as not Failing the Cure of above in all."[65] In each of these advertisements, Read is given the title "Oculist and Chyrurgian Operator." Then, as though he had officially passed the test before Sir Edmond King, the next two advertisements placed in the *London Gazette* for 24–27 and 27–31 July 1704, give his title for the first time as "Her Majesty's sworn Oculist in Ordinary."

However, in the same advertisement Read also repeated the names of the people he cured in Oxford from "Post nubila Phoebus, nihil absque Deo."[66] It is exactly this sort of repetition of the names of former patients that gives weight to the suggestion that Read was a quack, and one can but wonder at his lack of awareness of what repeating advertisements of the names of those he cured many years previously might have on his reputation. However, it must also be borne in mind that it was the naming of his former clients that had gained him the title of queen's oculist, added to the examination by Sir Edmond King, which Read might easily have regarded as similar to the operations he had carried out at Oxford University before the chancellor. Such ad hoc qualification might make us quail at the thought of Read's ability to operate on eyes. However, like he and Edward Hannes, Sir Edmond King had no formal qualifications, nor even an apprenticeship to his profession, and had been accepted into the Royal College of Physicians because of a change made in their charter by James II.

Affidavits for Cures

After Read's appointment as "Her Majesty's sworn Oculist in Ordinary," his career altered dramatically, and his placement of advertisements doubled between 1704 and 1705. At this point in his career it might well be argued that his self-presentation had begun to resemble the accusation made by Emilie Savage-Smith that "Sir William was a more effective self-promoter . . . than he was an oculist." An advertisement in the *Daily Courant* of 3 November 1704 claims he had "cured above a thousand since New-Years-Day last,"[67] which figure would suggest he had couched one thousand people between 25 March and 1 November. However, if the claim is compared with the detailed claim of 563 cured between Christmas 1703 and 27 April 1704,[68] the number is not out of the question, amounting in each time period to 4.5 people treated each day. If it is borne in mind that each couching operation took no more than ten minutes, this is not a heavy workload, even if, as Read claimed, "the Poor that are Blind . . . appear by hundreds that resort to his House and have found relief since Christmas last."[69]

But curing poor people was as fraught in the eighteenth century as it is now with the question of who pays and who is entitled to free care. The advertisement giving details of the numbers of those cured suggests that about one-third of Read's patients were "Persons of Name" who presumably paid for their treatment themselves,[70] and in many advertisements, such as those for John Blowes and Mrs. Payne, the cured person demonstrates their ability to pay Read if only by paying for the advertisement as well. But for the poor, it was necessary for someone to bear witness to their worthiness to be cured before the event. The mechanism of what exactly took place is never thoroughly explained, but some advertisements tell us that churchwardens and elders of a poor person's church acted as guarantors to the entitlement to treatment, though it would appear Read gained no recompense for his services.

There are many such advertisements, but I will explore just one which covers the issues recognizable in the twenty-first century as health-care tourism and access for the poor to care free at the point of delivery. In the *Daily Courant* of 24 March 1704, we read:

> Whereas we the Ministers and Elders of the French Church in *Threadneedle-street, London*, do certifie that Mr. *Joseph Fournalis* a Spaniard, converted to the Protestant Religion, who is a Member of our Church, hath been afflicted with a Cataract, whereby he lost the sight of his Left Eye, and that Dr. READ the approved Oculist, living in *Durham-yard* in the *Strand*, hath couch'd the said Cataract, and restored him to his perfect Sight in a Minute, without any pain or very little Confinement. This we thought fit to publish, not only to acknowledge Dr. *Read's* Charity toward this poor Man, from whom he could expect no Recompense at all, but also for the Encouragement of others in the same Affliction. Witness our Hands *March* 20. 1703-4. *D. Primerose. T.Hestal, James Saurin, Ch.Bestheau* Ministers of the said Church, *John Ramett, John Dencio* Elders.

The French Church in Threadneedle Street was the largest of twenty Huguenot churches in London, and dated from 1550, when Edward VI granted Protestant refugees freedom to worship by Royal Charter.[71] After the revocation of the Edict of Nantes in 1685, the Huguenots made up about 5 percent of London's population, specializing in textiles, gun making, silversmithing, and watch and clock making. Fournalis, being Spanish and poor, would appear to be an employee in one of these trades, whose sight was integral to his work. Only two of the guarantors come down to us in any historical detail. "D. Primrose," presumably David Primrose of the line of Gilbert Primrose, principal surgeon to James VI of Scotland, came from a background of religious controversialists in France, and another Gilbert Primrose (who was survived by a son David) was chosen as one of the ministers of the French and Walloon refugee church in London in 1623.[72] James Saurin was briefly preacher at the same church, between 1703 and 1705, before removing to The Hague, where he served in another French refugee church at the palace of the Prince of Orange.[73]

Despite being from a wealthy community, the advertisement does not suggest that the French Church paid William Read for the treatment of Joseph Fournalis. The church is gracious in its thanks for Read's "Charity," and they encourage others to take up his offer of free care, but the advertisement appears to have been placed in lieu of a fee. To be sure, in 1704 Read was still in the throes of gaining acceptance as the queen's oculist, and this advertisement is appended with a note from the oculist himself: "The said Dr. Read will freely continue his Charity in helping the Poor so long as he lives, . . . and have cured above 100 poor People *gratis* since *Christmas* last of Cataracts and other Distempers incident to the Eyes."[74] However, when Read opened up two further avenues for gaining business after receiving the title of queen's oculist, there is no suggestion that either brought him any money. In April and May 1705, a number of advertisements were published naming soldiers and sailors cured, for example, Richard Geary, sailor,[75] and Richard Murray, soldier.[76] Although some of these advertisements featured the names of the officers who attested the cures rather than those of the patients,[77] they all note that Read "perform'd the said Cures gratis, without the expense of the medicines to the Patients." As a tactic for gaining a knighthood to add to the title of "Oculist in Ordinary to Her Majesty," it succeeded, and the citation in the *London Gazette* of August 1705 states it was "a Mark of Her Royal Favour for his great Services done in Curing great Numbers of Seamen and Soldiers of Blindness *Gratis*."[78] But despite the increased fame, Read was not making any money out of the practice. In January 1709 Read began to make a sales pitch out of his free treatments when he published the first of many advertisements: "The Invitation, or New Years Gift to the Poor, that are Blind of Cataracts and other curable Distempers, relating to the Eyes, from Sir William Read, her Majesties Oculist, who will generously cure all such as are recommended to him, either by the Ministers or Churchwardens of any Parish, for Charity, as well, her Majesties Seamen and Soldiers, . . . at any time from the Publication of this advertisement till 25th March next."[79]

If Swift was repeating true gossip that guests ate from "golden vessels" at the Reads', the oculist was not buying them from money made out of the bulk of his practice. If the title queen's oculist brought a stipend, it might have been £300 a year if it was at the same level of the stipend earned by William Cheselden for service to the Crown thirty years later. But there is no record of any money coming with either the title or the knighthood, and evidence suggests that Read had to make money by other means.

Tour Itineraries

The problem with having a static practice working largely on one procedure is patient shortage, or at least for Read, a shortage of paying patients from which to finance his much larger gratis practice. If he attended 166 paying cases in four months,[80] and they all paid the going rate of 6s 8d charged at St. Bartholomew's Hospital when John Freke was put in charge of eye operations in 1727, he would have had an income of about £100 per quarter, which would not have been enough to finance a new house and "golden vessels." William Cheselden charged as much as 200 guineas for a private consultation and "cutting for the stone,"[81] but there is no record of what Read charged for couching a cataract. Either he had to work out a method of making his gratis practice pay, of which there is no evidence he succeeded in doing, or find other sources of income. The easiest way to supplement his London income was to find more paying patients, and

Read toured extensively throughout England. Sadly, this is another source of the idea that he was not skilled at couching since he might "cut and run," that is, operate and leave the town before the bandages had been removed from the patient's eyes. As Roy Porter argued, "It made better sense for the irregular doctor to be itinerant (mobility . . . gave the unscrupulous the advantage of being able to make himself scarce before his failures became obvious to all)."[82] However, the evidence of the foundation of Read's career as the queen's oculist must give the impression that it was unlikely that he could hide by running away: he was too large a target. And nor did he. It is likely that London had run out of paying patients with ripe cataracts to couch a year after Read's knighthood, when he took to the road, advertising in May 1706 where and when he would be available for consultation: "Being sent for by several Persons of Note to Shrewsbury and Manchester, [Sir William Read] designs to continue at Shrewsbury to be advised withal from 6th of June to the 20th, and at Manchester from the 25th to the 10th of July. He intends to be in Worcester the 26th Instant [May], in his way to the Places above-mentioned."[83]

Remaining two weeks in each destination gave adequate time for initial problems in his work to have begun to show themselves, and although Read did not name her, he mentioned couching "a young Gentlewoman who was born Blind, [on] the 13th Instant [June 1706]."[84] On the same tour, in October, "Edward Calvert of Beckles in the County of Suffolk" placed an affidavit to his cure, attested by "J. Elmy, J. Harber Jun., J. Elmy Jun., Wm. Randal."[85] Calvert's advertisement bears the NB, "Sir Wm will be at his House in Durham-yard the 10th Inst. [October 1706]." The only other surviving advertisement for the tour suggests that after Worcester, Shrewsbury, and Manchester, Read visited Chester and Knaresborough before ending up in Suffolk, but with the loss of so many local newspaper runs, it is impossible to know in more detail where Read was on this four-month tour. Read carried out some operations on soldiers and sailors on the tour, but the two named cures I have found would probably have been paying clients.

Read undertook a similar tour in 1707, beginning earlier in March of that year and in the West Country: Exeter, Bath, and Bristol. Once again there are very few advertisements remaining which give details, but those which still exist tell where and when he can be consulted, and one explains that though it is in one of the capital's newspapers, the tour "is designed for the Advantage of those that live remote from London."[86] Once again Read advertised the names of those who paid for his cures, Mr Chapman, a shoemaker in Bath; Mrs. Jeffries and Mr. William Norris of Exeter; Mrs. Parsons of Wraxel near Bristol.[87] Read did not return to London that winter because he was ill, and although it was reported that he was dead,[88] an advertisement in the *London Gazette* for 17 November 1707 explained that far from being dead, he was to be consulted in Birmingham and Stafford.[89]

The same advertisement states that Read had left his brother-in-law, Mr. Brinsden, in charge of his practice in London, something necessary to keep his business alive while he was away. But it did not turn out to be a good move. I cannot locate any advertisements after the retraction that Read was dead until November 1708, suggesting that until that date Read continued his tour of England, perhaps going to Scotland or maybe Ireland. But when he returned to London and placed an advertisement that he was back at Durham Yard,[90] the next day his brother-in-law placed another advertisement declaring "Sir Wm. Read's Brother, Mr. Brinsden, Oculist and Surgeon," had moved his business to Bedford Court, Covent Garden.[91]

Warnings against Imitators

Throughout his advertising campaign Read warned his readers against imposters, but the split between the two men suggested that Read had discovered there was an imposter in the bosom of his own family, and Brinsden was rooted out forthwith. Even in the advertisement that he was being tested by Sir Edmond King for the role of oculist to the queen, Read warned: "The said Dr. Read daily gives Advice, and cures all curable Distempers incident to the Eyes, and several lately that have been injured by Women, and such like Impostors, as appears by daily Complaints."[92] Likewise in the advertisement about the cure of Joseph Fournalis, Read adds: "The said Dr READ will freely continue his Charity in helping the Poor so long as he lives, that People may not be imposed upon by Women and such-like Intruders to that curious Art."[93]

I can find no advertisements placed by women oculists until 1715, when Mary Cater began a successful advertising campaign for eyewashes and eye cures without needles, which will be the subject of the next section of this chapter. Nor were all the "Imposters" women. While on tour in 1706, Read advertised that "to prevent Counterfeits . . . he must make use of his Name, particularly one William Burner, a Fellow about 19 years old, a Seaman late of the Triumph, Capt. Edwards Commander, and since a Soldier in Gloucester: He goes sometimes by the Name of Read, and a Relation of Sir William's, which is false and groundless."[94] There can be little doubt that Read's warnings were placed to protect his own business from other practitioners who undercut him in price, but the result of his brother-in-law's behavior toward him is interesting in terms of Read's attitude toward women as medical practitioners.

Brinsden was first mentioned in the advertisement of May 1706 giving Read's tour itinerary, which ends: "He [Read] has left his Brother [Mr. Brinsden] at his House in Durham Yard in the Strand, London to couch Cataracts, attend patients, and take Care of Her Majesty's Seamen and Soldiers, with an Apothecary to assist him."[95] With Read on tour for the whole of 1707 and 1708, it is likely that it was Brinsden himself who had placed the advertisement that Read was dead sometime before the retraction of November 1707, in order to bring in patients who might be waiting for Read's return to London for the winter. It would appear to be the discovery of Brinsden's treachery that precipitated the split between the two on Read's return to London in October 1708. Negative advertising was not unknown in the medical world, and in 1715, Peter Kennedy complained that it had been "maliciously given out or insinuated, that Peter Kennedy, Author of Opthalmographia, or Treatise of the Diseases of the Eye, has left the Town," which his advertisement was designed to correct.[96] But whereas Kennedy did not know who had advertised against him, all Read had to do was ask the publisher of the paper who had advertised that he was dead. The result was twofold.

First, Read changed the newspapers in which he advertised, eschewing the *London Gazette* and *Post Man and Historical Account* in favor of Abel Boyer's *Supplement,* Daniel Defoe's *Review,* Addison and Steele's *Tatler,* and ending up his career with advertisements almost exclusively in Abel Boyer's *Post Boy.*

Second, Read trained his wife to couch cataracts and during future tours advertised that she would remain at the Durham Yard house while he was away on tour. In one of his last advertisements in the *London Gazette*, Read notes that since he "is obliged to Couch for Cataracts some Persons of Note, and others in or near Canterbury . . . and then return to his House in Durham-Yard in the Strand, London, where his Lady constantly gives advice in all Distempers of the Eyes, and Couches Cataracts with good Success; Sir William having instructed her in this Art for the Benefit of the Publick."[97]

Thereafter, most of Read's advertisements were rounded off with the phrase "and by my Lady Read in his absence."[98] Furthermore, in 1712, when Read was advertised as being on tour in East Anglia,[99] Lady Read placed a long advertisement in the *Post Boy* where she drew attention to her own skill:

> This is to satisfy, That Sir WILLIAM READ, Her Majesty's Principal Oculist, has, for the Service of the Publick, instructed my lady Read to couch Cataracts, which she performs with as much Dexterity and Success as has been known by any: Sir William has also instructed her how to prepare his Medicaments for Strengthening, Clarifying, and Preserving the Eyes, as appears but the great Success my Lady Read has had upon many Cures she has lately perform'd in the most difficultest Distempers relating to the Eyes. She is always to be advised with at Sir William Read's House in Durham-yard in the Strand, London; where is only sold, and by himself, his renown'd Stiptick-Water for stopping of Blood external or internal, and for curing Fistulas, Cancers, Scrophulous Ulcers, or others. NOTE, My Lady Read gives Advice in all Distempers incident to the Eyes, and couches the Poor of Cataracts *gratis*. 36 Years Practice both at Home and Abroad, must qualify Sir William to give any body a greater Insight in his Business than those that never had the same Experience.[100]

As a woman, Augustina Read (presumably née Brinsden), would have been excluded from medical education by any formal route, but her advertisement demonstrates that she had trained as her husband's apprentice, a method common in the seventeenth and eighteenth centuries for male doctors. Emilie Savage-Smith suggests that after Read's death, "It is said that his widow . . . continued his business in Durham Yard, presumably selling his various proprietary potions." This is not entirely correct. My lady Read did continue her husband's business after his death, but the advertisements she placed tell us that she continued to couch cataracts and perform the other operations she had learned from her husband: "The Lady Read in Durham-Yard in the Strand, London, having obtain'd to a peculiar Method of Couching of Cataracts and Curing all Diseases of the Eyes by Sir William Read's Method and Medicines, and having above 15 Years Experience, and very good Success in Curing Multitudes of Blind and defective in Sight, particularly those born Blind. She may constantly be advised with at her House as above, where the Poor and Her Majesty's Seamen and Soldiers may meet with Relief as formerly, gratis."[101]

Product Placement/Other Operations

However, Lady Read's advertisement continues: "Note, Sir William Read has left only with his Lady the true Receipt of his Styptic Water, so famous for stopping all Fluxes of Effusions of Blood, and of all the other Medicines he frequently used in his Practice; which may also be had at the Place abovementioned." William Read's "Styptic Water, Balsam and Pills" had been counterfeited since they were first advertised in 1699.[102] But patented remedies are another source of the idea that Read was a quack. In fact, history transforms many doctors who sold a patented cure into a quack, although the reason for this can sometimes have little or nothing to do with the effectiveness of the medicine and much more to do with the struggle at the heart of the medical profession between physicians and surgeons.

An example of a fully trained doctor whom history has turned into a quack is Paul Chamberlen (1635–1717) of the "Asclepiad-family" of doctors of that name. Grand-nephew of Peter Chamberlen the elder (1560–1631), who attended the queens of James I and Charles I, and the son of "Dr. Peter" Chamberlen, who tried to organize midwifery into a college in the seventeenth century, Paul invented a number of remedies, including the anodyne necklace, and also advertised a "Chrystal Cosmetick" which "cures all red faces" and acne.[103] While for the most part the rest of the doctors in the *ODNB* entry for the "Chamberlen family" are treated seriously, Paul is dismissed as "a quack doctor living in Great Suffolk Street" because of his patented cure. However, there is a subtext in the article which suggests other levels of complexity in the way each family member came to be treated in history.

Peter the elder, a barber-surgeon, was fined by the College of Physicians in 1609 because of his "reluctance to restrict his activities to surgery." No hint of the basis of the college's accusation is mentioned. Dr. Peter, a member of the College of Physicians, was expelled from the college in 1649, when "the college became more conservative and began to take action against empirics and others challenging its authority." In this case, the *ODNB* article suggests it might have been the "family secret" which was Dr. Peter's downfall. Either Dr. Peter or Paul's brother Hugh tried to sell to the Crown the "family secret," which is hinted at to be forceps for the delivery of children obstructed in birth. However, all the family of Chamberlen doctors did, which set them all at one time or another beyond the pale, was to be at once surgeons and physicians. We must surmise, but the evidence of the *ODNB* article suggests that Peter the elder was fined by the College of Physicians for using medicines in his attendance at births. Dr. Peter, by reverse fortune, was expelled from the College of Physicians when it became more conservative in its actions and perhaps for using the "family secret"—forceps, a surgical tool.

The parallel between midwifery and ophthalmology is compelling. Both were traditionally the concern of women, and it will be remembered that Read warned against women as "Imposters" and had no compunction about training his wife in his procedures. Both used methods which fell between the medical men's separate roles of physician and surgeon, applying eyewashes and other chemicals, and also invasive measures with needles and blades. And both were in the process of being taken over by "trained" "professional" men.

In comparison with the Chamberlens, therefore, William Read could not but be recorded by history as anything other than a quack because he too did not separate his medical work into the two professional fields and acted at once as a physician (providing stomachic medicines, cephalic snuffs, etc.) and a surgeon (couching). But this was because he practiced in the period when his field was changing from an area of traditional practice to one that was taken over by the medical profession.

That said, Read was more like his surgical brethren than might at first appear because he was a general surgeon, performing many more than just couching operations—but unfortunately, he was helped by his styptick water. The use of alum-based preparations to stop bleeding is recorded in pharaonic Egyptian history and appears regularly in sixteenth- and seventeenth-century medical handbooks, such as *A needeful, new, and necessarie treatise of chyrurgerie*[104] by John Banister, who trained his nephew Richard Banister, whose *Breviary of the Eyes* was claimed to have been plagiarized by Read. By the end of the seventeenth century, however, the use of styptic preparations was no longer in fashion with the Royal College of Physicians, probably because of its association with staunching the blood from small cuts during barbering. In 1703, Robert Pitt wrote against styptics in *The Crafts and Frauds of Physic Expos'd*,[105] attacking the Apothecaries' Company for selling styptics. And when Robert Eaton attempted to present his Styptick Balsam to the College in 1723, "regardless of what fashionable Systems may be discredited,"[106] he was met with total rejection by Dr. C. J. Sprengell, who presented a paper against Eaton's preparation to the Royal Society in 1724, in which John Ranby cut an artery along its length for half an inch (cutting across an artery being said to be "the old trick"), and Eaton's styptic failed to staunch the flow of blood.[107] Ranby was a military surgeon who presumably would have appreciated the help of the sort of styptic agents that are now used on the battlefield, but in 1725 he was in the process of separating the Company of Barbers and Surgeons to form a Company of Surgeons in order to professionalize surgery so cannot be wholly believed as he had too much to lose. When he finally brought about the split, he was created the first master of the new Company of Surgeons. William Cheselden, the second master of the new company, never used the word "styptick" in any of his publications about surgery and so perhaps did not use any chemical to staunch blood flow, though he mentions tying blood vessels.

But the sort of operations that Read advertised where his styptic had assisted did not cut along arteries. The *Daily Courant* of 10 March 1705 reports that Read used his "*Aqua Styptica Celiberrima*" when he "took off a mortified Leg from Mrs Anne Crook,"[108] the stopping of blood flow from a transversely cut artery would presumably be thought of as a cheat by John Ranby. Read also staunched the blood flow from "a Soldier from Scotland-yard [who] receiv'd a very large Wound in his Head, given by a Grenadier with a broad Sword.[109] The same advertisement also suggested the styptic staunched blood flow in cases of "cancerous Humours, King's-Evil or Leprosy of the Blood . . . [and] ulcerated Cancers of the Breasts without cutting." Understood from a twenty-first-century perspective, this is nonsense, and to be sure, the relief offered in any of these cases could only have been the drying up of the "unnatural Juices" produced by tumors.[110] Read carried out other operations for harelip and wry-neck,[111] using his styptic water to reduce bleeding. It can be no surprise that Richard Banister, from whose book Read learned his trade, also carried out like operations using a styptic, but in the seventeenth century when its use was still in fashion.

Quackery or Simple Economics?

When we question William Read, we find many other reasons for his afterlife as a "quack" than poor medical practice: political, professional and contextual. If these are considered, "It is [less] difficult to assess the validity of Read's claims . . . to have performed many cures." Sir William Read comes across as a serious medical practitioner, and one who made a success out of his practice, rising to the highest honors possible in his day by advertising his skill in newspapers. It is no surprise that in January 1715, the year of his death, he was sworn oculist to George I.[112]

More importantly, Read had begun to formalize the link between private practice and practice that was available to the poor free at the point of delivery. But it would be thirty-five years before what is now standard economics for doctors was properly financed, and it would take two eye specialists to do it—one to go on tour, and one to remain in London. Both were called John Taylor, and they will be the subjects of chapters 5 and 6.

Mary Cater: Complementary Medicine and the Attitude to Professional Eye Care

With eerie timing, on 21 May 1715, the same date that William Read's death was announced in the *British Weekly Mercury*,[113] Mary Cater placed the first in what was to become a long series of advertisements for her "Eye-Water" in the *Weekly Journal with Fresh Advices Foreign and Domestick*.[114] Perhaps it was not so eerie since the next week's number of the *Weekly Journal*, which carried Mary Cater's second advertisement on page 126, also noted the death of Willian Read "at Rochester in Kent, on his Peregrinations" two pages earlier.[115] Perhaps Mary Cater, whose advertisement claimed she had "above 100 Certificates for Cures perform'd by her, of most Distempers of the Eyes" believed she, as one of "the Women" imposters, was finally able to advertise her "Eye-Water" free from harassment by "his Majesty's Oculist in Ordinary."

Mary Cater's advertisements are almost identical to each other and show only a slow development over the twenty-six years she advertised her cures, which will be the subject of this analysis. They learned a lot from William Read's, in terms of self-presentation, naming the person cured, and giving their address, explaining the cure that had been successful, giving her name and address, enumerating her other cures, and advertising patent remedies. But she added two extra items: a readily recognizable visual symbol that appeared in all her advertisements and, early in the series, numbers. Her first, for "John Lothen living in Bull Court in the Strand," bears the hand and eye visual but no number; the second, for Elizabeth Jones, is numbered 2.

Mary Cater's address, Castle Court, now called Bengal Court, is one of the few present-day survivals of eighteenth-century London, although it was at the center of the fire on Friday 28 March 1748 so has been rebuilt since Cater's occupancy. Ironically, the fire burned down the London Insurance Office, so contemporary maps giving the details of the businesses carried on in Castle Court are available from an insurance map listing the destroyed houses (see fig. 3). Thus, we can readily know the sort of neighbors Cater is likely to have had: notaries, alehouses, coffee shops, barbers,

96 MEDICINE

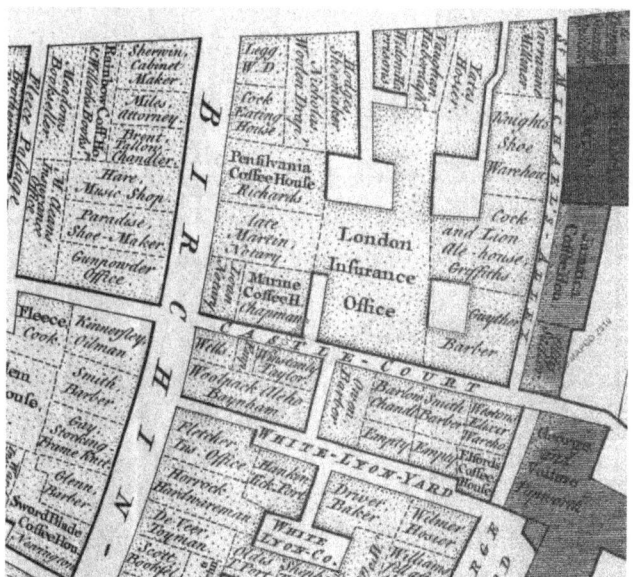

FIGURE 3. Insurance map showing the site of Mary Cater's "Hand and Eye" in Castle Court off Birchin Lane.

Winstanley the Taylor, Barlow the Chandler, and the curious Warton's Elixir Warehouse. Whether her business was carried on from the building marked "Wells." or "shop" is tantalizing, though she died ten years before the fire, so we shall never know exactly.

However, since her visual, a hand pointing to an eye, remained a constant in her advertising, it is safe to assume that she had the same visual displayed over her shop in Castle Court, a narrow alleyway no more than two yards wide, so that passersby in Birchin Lane could readily find her place of business.

My father, a soldier in the Indian Army, used the expression "That's eye-wash!" throughout his life in a metaphorical sense, meaning that what had just been said was nonsense. A wider definition is given in the *OED* as "Actions, behaviour, statements, etc., intended merely for outward show, or to obscure or conceal actual facts or motives; (Mil. slang) unnecessary attention paid to appearances, ceremonial, etc." Whether or not Mary Cater's eye water was at all effective, she made enough of a living out of it to place above six hundred advertisements between May 1715 and August 1741.

And if Sir William Read's life in advertisements gives us an example of the effects of the changeover from traditional medical practice concerning eyes to professionalization, Mary Cater's gives us something of a sense of what happened to traditional medicine and how it survived as a specialism alongside the drive to modernization, much as complementary medicine still survives today.

Eye Water

We need look no further than John Banister's *A needefull, new, and necessarie treatise of chyrurgerie* of 1575, to find a traditional eye treatment based on the plant "eye-bright," "Eufrasia, Eie bright, hoate & drie, it quickeneth the sight and memorie."[116] A year later George Baker translated Konrad Gesner's *The newe iewell of health wherein is contayned the most excellent secretes of phisicke,* which gave two more detailed recipes for eyewashes:

> A most syngular water, helping the spottes of the eyes: Take of whyte Hony two pyntes, of Antymonie, of Titia prepared, and of Sugarcandie, of each thrée drams, of the best Aloes halfe a dram, of Celondine, of Rue, and eye bright, of each halfe a handfull, these grosse beaten and myxed togyther, distyll in a Lymbecke.

> A water of Tutia prepared: take of the eye bryght water, of Fennell water, of the Hony suckle water, of eache halfe a pynt, of Rosewater two pyntes, of Tutia prepared two drams, of Aloes halfe an ounce, of whyte Coperase halfe a dram, of Camphora one dram, all these laboured and dilygently myxed togither, distyll according to arte: For this is a notable water, experienced sundrys tymes, against the spottes of the eyes: this borrowed out of the learned practises of Arnoldus.[117]

The two "Eye-Waters" both contain ingredients that had been known for centuries as salves for sore eyes:

- Titia/Tutia or Tutty, "an impure oxide of zinc"[118] was known as a salve for eyes from Galen to Marco Polo,[119] and is mentioned in contemporary preparations by Benedict Duddell.[120]

- Honey is now known as an antibacterial.
- Fennell contains "anethole" an oil which reduces inflammation and is also mentioned by Duddell.
- Aloes were known from antiquity to relieve the skin.
- Celandine boiled in milk was thought to remove cataracts.[121]
- Camphor is a local anesthetic.

Whatever was in Mary Cater's "Eye-Water," it could not have been dangerous to use since it was advertised over so many years and used on so many people. But how she was able to get away with practicing as an herbalist without the censure of the College of Physicians is a little hard to explain.

Both of the texts from which the recipes above came were the productions of barber-surgeons, and both John Banister and George Baker were denounced by the College of Physicians on 5 July 1588 for practicing illegal medicine since neither was licensed by the college.[122] It may just be because she was so vehement that she did not use surgical techniques that Cater was left unhindered to sell her "Eye-Water," her "Ointment for Rickety Children," and her "Powder for Ruptures." Furthermore, there was a long tradition of selling eye waters, though few advertisements remain in the archives. I have located one for an eye cure in *Kingdome's Intelligencer* of 3–10 June 1661, which speaks of "Rare Pills against . . . defluxions of the eyes." In the next surviving advertisement, dating from 7 June 1695 in *Collection for Improvement in Husbandry and Trade*, we find "The Chinese Eye-water, being the best in the World, which has done more Cures than any, and many of those extraordinary, is sold by Mrs. *Hope*." Two things are important here, first, for this "Eye-water" (and it soon lost its epithet "Chinese") to be the best in the world there must have been others; second, it is sold by a woman.

As a practitioner with medicines, in effect an apothecary, it is likely that Cater might at least have come under the lash of some satirical effusion from a physician such as Samuel Garth, whose *Dispensary* accused apothecaries of fast practice and selling medicines at high prices.[123] The longevity of the run of Mary Cater's advertisements argues that she may have been protected by some benefactor, and as we shall find, her advertisements were all placed in Jacobite journals which points where her help lay.

Until she explained her practice at the very end of her career, it was difficult to work out what method Cater used to treat her patients from her advertisements, but those she claimed to cure fell largely into four categories: those with films over their eyes, usually caused by smallpox or scrofula; those with "a great Cold"; those suffering after blows to the eyes; and those "having no eyes," presumably due to swollen eyelids, or from imposthumation (abscesses). Other conditions treated that are mentioned once or twice each over her career were "blind by the humour" (presumably with cataracts or what was then known as glaucoma),[124] measles,[125] and gutta serena.[126]

After advertising cures of John Lothen and Elizabeth Jones, both from films over their eyes, Cater's third advertisement claims a cure of "The Daughter of *John Giffard*, Brick-maker, at the Pindar of Wakefield, near Pancras, having been blind by the Evil,"[127] and her fourth of "*Elizabeth Hope*, Wife of *Anthony Hope*, in Duke's Place, a Shoe-maker, was afflicted with a thick Film that grew on both Eyes, occasioned by the Evil,"[128] presumably the King's Evil, scrofula.

The nature of the blinding cold is more difficult to understand. Cater treated "*Thomas Miles*, living in Cock-Yard near Red-Lion-street, by the Whittington's Cat, in White-Chappel, Penny-Post Man, [who] . . . laboured for some Time under a sore Distemper in [his] Eyes, occasioned by a desperate Cold,"[129] which would appear to mean he suffered from overly watery eyes. Without offering a retro-diagnosis, the case of "Henry Middleton, Staymaker, living in the Round Court in the Strand" offers us a suggestion of a more unpleasant condition caused by the cold. He describes himself as "being for a long Time very much afflicted in my Eyes, occasioned by an extraordinary Cold, insomuch as I was in great Danger of being quite blind, being in continual Pain."[130] If Cater's eye water did no more than take away the pain, she would have relieved the panic of incipient blindness from someone who worked with his hands and eyes. Of all of her patients, those treated for the "Cold" were the most numerous, and when her business was so well established she could place the same advertisement once a week for several months, those used in the winter were usually affidavits for treatment for this complaint. Thus, "Mary, Daughter of Thomas Hammet, of Barn Elms in the County of Surrey, Yeoman," whose advertisements ran from 30 September 1721[131] until 7 January 1722,[132] and "Alice Sturgis, servant to Mrs. Elizabeth Sparks in Westminster Court in Dunnings Alley without Bishopsgate," whose advertisement was placed seven times between 8 December 1722[133] and 26 January 1723.[134] If this is an example of seasonal advertising, then it is a very early one.

Black eyes, and inflamed and swollen eyes, caused usually by work-related accidents, were a regular problem. As with the condition caused by the cold, those who advertised their cures resorted to Mary Cater because they were unable to work. Thus, "Stephen Phillips, at the Swan in Friar-street, Black-Friars, having had the Misfortune to have a Blow with a Stone fall on the Sight of my right Eye; which said Blow affected the other Eye which rendered me incapable of my Business . . . [was] advised to Mrs Cater [and] in eight Days I could read the smallest Print."[135] Likewise, "John Berwick, Wyer-Drawer, living with Mr. Bright, in Crooked-Lane, at the Blue Boar's Head near Cannon street, London, having had Sand or Gravel threw into my Eyes, which by rubbing them with my Hands or Fingers, occasioned so great an inflammation and Films over both Eyes that I could not see to go about my Business . . . [was] advised to Mrs Cater . . . who at first Sight not only promised Cure, but performed the same in as short a Time as in Reason could be expected, to my great Satisfaction."[136]

Such treatment for inflammation or swelling is probably the same as the fourth category of cure for those with no eyes. Thus, "Peter Otter, who may be heard of at Mr. Andrew Jurgen's, a German, at the Sign of the Ship called the Nonsuch, in Bow-street, Covent Garden," who was described as "being blind insomuch as there was not an Eye to be seen," was "brought to Sight in both Eyes, without Spot or Blemish, notwithstanding the Opinion of Many, that he would never see more in this World."[137] A much worse case was "Ashley Fox, Coachman in Garland-alley without Bishopsgate, being quite blind with one Eye by an Imposthumation in my Head, which breaking the Weight and Virulency of the Corruption fell into my Eye, the Anguish of which was such that I never expected the Light of the World again, and the Misery I was in made me desire Death rather than to live in such Torture, my Eye being sunk into my Head, and to all that saw it appeared like unto rotten Liver."[138] So bad was the situation that it took Mary Cater six weeks to help Fox "recover his Sight and Health," but whatever she did, which was no more than apply antiseptic, antibacterials, local anesthetic, and skin salve, it should perhaps be argued that her success lay in the fact that Mary Cater offered an alternative to contemporary medicine. All her advertisements include some form of words that suggest her patients had sought treatment elsewhere first, and most claim that she "cures without the help of an Instrument."[139]

"The Hand and Eye"

Mary Cater's regular visual symbol, which she called "the Hand and Eye," evokes the surgeon's motto "Consilio manuque" (By using the intelligence and the hand), but for the professional brethren this meant the manipulation of blades and needles whereas Cater's hand is empty (see fig. 4). I have not found the image used by other advertisers, but minor variations in the image suggest that the printing block was not owned by Mary Cater herself (see fig. 5). But she did exercise control of the image used. When Cater placed the same advertisement over several months, it usually remained set with the same image as though a block was made for the whole advertisement once and reused. However, when an instrument appeared in the first two prints of an advertisement for the cure of the baby of Nathan and Elizabeth Walker,[140] it was replaced two weeks later by a reset version of the same advertisement with no instrument.[141] Oddly, and perhaps accounting for the inadvertent use of the image with the instrument, the wording of the advertisement for the cure of the Walker baby does not include the usual statement that "no instrument was used in the cure."

However, when Mary Cater moved to the *Craftsman* in May 1729, all

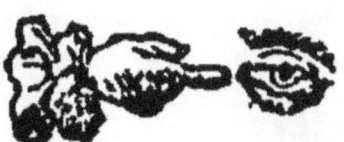

FIGURE 4. Mary Cater's "Hand and Eye," version 1.

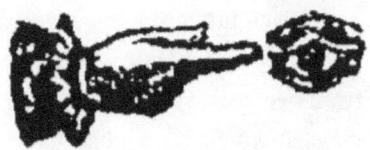

FIGURE 5. Mary Cater's "Hand and Eye," version 2.

the early advertisements included the statement that she cured without an instrument although all advertisements were surmounted by a hand holding some sort of an instrument.[142] Perhaps in anger at the intransigence of the publishers of the *Craftsman,* Cater removed her advertisements from 13 September 1729,[143] to 14 February 1730,[144] and when her advertisements returned, the image no longer included the instrument. Cater placed her advertisements in the *Craftsman* less and less regularly until her last, placed on 1 August 1741, in which she finally explained her procedure with some humor:

> The said Mrs Cater humbly offers to the Publick the following Quere, viz. How is it possible! for a Film to be taken off the Eye by violent Liquid Snuff snuff'd up the Nose? It always has been, and will ever be her Practice, to apply her gentle Medicine to the Eye; whereof (through the Blessing of God) she never fail'd of the best Success.—Moreover, she gives leave, for any Person to be present at the Time of her Dressing and promises to take off part of the Film in five Minutes done. She also, is sorry to think the afflicted, (as if vic of all Reason) suffer themselves to he so imposed upon; when it would be as probable, for them to be persuaded, the Cure of a Film in this Eyes, might be obtain'd, by bathing their Elbows.[145]

How her eye water worked when it was dropped into her patients' eyes is not my concern, but the fact she used a remedy was in contravention of the code of the College of Physicians even if she avoided breaking the rules of the Surgeons' Company by not using any instrument.

There are gaps in her runs of advertisements such as that mentioned above, which might be accounted for by her being called to appear before the court of the College, but when she disappeared between 9 March[146] and 25 May 1728, she advertised that she had been ill and "her Physicians, directed [her] to go to the Country for the Recovery of her Health, which hath given birth to a Report that she is dead."[147] The same technique had been used on Sir William Read, which suggests that she was under attack from her rivals such as Lucerna Lucis, an unnamed advertiser in the same magazines who claimed both to use eye waters and to couch cataracts.[148] In this case, Mary Cater had to advertise outside her usual weekly magazines to get her business up and running again, and took to the *London Evening*

Post four months later with the same advertisement stating that she was not dead.[149]

The magazines in which she advertised might be the key to her running an advertising campaign over so many years and remaining unmolested by the authorities. Mary Cater advertised in Jacobite journals: Nathaniel Mist's *Weekly Journal or Saturday's Post, Mist's Weekly Journal, Fog's Weekly Journal,* and the *Country Journal or the Craftsman.* If this suggests that Mary Cater had friends in high (if politically dangerous) places, the advertisements give further evidence. For example, Dr. John Radcliffe, whose Jacobitism was noted above in this chapter, advertised with Mist the sale of his "Cordial Tincture . . . [whose] Virtues are more general than in any Stomachic extant, being composed of the most rich and effective Cordials that recruit and strengthen decay'd Nature, and is the most excellent Bitter hitherto discover'd."[150]

The political nature of her practice is further borne out by her humor. Many of her advertisements in Mist's *Weekly Journal or Saturday's Post* bear the added paragraph: "Note, She likewise hath a never-failing Remedy for Agues of all Sorts, that hath cured many Hundreds, and never knew once to fail, being without the least Grain of Cortex, or what they call the Jesuit's Bark, at five shillings the Vial, which is sufficient to make a perfect Cure, if of ever so long Standing."[151] Jesuit's Bark, the name given to Peruvian Bark, or Cinchona Bark, was discovered in 1650 by Sebastian Bado, and a monopoly of the Spanish trade from South America. It is a source of quinine and effective in malaria, so was thought to be something of a cure-all in the early eighteenth century and is mentioned in Thomas Sydenham's *Observationes,*[152] where it caused something of a rumpus in the medical world since Sydenham believed he had been plagiarized and lost a lot of money on its use.[153] Cater's refusal to use it both suggests her knowledge of contemporary medicine and wryly mocks those who might have thought she were a Catholic.

The evidence suggests that Mary Cater retained a strong hold over a niche market for curing eyes without the use of instruments that William Read had made fashionable. Her status as a woman herbalist links her with the ancient traditions of wise women. The fact that she worked only on the surface of the eye places her outside the new fashion of cutting into eyes, but that all her affidavits were for eye cures places her as working within a specialism despite the other cures she advertised. In the next chapter we shall explore how surgery began to gain the ascendency over medicine which it still has today. In this narrative, Mary Cater represents the complementary medicines in all their gentle effectiveness, signified by her use of the epithet "By the Grace of God" throughout her career to describe the help she had. Furthermore, she was helped by her knowledge of hygiene and antiseptics, something which the medical world would not learn about until the next century.

5

OFFICIAL EYE CARE

William Cheselden and Peter Kennedy

William Cheselden

If "quacks" were an easy target for the satirist's pen, official doctors were easy heroes. William Cheselden, F.R.S. and Surgeon to Her Majesty, and to St. Thomas's Hospital, was so famous for his eye operations that he became synonymous with them in a poem by Alexander Pope:

> Weak tho' of limb, and short of sight,
> Far from a Lynx, and not a Giant quite,
> I'll do what Mead and Cheselden advise,
> To keep these limbs, and to preserve these eyes.[1]

Nowadays, Cheselden is probably known most for his 1728 report to the Royal Society on "a young Gentleman, who was born blind, or lost his Sight so early, that he made no Remembrance of ever having seen, and was couch'd between 13 and 14 years of Age."[2] The boy's inability to comprehend the relative sizes of a real face and a miniature portrait was taken to act as a final statement on George Berkeley's question of the visual perception of depth and size. In fact, it spawned in Chelselden his interest in eye surgery since he had hitherto been famous for his remarkable success rates in lithotomy, the operation to remove bladder stones, an aspect of his work about which Pope knew but only mentioned in a letter to Swift rather than trumpet it about in a poem.[3]

Cheselden carried out experiments into a wide range of subjects, and the papers he published in the *Philosophical Transactions* demonstrate an interest in anatomy, tumors, bones, fractures, and eclipses.[4] He was also committed to teaching medicine at St. Thomas's Hospital,[5] and in 1713 he published *The anatomy of the humane body*, a students' textbook (in English) with plates, of basic physiology, anatomy, and operative surgery.[6] The book probably served as the background reading to the lecture series Cheselden gave for students as part of their general medical training and so described all parts of the body. It was successful, probably from sales to medical students, and made thirteen editions in Britain, and two in the USA, although it was a victim of its compendious nature, and the chapter on the eye, for example, is so short (at less than three pages) as to be of little use other than as a piece of descriptive anatomy: there is no plate of the eye in the early editions.

Germane to the present comparison between the unofficial and official practice of eye care is the number of advertisements for the book which Cheselden placed within a year of its publication, amounting to nine,[7] which is similar to the number of advertisements placed by William Read over the same months.[8] It could be argued that the difference between the two was that Cheselden advertised his books where Read advertised his services, but in February 1714, when William Salmon advertised the publication of *Ars Anatomica, or, The Anatomy of Human Bodies*,[9] a book similar to Cheselden's *The anatomy of the humane body*, either he or his publisher began vigorously to readvertise.

Furthermore, when Cheselden was appointed queen's oculist in 1727, eleven years before Pope's poem was published, like Sir William Read, he used the title in his self-presentation as a doctor. Thus, when an apprentice tailor was struck blind by lightning, "His Master sent immediately for Dr. [James] Douglas, Mr. Cheselden, the Queen's Oculist, and several other able Surgeons, and they all agreed that it was impossible to retrieve his Sight, the Optick Nerve being perished."[10]

With the weight of this evidence, we might begin to ask ourselves just how different was William Cheselden's practice and self-presentation from William Read's. It will be remembered that Emilie Savage-Smith's opinion of Read was that he "flamboyantly advertised his medical and surgical skill" and in the same way, a close analysis of the alterations Cheselden made to his *Anatomy* as it went through subsequent editions demonstrates that beneath its benign exterior of being a "text-book" for students, it began to sell Cheselden's skill as a surgeon.

The additions made between the third edition of 1726 and fourth of 1730 (which were published separately as an *Appendix* "for the Use of those who have the former Editions")[11] included "A short historical account of cutting for the stone." The chapter is brief but gave Cheselden the chance to append a list of the names of forty-six patients on whom he had successfully operated by a new "Lateral" method for removing bladder stones with minimal invasion time, and an incision that healed without stitches. Although Cheselden claims to "scorn to use any fallacious way of representing my success," the way the names are given with the dates on which they were operated is so similar to the advertisements placed by William Read that I will, once again, name names:

March 27. 1727.
Robert Kason	aged 4
Henry Webb	5
Francis Willmore	15

April 12. 1727.
Hannibal Basketfield	aged 3
Thomas Hull	4
Alexander Montgomery	8
Henry Cope	44

May 15. 1727.
Thomas Nailer	7
John Letheridge	8
Daniel Bezely	9

April 8. 1728.
Walter Bromingham	4
William Jersey	4
Thomas Kennet	13
April	
William Davis	4
Thomas Ellis	5

| William Adams | 6 |
| James Bond | 10 |

May 9. 1728.

John Parson	5
William Chater	11
Wilfrey Peale	40
William Hassenden	67

May 25. 1728.

| Joseph Godwin | 3 |
| Ellis Bakewell | 5 |

March 21. 1728/9.

William Ward	aged 10
John Edwards	15
Thomas Warren	17 died
Isaac Wood	25

April 21. 1729.

John Payne	4
Thomas March	6
Robert Caruthus	10

April 29. 1729.

Gabriel Forster.	21
Simon Sutcliffe	36
John Miles	42

May 1729.

Four cut in the presence of Mons. Morand, one of which, named Money, died. The names of the other three I have lost.

July 1. 1730.

Henry Hall	4
Walter Scott	4
John Tooting	7
John Paxter	11
Edward Eilding	13

July 31. 1730.
Joseph Wright   6
Joshua Philips   7
Richard Mitchell   10
Daniel Hall   14
In all 46.

At the end of the list Cheselden notes that he operated on many more than this, but states: "I cannot take the liberty to mention the names of private patients, therefore I will give detail of those only which I cut this way in the hospital, where the first twenty five recovered, to the truth of every one of which I had above twenty witnesses, and I do believe these patients are all living at this time."[12] Cheselden does point out that "Many of the children had the small-pox during their cure, and some the measles."[13] But considering the operations were done without anesthetic or antiseptic, this death rate is truly remarkable, and the sort of rate which surgeons are proud to advertise even nowadays.

As a further mark of Cheselden's skill and success with the new "Lateral" operation, the *Appendix* also prints ghoulish pictures of the "Thirty three stones taken out of William Hassenden, in the sixty eighth year of his age"[14] and "A stone which weighted eleven ounces, and measured ten inches round, taken from John Miles, who is now living in Reading."[15]

The same *Appendix* also draws attention to Cheselden's new skill in eye operations. A second brief chapter gives a full version of the paper he presented to the Royal Society about the "young Gentleman who was born blind," followed by "Three figures of eyes to explain an operation which I invented some years ago, and printed a short account of in the Philos. Trans. and have often practised with success."[16] The operation, a method of making an artificial pupil by incising the iris of a patient whose pupil has closed up or who was born without one, is described as "a pioneering procedure" by Rutson James and in the *ODNB*. The "short account," "An Explication of the Instruments Used, in a New Operation on the Eyes,"[17] was published on 1 January 1727, so although the operation may have been invented "some years ago," the publication was right up to date in its advertising of Cheselden's skill.

Together, the two chapters of the *Appendix* along with its separate publication suggest that Cheselden was taking the opportunity of the success of his medical text book to advertise his talents to a more lucrative private practice. Another sign that Cheselden's practice was becoming more remunerative was the fact that the third and fourth editions of *The anatomy of the humane body* and the excerpted *Appendix* were printed by William Bowyer (father and son of that name were both alive and working together), who became the most important printers of the century and eventually printed the *Philosophical Transactions* for the Royal Society. The Bowyers were also working at this time on the crowning glory of Cheselden's publication career, the *Osteographia*,[18] a series of drawings of the human skeleton, described by Allister Neher as "universally recognized as one of the most important and beautiful books in the British anatomical tradition."[19]

Adding to Cheselden's sales pitch, the quote above from the lithotomy chapter reminds his private patients that they will not be operated on in public and their names will not be added to his lists of successful operations. In its turn, the description of the eye operation, which accompanies the "Three Figures of Eyes," explains a very simple operation where a single-sided blade makes a single cut through an occluded iris as it is drawn out of the eye. What is described would have been a much simpler procedure than the couching which restored the sight of the "young Gentleman who was born blind." However, couching, the cutting around of the lens and pushing it back into the aqueous humour of the eyeball to remove the occlusion of a lenticular cataract, was an operation that had been in the public domain for three thousand years, while Cheselden, in effect, patented his operation for making a new pupil where the iris caused the occlusion. In making public the facts of the operation, he was advertising his skill, or at least his experience in performing it. The *ODNB* notes that Cheselden performed his "Lateral" operation for the stone privately for a fee of 200 guineas, and we can but wonder how much he charged to cut a pupil.

The fourth edition of *The anatomy of the humane body* (1730), which included the appendices giving the sales pitches for Cheselden's skill as an operator on bladder stones and eyes, also marked a turning point in his career. The *ODNB* tells us that at this time Cheselden sought an international aspect to his reputation: "In 1729 he became a corresponding member of the Académie Royale des Sciences de Paris, and in 1732 he was elected the first foreign member of the newly founded Académie Royale de Chirurgie in France." The same account of his life then notes that "Suddenly, and without explanation, he resigned his hospital appointments in 1737 to take up the post of resident surgeon in the Royal Hospital, Chelsea," where his duties were largely administrative.

There are several reasons we might give to explain why Cheselden might have made the split with St. Thomas's Hospital, some less charitable than others. The first is that the appointment as queen's oculist began to command a stipend of 300 guineas a year.[20] Along with this income, since Cheselden kept on his private practice while at Chelsea, he might have regarded the move as economically advantageous: he need only operate on a few private patients at 200 guineas to make up the annual hospital stipend of £49 plus £5 for each public lithotomy. To be fair, the fee for private operations also had to pay for the theater and assistants; however, since each operation lasted only a couple of minutes, he could fit at least four into a working day, as the list of operations in the *Appendix* demonstrates.

To give a more generous account of the split with St. Thomas's Hospital, we might explore Cheselden's association with the Académie Royale de Chirurgie in Paris. The Académie was set up specifically to train surgeons and saw a number of remarkable developments in surgery: the evacuation of a brain abscess hematoma by extradural incision; tracheotomy in cases of diphtheria; removal of an infected kidney stone; removal of the whole lens (rather than couching) in cases of cataract. Its motto, "Consilio manuque" (By using the intelligence and the hand) made a link between manual dexterity and intelligence which was manifest in the new successes and the wider range of conditions which could be operated on, as well as the lower death rates after surgery noted above.

The Académie Royale de Chirurgie had been set up as an offshoot of the Académie Royale des Sciences by two surgeons whose lower-middle-class backgrounds were similar to Cheselden's. Georges Mareschal was the son of an amputee army officer turned hotelier and was apprenticed to Paul Knopf, "chirurgien-barbier de Gravelines." Mareschal made his fortune by being a surgeon to the military wounded and became "chirurgien et confident du roi Louis XIV."²¹ François Gigot de Lapeyronie was the son of a barber from Guyenne, who was apprenticed as a barber-surgeon and then studied under Mareschal in Paris. Lapeyronie likewise made his fortune by being a surgeon to the military wounded and became "chirurgien et confident du roi Louis XV."²² Lapeyronie gave Cheselden a further model for the changes that he would effect in Britain, in that the French surgeon, using his close association with Louis XV, was the origin of the royal ordinance that made the definitive separation between barbers and surgeons in France on 23 April 1743. William Cheselden needed the assistance of John Ranby to bring about the equivalent changes in Britain in 1745, but they were brought about in a single stroke.²³

Ranby was the son of an innkeeper. He was apprenticed to Edward Barnard, foreign brother of the Company of Barbers and Surgeons, and admitted into the Company in 1722, ten years after Cheselden. But where Cheselden's expertise was confined to urban practice, Ranby's was military. First surgeon-in-ordinary to the king's household (1738) and then sergeant-surgeon to the king (1740), Ranby gained royal notice after becoming principal sergeant-surgeon to the king in May 1743, whence he tended to the bullet wound of George II's son, Prince William, Duke of Cumberland at the Battle of Dettingen (27 June 1743).²⁴

Following the French example,²⁵ Ranby used his influence with the king in Parliament to incorporate a new Company of Surgeons. This was brought about using the same move made by Lapeyronie as it separated the Company of Barbers and Surgeons, an amalgamation effected by Henry VIII in 1540.²⁶ Ranby was nominated as the first master of the newly founded company, though he had held no office in it. Joseph Sandford, the senior warden of the Company of Barbers and Surgeons, and William Cheselden, the junior warden, took office under him as the first wardens. Cheselden was the second master of the Company of Surgeons in 1746, which suggests that he was also influential in the separation.

There were three job descriptions (barbers, surgeons, and physicians) at stake in the formation of the Company of Surgeons. The first two, and the most obvious, concerned the components of the Company of Barbers and Surgeons: the new and complex surgery being undertaken in Paris and London was radically different from cutting hair, shaving faces, or letting blood. But the job description was also undergoing radical change between surgeons and physicians. The superficial difference between them was that surgeons performed operations to cure patients, whereas physicians used drugs. What this hides is that the physicians[27] were originally incorporated in 1518 as a Royal College and required a medical degree as minimum training. The new Company of Surgeons licensed apprenticeships for surgeons and no degree, but rather manual dexterity was required and tested.[28] Both surgeons and physicians cured patients but by different and incompatible methods and with different and incompatible standards of skill, and also with different rates of recompense. As queen's oculist, Cheselden received 300 guineas a year, whereas her physicians received 500.

Thus, when Ranby and Cheselden effected the separation between the barbers and the surgeons, they also set up the Company of Surgeons in opposition to the Royal College of Physicians as part of their bid to be recognized equally for their contribution to medicine. We find this aspect of the project in the publication of Ranby's *Narrative of the last illness of the Earl of Orford, from May 1744 to the day of his decease, 18 March following*,[29] which is a sustained attack on the competence of physicians to diagnose and treat the different cases of kidney and bladder stones. It is noted across most of the standard biographies of John Ranby, the surgeon, and Dr. James Jurin, the physician, who tended Robert Walpole in his last illness, that Ranby accused Jurin and his fellow physician Sir Edward Hulse of poisoning the former prime minister by prescribing doses of concentrated lixivium lithontripticum[30] pursuant to their diagnosis of kidney stones. Throughout the *Narrative*, Ranby highlights the brownness of Walpole's tongue, the dryness of his mouth, and his coffee-colored urine,[31] which together would suggest poisoning. It is therefore apparently with some triumph that Ranby notes that Walpole's autopsy showed "No Defect was ... discoverable in the Kidneys, nor *Ureters*,"[32] his diagnosis of bladder stones, which could have been removed by lithotomy, was vindicated.

While Walpole was still alive, and in hope that his diagnosis would be accepted and the lithotomy undertaken, Ranby called in William Cheselden. Although there can be little doubt that his services were called upon to perform a lithotomy, the *Narrative* states that he was called in to help insert a catheter.³³ However, there was little chance that Walpole would undergo the operation, even with the best lithotomist in the country, since in the entry for November 1744 (that is, very early in Walpole's final illness) Ranby notes that Jurin and Hulse were called in because "his Lordship at the same Time fixed in a Resolution not to be Cut."³⁴ In the event, the plate in the *Narrative* showed twenty-eight stones, and one large stone that blocked Walpole's urethra is less dramatic (perhaps on purpose) than the plates of stones removed from others of Cheselden's patients. Nevertheless, the autopsy also showed that "The Prostate Glands were enlarged, and become harder than they commonly are."³⁵ Whether Walpole died of the stone, poisoning, or of prostate cancer will forever remain a mystery, but the intention of Ranby's *Narrative,* in "Fulfilling the Will of the Dead,"³⁶ is to recommend the advice, diagnosis, and procedures of surgeons over the potentially poisonous medicines of physicians. James Jurin's reply, which concedes the correctness of Ranby and Cheselden's diagnosis and recommendation of surgery, turns to the ethics of the press for vindication. In the opening statement of *An epistle to John Ranby,* Jurin claims that "abusing the Living by Invectives, under the specious Pretext of inviolably performing the Will of the Dead, has been detested by all Mankind, into whom have been instill'd even the first principles of Morality."³⁷

Benedict Duddell and Peter Kennedy

If we have come a long way from oculists and their practice, which shall be remedied forthwith, I can but claim that the foregoing was necessary in order to give an exposition of the changes that were fissuring the medical profession at the beginning of the eighteenth century in order to explore the new and developing specialism of oculist. For if Cheselden has come to be known as the greatest English oculist of the early eighteenth century, it has to be argued that the claim to the title owes less to the "pioneering procedure" he devised to cut a new pupil, and even less to the paper read to the Royal Society about the "young Gentleman, who was born blind," and rather more to his being one of the three who set up the new Company of Surgeons. At least this is what two specialist oculists of the period tell us.

Benedict Duddell, calling himself "Surgeon and Oculist," began with a veiled attack on Cheselden's lack of skill in eye surgery that was designed to avoid a charge of libel in his *A treatise of the diseases of the horny-coat of the Eye* in 1729,[38] a year before the publication of the fourth edition of Cheselden's *Anatomy*. Duddell claimed to be a generalist like Cheselden but tells us he was moved to specialize in eye surgery after having blinded a poor man in Worksop in Nottinghamshire who came to him for treatment. He retrained in Paris, returned to England, and set up practice in Hammersmith, where as a Catholic he could worship at the Convent of the Institute of the Blessed Virgin Mary in Hammersmith Road, which was active between 1672 and 1792. His preface first turns to difficulties he has with John Taylor's *An account of the mechanism of the eye* of 1727 (of which more in chapter 6), then to Cheselden under the guise of "several Surgeons in London, who . . . go under the Notion of being Anatomists."[39] Duddell is damning of Cheselden's lack of skill as well as his arrogance and condemns him for thinking himself "entitled to perform all Operations on the Eyes, without having learnt them from Persons capable of giving them a true Insight into this Master-Piece of Nature." A Gentleman of my Acquaintance," Duddell continued, "ask'd one of these conceited Anatomists, how he did to know the different Natures of the Distempers of the Eye. His Answer was, that he undertook all. If his Operation succeeded, so much the better; if not, the Patients could be Blind, or in danger of being so, as they were before. And thus the Publick suffers for these Gentlemen's Experience."[40] There can be no doubt about the target of Duddell's attack after the publication of Cheselden's *Appendix to the* [fourth edition of the] *Anatomy* in 1730. Duddell's *Appendix to the treatise of the horney-coat of the eye* of 1733[41] is subtitled *With an answer to Mr Cheselden's appendix, relating to his new operation upon the iris of the eye,* and much of the book is directed at Cheselden's failures in operating technique. I shall not enumerate them since they had little or no effect on Cheselden, probably because Duddell was a Catholic.

The same was not true of Peter Kennedy's attack. In *A supplement to Kennedy's Ophthalmographia* of 1739, Kennedy, an eye specialist, published an attack on Cheselden for plagiarism, his too brief anatomy of the eye, failures in surgical procedures on the eye, and an inadequate theory of vision.[42] Kennedy never directly calls himself an oculist, but an advertisement which appeared in the *Daily Courant* in 1715 stated: "Whereas some pretending Practitioners to the Diseases of the Eyes have maliciously given out or insinuated, that Peter Kennedy, Author of Opthalmographia, or Treatise of the Diseases of the Eye, has left the Town, he thinks himself obliged to give Notice to the Publick of the contrary, and that he is to be spoke or advised with at his Lodgings [at] the Sign of the Peacock in Loathbury [sic], near the Royal Exchange."[43]

The advertisement suggests that Kennedy was specializing his medical practice in eyes and that other oculists had tried to steal his practice. Kennedy's title of the *Supplement* reminds his audience that he was the author of *Ophthalmographia, or, a treatise of the eye*,[44] which he published just before[45] the first edition of Cheselden's *The anatomy of the humane body*. If the *Supplement* was nine years late in attacking the third and fourth editions of Cheselden's *Anatomy*,[46] the reason would appear to be associated with, among other things, the separation of the Company of Barbers and Surgeons and the animosity this exposed between surgeons and physicians. Kennedy begins:

> I know not whether (in a great measure) I may not have been consider'd as *one dead* or *asleep*, these many Years by-past; . . . I know not, I say, whether, during this my *Quietude*, some *nocturnal* or *other Birds* may have made a little over-free with some of *my Feathers*, to deck themselves with. However, I must now own, that on hearing the *melodious Songs* of a *celebrated Nightingale*, in the praise of his *Eye Curer* . . . the *enchanting, warbling Notes* of this *melodious Bird*, I say, *roused me more than all the Noise and Bustle* of those of the College of [Physicians] or those of the *S[urgeons'] hall*, in running after our clamorous, vain, pretending *Occulist T*[aylo]*r*. I must nevertheless, at the same time say, that to judge right, and truly well, such who pretend to make a proper Judgment of a Person's Knowledge in any particular Way, they ought to be more learned in that Way than those they pretend to judge of, or at least very near as much; otherwise they will not only be very liable to the being *deceiv'd themselves*, but by such means also most ready to *impose on others*.[47]

The date of the publication of Alexander Pope's "First epistle of the first book of Horace imitated" in 1738, and the publication of the *Supplement* in January 1739 suggest that Kennedy's reference to "the *melodious Songs* of a *celebrated Nightingale,* in the praise of his *Eye Curer*" are the lines already quoted above:

> Weak tho' of limb, and short of sight,
> Far from a Lynx, and not a Giant quite,
> I'll do what Mead and Cheselden advise,
> To keep these limbs, and to preserve these eyes.[48]

That Kennedy believed he needed to correct Pope's endorsement of the idea that Cheselden was a satisfactory eye specialist says much for the popularity of the poet. The fact that the context of Kennedy's citation of Pope suggests that neither the College of Physicians nor the Company of Surgeons was competent to criticize John "Chevalier" Taylor, the most well-known eye surgeon in Europe, whose career will be addressed in chapter 6, says even more about Cheselden's lack of competence.

This time, after Peter Kennedy's attack on Cheselden, two new editions (the fifth and sixth) of *The anatomy of the humane body* appeared in quick succession in 1740 and 1741, with changes made to the material on the eye. But it must also be noted that Kennedy's attack specifically mentioned Cheselden's part in the separation between the role of surgeon and physician, and of the development of the role of the specialist doctor.

The titles of the sections of Kennedy's *Ophthalmographia* are integral to his concept of medical practice.

- Part I. Containing a New and Exact Description of the EYE; as also the Theory of the Vision considered, with its Diseases.
- Part II. Containing the Signs, Causes, and Cure of the Maladies incident to the EYE.

That is, one needs first to know the structure of the organ under consideration, and second, one must have an idea how the organ works; only then can a practitioner describe malfunctions and suggest cures. This model of medical practice, which has now become standard, questions the separation of surgery and medicine. For a personal statement about how

Kennedy understood himself as a doctor, we may turn to his second book, *An essay on external remedies:* "As to the Name, or Distinction, upon the Title Page, of *Chirurgo-Medicus,* I doubt not but that it will appear somewhat new, and uncommon to us; tho' all the best of the Antient Writers were such . . . they were both Physician and Surgeon."[49]

Kennedy also reminds his readers that Zamboni and Archisi in Florence, Rau in Amsterdam, and Pitcairn in Edinburgh all used the mixed title. But if Kennedy elides the job descriptions of surgeon and physician, he does so to elide "experience, observation, and practice" into practice and theory as the foundation of the whole medical profession: "One good Observation is worth twenty bad ones, and that this Treatise contains the Practice with the Theory, or the latter is founded upon the first; for where is altogether Practice without Theory; it might then properly be called Empiricism or Quackery."[50] Thus we find the reason why Kennedy separated his *Ophthalmographia* into two sections: to avoid the charge of "Empiricism or Quackery," and why he attacked Cheselden for having too brief a theory to support his practice.

The dedication of *Ophthalmographia* to John Arbuthnott [sic] sets out Kennedy's understanding of the state of the medical treatment of the eye at the beginning of the eighteenth century, suggesting it was "a Subject not much Studied, and perhaps for this Reason undervalued, because it is mostly pretended to by ignorant People, to the sad Misfortune of such as labour under Diseases of the Eyes."[51] Kennedy claims to have published *Ophthalmographia* since he believes that "the more knowing World must allow it to be one of the most curious Branches of Philosophy, Physick and Surgery."[52] And he explains to his readers in *An essay on external remedies* that his knowledge of the "knowing World" was gained in an extensive medical training in Italy, Paris, and Amsterdam. But this is not to say the *Ophthalmographia* is a translation (and it is certainly not a plagiarism) of earlier books on the eye which Kennedy quotes, such as Antoine Maître-Jean's *Traité des maladies de l'œil,*[53] or Pierre Brisseau's *Traité de la cataracte et du glaucoma.*[54] In fact, *Ophthalmographia* lives up to Kennedy's claim that "The Reader will find a great many new Things in the Description of the Eye, as likewise in the Theory of Vision, consider'd with some of its Diseases, also in the Method of Cures, which many Observations in my own Practice, not at all taken notice of by Galen, Plempius, Briggs, Maitrejean, Brisceau, or any other Latin, French or Italian Author."[55] Kennedy's *Ophthalmographia*, which is based on how the four humors affect the eyes, nevertheless develops the ancient ideas. His remedy, for example, given for "Pterigium, Unguis *or* Ungula" (a liquid incursion between the conjunctiva and the cornea) presents the choice between surgery: a complex and briefly described operation, or, if the condition is caught early enough, medical: powders consisting of *"Aerugo, Alumen ustum, Vitriolum album,* Sugar-Candy, &c."[56] The staged combination of approaches confirms that Kennedy believed it was not possible to support either side in the debate between the surgeons and the physicians as both roles had to be combined in the role of the specialist.

The substance of Kennedy's attack on Cheselden is that, in terms of the eye, his theory is inadequate and what is there is plagiarized from his *Ophthalmographia*, while his practice is ill-thought-out and supported by unsubstantiated claims of success. The section on Cheselden is the longest in the *Supplement* and begins with a set of complicated arguments about how in Cheselden's "Accounts of *the Eye* . . . the *drift* in *several Parts,* if not *in the whole,* seems plainly enough *to squint towards me*."[57] Dropping the metaphor, Kennedy suggests that if Cheselden is *"guilty of filching* of any thing from any *such Person's Performance . . . without the* least *Apology for so doing,* what must we think?"[58] The first accusation of plagiarism Kennedy makes against Cheselden is that he has stolen the *"Figure on Vision,"* that is, the "Three Figures of the Eye," a diagram of how light enters the eye, suggesting it is "as is contain'd in mine [the *Ophthalmographia.*]"[59] While Kennedy points out that all figures of light entering the eye appear similar, the force of his argument lies in the fact that William Cowper, Cheselden's anatomy teacher, had been accused of plagiarizing, or at least of borrowing without acknowledgment, Gerard de Lairesse's plates taken from Govard Bidloo's *Anatomia humani corporis*[60] for his *Anatomy of Humane Bodies*.[61] The suggestion is that William Cheselden had engaged in the same practice of borrowing without acknowledgment in his *The anatomy of the humane body,* but as far as Kennedy's arguments about Cheselden's theory go, they remain suggestions for improvement, since he "cannot by any means imagine, no more than some of his [Cheselden's] best Friends, who seem ready enough to allow, that this Part is not his *greatest* or *best Talent*."[62]

In the part that is Cheselden's greatest and best talent, surgery, Kennedy is more censorious of Cheselden's bogus claims and poor technique when treating eyes. Concerning the operation for the contracted or absent pupil, Kennedy begins: "And this *singular Operation* he has . . . been at great pains accurately to describe in the *Philosophical Transactions*, . . . But, methinks, on his so obligingly acquainting us with the Discovery of this so very *ingenious Operation,* it had not been amiss, I should imagine, that he had at least also inform'd us somewhat more particularly of *the Nature of these Parts,* and *when in their preternatural State?* More especially when most necessary to perform this *excellent Operation?*"[63] In his practice, Kennedy had never seen a closed pupil, or if he had, then not one which was forever closed, and so, apt for Cheselden's operation.

> The Distemper, says he, for which this Operation is perform'd, is either a total Closure of the Pupil, which is sometimes natural, and sometimes happens from Inflammation. The first, methinks, of the total Closure of the Pupil, appears to me to be a very unnatural State; and very rarely, if ever, fit for any such Operation; and as to the other kind, which, sometimes, quoth he, happens from Inflammation, there this notable Operation seems to me to be full as unnecessary and improper, since either the Inflammation will, with time, of itself, or by proper Methods, go off, or it will not, by that, or by any other Means.[64]

Nor does Kennedy believe that the operation itself is advisable or its results efficacious:

> And is it then the best Practice, or was it ever hitherto practiced, to separate or cut a Muscle (or Sphincter) to pieces, so to render it useless, by way of the best Cure for an *Inflammation thereof?* . . . But in spite of all this or any other such little Observations, or trifling Difficulties, our Author can still go *boldly on* to perform his so *successful Operation;* thus making his *notable Slit,* or *new Pupil,* which, tho' not performing the Office of *contracting* or *dilating* (as natural *Pupils* do) yet the Patient, as we are inform'd, will nevertheless *see very well;* such *Contraction to Dilation,* (according to our present Author)

being, it would seem, with him, *a meer matter of Moon-shine,* of little of *no consequence or use.*[65]

Nor was Cheselden happy to tell Kennedy on whom the operation had been performed: "I judged it the best Method to enquire of Mr *Cheselden himself,* where the Generality, or several of such People were to be seen or heard of, on whom he had *so often practised this Operation with Success?* . . . But upon my Enquiry into these Particulars he acquainted me, that he could not pretend to inform me where several of such People were, or what might become of them."[66]

When Kennedy pressed Cheselden, in the presence of another doctor, he was given the name of a single patient, the wife of a musician called Crome, living in Deptford, on whom the operation had been performed ten years previously. The woman gave Kennedy an account of her pupil closing up due to smallpox, which took her other eye, and how grateful she was for the operation as her husband would not have married her had she been totally blind. As to the operation and its result, Kennedy remarks: "There could be little risk in opening it; yet why it should not rather (in this Case) have been open'd in the very middle of the *Iris,* so the better to represent and do the Office of the *Pupil,* is what I cannot comprehend."[67] The new pupil cut by Cheselden, Kennedy describes as "being twice the Largeness of the *natural one,* and is consequently twice as large as *truly necessary;* a very great prejudice on several accounts; particularly, that of not *seeing Objects tolerably,* if at all, at any great, or even at *a moderate Distance.*"[68] When Kennedy tested Mrs. Crome's vision, she could only with difficulty distinguish a four-inch-long key. His disgust at Cheselden's fraud is palpable: "'Tis pity but that he had a *particular Patent granted him* from the *Crown;* or an express *Act of Parliament* for the making of *new Pupils,* to all his *Friends* (when they've the Occasion) as well as to all others who like it."[69] In a footnote, Kennedy gives further information about the "Woman of *Deptford*," explaining:

> I lately spoke to Mr Cheselden, acquainting him, That I had seen his Patient; and that I observed a *transparent Body* lying behind the lower Part of the *Iris:* He readily owned it to be the *Crystalline,* as I judg'd it to be. Well, but said I, I never saw *a Cataract like that,* To which he reply'd, *They were of all*

Colours. Yes, said I, but not *quite transparent as this is*. To which he made no Reply, but went away. This sufficiently confirms me in my foresaid Opinion, of there having been more done in this Operation than necessary; and it appears no manner of Question to me, that were that same *transparent Body* or *Crystalline* in its proper Place, she would consequently see much better than she does at present.[70]

The substance of Kennedy's accusation is that Cheselden had not only cut a new and too large pupil but that he had also couched Mrs. Crome's eye, both of which procedures reduced the acuity of her vision. Kennedy's search for other evidence of Cheselden's success with the same operation is in vain: "In a word, as to the further Particulars of this *Operation, so newly invented by our Author,* as he is pleased to acquaint us, Mr *Serjeant Amyand* told me, that he saw him attempt it twice, in *Guy's Hospital,* which he very quickly perform'd, but *without any,* or *the least Success.*"[71]

What disgusts Kennedy most about Cheselden's claims for his pupil-cutting procedure is his self-justification: "But it is certain, that this same Practitioner here mention'd, is somewhat ready to advance that it is no way necessary to satisfy the rest of Mankind on any such-like Subjects, provided that they the *Practitioner* concern'd therein, be *themselves satisfy'd.*"[72]

Whereas Benedict Duddell's attack on Cheselden for the same failings had elicited no response, Kennedy's produced discernible, if not dramatic, changes in Cheselden's *Anatomy*. In the "Theory" section, Cheselden adds but one sentence to the end of his chapter on the eye: "In all inflammations in the eye, the utmost haste should be made by bleeding, purging, abstinence &c. to get rid of the inflammation, because a continued inflammation seldom fails to make white opake scars on the cornea, which cause dimness if not blindness; and no eye-water with powders in it should ever be put upon the eye, because none can be made fine enough."[73] The statement counters Kennedy's medical remedies, which we saw above used powdered medicines in the eye and must be argued to be more the ideological statement of a surgeon rejecting medicines than an attempt to discover best practice.

The more obvious responses to Kennedy were made to the "Figures of the Eyes" and tables 32 and 33 of the fourth edition, which had been plagiarized from *Ophthalmographia*. These were substituted with a new table 34, which shows a different technique for the pupil operation, as well as the cutting of the new pupil in the center of the iris. Below these images on the same table were two new pictures of light entering the eye and light being unable to enter the eye due to cataract. These latter were smaller versions of the original table 34 in the fourth edition.

The description of the lens operation is also significantly changed. Gone is the swaggering statement of the fourth edition: "Three figures of eyes to explain an operation, which I invented some years ago, and printed a short account of in the Philos. Trans. and have often practiced with success."[74] The replacement description is much more careful, and even contains a warning: "This operation I have perform'd several times with good success; indeed it cannot fail when the operation is well done, and the eye no otherwise diseased, which is more than can be said for couching a cataract. In this operation great care must be taken to hold open the eye-lids without pressing upon the eye, for if the aqueous humour is squeez'd out before the incision is made in the iris, the eye grows flaccid, and renders the operation difficult."[75] The new description of the technique also gives an entirely bogus response to Kennedy's charge that Cheselden had done more than necessary in the case of the "Woman of Deptford," suggesting that her detached lens was an artifact of cutting the pupil: "The operation being thus done, the crystalline humour [the lens] immediately falls out; and in a few days the lips of the wound unite."[76] It is impossible that the lens would fall away from the ciliary muscles if only the iris was cut. The only explanation for Kennedy's description and this cover-up is that Cheselden had attempted an unnecessary couching on the near-blind "Woman of Deptford," and he was trying to pull the wool over his readers' eyes, who, being largely his medical students, would hardly disagree with him.

What does not change between editions four, five, and six of Cheselden's *Anatomy* is the inclusion of the *Philosophical Transactions* account of the boy born blind, except that in the two new editions, brought on by Kennedy's attack, it is moved to the main body of the text below the chapter on the eye and out of the appendix. It must be argued that any pride Cheselden might have had in the paper was based in the philosophical rather than the surgical importance of the observation, since in his *Supplement,* Kennedy is, if anything, more dismissive of Cheselden's claims about the boy than the pupil operation. From his very first footnote, Kennedy mocks Cheselden's assertion that the boy was not truly blind as with a cataract he could still make out colours:

> Cheselden: Tho' we say of the Gentleman that he was blind, as they do of all People who have Ripe Cataracts, yet they are never so blind from the Cause, but that they can discern Day from Night; and for the most Part in a strong Light, distinguish Black, White, and Scarlet; but they cannot perceive the Shape of any thing.[77]

> Kennedy: As some have been bold enough to assert, that the best Poets have been blind . . . which . . . is proved by the Improvement of our Reason, when we are not diverted by Outward Objects: . . . methinks it would be worthy his [Cheselden's] Enquiry . . . to know, or find out, what sort of *Blindness* it might be that *Homer* in particular was afflicted with; because, if it was of the *Cataract Kind,* (especially of the proper sort) he then, as our Author observes; being able to *distinguish Colours,* could not be so well said *to be blind.*[78]

As he had with the "Woman of Deptford," Kennedy visited the boy whom Cheselden couched, finding him in a worse condition than Cheselden suggested in the paper:

> As to the young Gentleman mention'd by *our Operator,* which he informs us gave those *singular Accounts* of the Representation of Objects, after his being couch'd, they are much the same with those of others, who have had the misfortune of being born blind, or very young when the Cataract first came on, and so thereafter have been couch'd. Now, as to this Gentleman's seeing, I am sorry to say for his sake, that it is still but very *imperfect,* and far from being about to read or write therewith; which, says our *Author, he thought only worth the undergoing an Operation for;* It seems even to be with considerable difficulty he can guide himself along with out some Assistance; and I am apt to believe, that he still knows *Puss* (whom our Author mentions) much better by *his feeling* than he does by *his seeing.*[79]

Kennedy also notes that six months after the operation on the second eye, the boy had an "Abscess of a total Suppuration, or purulence of the Crystalline Humour" due, presumably, to complications from Cheselden's couching operation.[80] The philosophical importance of Kennedy's criticisms of Cheselden were discussed in chapter 1, but apparently Cheselden himself was not bothered by the quality of his operations on the boy and believed that the observations about the perception of dimension and distance he gleaned from the "boy born blind and made to see" were valid however poor his sight, which might account for the pride of place of the paper in the fifth and sixth editions of the *Anatomy*.

All Kennedy's criticisms might, of course, be explained as a venting of the disappointment of a doctor whose practice had suffered as Cheselden's reputation rose. We saw something like this in Kennedy's advertisement in the *Daily Courant* of 1715 saying he was still in London when his detractors said he was abroad. However, Kennedy does not merely attack Cheselden's failures in eye surgery. He also praises his skill in lithotomy: "Now, if after what has been advanced, it be as yet alledged, that whatsoever Faults I may pretend to have found in relation to our present *Author*, here mention'd, Mr. *Cheselden* his Knowledge, or the operative Part with regard to the Eyes; yet that I cannot certainly, with the least good Ground, have any other Remarks to make than that the highest Success, in the *Operation of Lithotomy*, which is so *universally agreed to*."[81] This is not to say that all of Kennedy's praise for Cheselden's bladder surgery is unalloyed, and he makes some tart comparisons with Italian and Dutch surgeons whose death rates are much lower. However, from the beginning of the *Supplement*, Kennedy repeatedly asserts that he was "no way *on the catch, or to criticise* for *criticising sake*, but merely for the *sake of Truth*."[82] At the same time, and more importantly for the present argument, Kennedy defines his method of attack in a way which promotes the idea of specialism: "The best, *most laudable*, and most effectual way of *playing the Critic* on any Performance or Book, is to write a better of our own. Now, as I have already writ *a Treatise on the Subject of the Eye*, it may, I think, freely enough be allowed me to take Cognizance of such as any way *treat of the like Subject*, tho' they treat not thereof in any distinct, *or particular Treatise only*, but accompanied with other Subjects."[83]

For Kennedy, the treatise on a single medical subject, such as his *Ophthalmographia,* is therefore to be preferred to the more general work, such as Cheselden's *Anatomy:* "I shall not, however, pretend or judge it in any other way necessary, to make Observations on his General, Anatomic Work, tho' the other [the work on the eye] be contain'd therein; especially, since I never have publish'd any such General Work, what'er I might once, or ever intended. Yet I shall now, I believe, hardly think of any such Thing."[84] As we saw in William Read's practice, for Kennedy, the performance of a single operation again and again was the most important element of a surgeon's training, so that the operator could become skilled in the procedure. This is not to say William Cheselden was a malign influence on surgery at the beginning of the eighteenth century. He was a loud voice in support of the "Hand and Intelligence" of the surgeon, and in the need for equality between physicians and surgeons to find the best cure for people. If he had a flaw, it was his belief that an intelligent hand could perform any operation: he simply did not understand how closely one had to specialize in surgical practice in order to be as good as he was at lithotomy.

In a footnote, Kennedy gives the details of another botched eye operation by Cheselden, where, as in the case of the "Woman of Deptford," Cheselden did too much but which, this time, Kennedy could repair: "I frankly own I a little suspect our present Operator to be full ready not to do less that necessary, probably some times more. He twice in a few days attempted couching a *Cataract* (before ripe) on a Servant to a Person of Distinction, which brought on a great Inflammation; yet would have attempted again: But I advised her to forebear, which she did, and now sees tolerably, which he hardly knows."[85] If Cheselden did not come up to Kennedy's high standards of specialism, we do not have, apart from the alterations to the fifth and sixth editions of the *Anatomy,* much sense of Peter Kennedy himself as an eye specialist other than from his own mouth. I have located eighteen advertisements for the *Ophthalmographia,* with an unusual rise in interest in the volume in 1738, just before the publication of the *Supplement.* Thereafter I have found seventeen advertisements for the *Supplement,*[86] all of which mention the *Ophthalmographia,* and one of which gives details of Samuel Sharp's failure properly to address the criticisms Kennedy made of his practice.

Nothing more is heard of Kennedy in the newspapers after 1739, until 1749, when Oxford University awarded one "Dr Kennedy" the Degree of Doctor of Physic by Diploma.[87] Whether this was our Peter Kennedy, or another "P. Kennedy" author of two *Discourses on Pestilence and Contagion*,[88] we cannot be certain. The *Discourses* argue that pestilence can be passed on by breathing bad air and are criticisms of Richard Mead's idea that pestilence requires a minimum of touch for transmission. "Pestilence Kennedy" resided in Lisbon for at least the 1720s and is noted for his role in reducing an unnamed contagion (probably cholera) in that city in 1723: "The Sickness in Lisbon is much abated, few Persons of any Note having dropt off, for it seems Dr Kennedy our Countryman is fallen upon a Medicine which effectually cures the Distemper, which has made such Havoc among the Poor of that City."[89]

The language of the *Discourses* is quite different from that of *Ophthalmographia* and *An essay on external remedies* and does not mention the author's European education nor his acquaintance with so many famous European doctors. But the final reason why I believe that there were two "Dr. P. Kennedys" is that the proposed compendious work on medicine mentioned and repudiated in the *Supplement* ("I never have publish'd any such General Work, what'er I might once, or ever intended. Yet I shall now, I believe, hardly think of any such Thing")[90] is also referred to in the preface to *An essay on external remedies:* "I shall only add, that having published this as a Specimen, or Part of a Work I formerly proposed for the Common Benefit of the Publick, it will be a very great Satisfaction, if this is found any way acceptable or useful; but believe it to be the best Trial or Approbation by doing the rest by Subscription."[91] Whether it was our Kennedy or "Pestilence Kennedy" who was award the doctorate in physic by diploma by Oxford University, each probably deserved it for his work on either eyes or cholera. But each Kennedy worked in the main and was successful in his own specialism. What is odd is that neither warrants an *ODNB* entry.

If Emilie Savage-Smith's assessment of William Read can still find adherents, I would like to make a similar but slightly modified accusation against Cheselden that "available [contemporary] evidence suggests that ~~Sir~~ William was a more effective self-promoter and plagiarist than he was an oculist." But what has become apparent is that if Cheselden was guilty of poor performance in his practice on eyes, the reason was his failure to understand the necessity to specialize in the manipulations necessary for so delicate an operation. After general training, he put too much emphasis on the intelligence of the hand above the particular requirements of a procedure such as a couching for cataract. It would take John "Chevalier" Taylor to alter the balance toward specialism when he set himself up in the "profession of Couching" in 1727.

6

A PROFESSION OF COUCHING

John "Chevalier" Taylor

A dynasty of oculist John Taylors was sired by one John Taylor, "surgeon and apothecary," of Norwich, who died in 1709. His son, John "Chevalier" Taylor, was the most successful itinerant oculist in Europe in the eighteenth century. His grandson John Taylor, set himself up as an oculist at No. 6 Hatton Garden, London, and although he did not travel, he did have a successful career. His great-grandson, the fourth John Taylor, was oculist to two King Georges. It would be next to impossible to separate four John Taylors out as historically distinct people; however, as we know little about the earliest, and the fourth left the profession to become a journalist, writer, and partial biographer of his forebears, we need explore only two.

Debate raged in the eighteenth century and still rages about whether "Chevalier John Taylor, Opthalmiater; Pontifical—Imperial and Royal" was a Doctor or a Quack, Pretender or Pioneer.[1] He was accused in his own lifetime of causing the death of J. S. Bach,[2] but could not have been involved as he did not prescribe drugs, which are known to have weakened Bach's already failing constitution, and the Chevalier was not in Leipzig the year Bach was operated on.[3] He was accused in his own lifetime of taking money from Handel in June 1758 for performing an operation that could not succeed.[4] The Chevalier himself records on 21 August 1758 that Handel was now resting in Tunbridge and that "Mr Handel's sight mends daily." Handel's sight was never restored, but the sight of many more was that day. The article in which this claim about Handel is made is typical of the sort of press release published throughout the Chevalier's career:

Tunbridge. Aug. 21. The Success which the Chev. Taylor continues to have here with all he undertakes, brings to him a Concourse of People for his Aid. Yesterday one received Sight, who was born Blind; another by Means of an artificial Pupil of a new Invention; but no Instance has given more Satisfaction to the Nobility who are daily witnesses of these Events than the Recovery of Mr. Owen, the Bookseller of Temple Bar, who now sees to the greatest Perfection, without having suffered the least Uneasiness. The many of Distinction here under his Care, and others which arrive daily for his Assistance, as well from Town as from other Parts of England, prevent his fixing as yet the Time of his return to his House in Leicester Fields for a Continuance. Mr. Handel's sight mends daily. On Tuesday last the Chevalier gave at the Rooms a Lecture on his new Manner of restoring Sight, at which attended the Chief of the Nobility.—On a Child born blind, who received Yesterday his Sight; all the Nobility present, by the Chevalier Taylor.

> **From Cure to Cure the Chevalier**
> Quick as his Tongue does Wonders here:
> Beneath his Hands with hideous Cries
> Thro' Fear, not Pain, an Infant lies;
> But in few Minutes blest with Sight,
> Now Starts astonished at the Light.
> The Light what as with Magic Pow'r,
> Presents a World unknown before;
> With painful Pleasure he sighs awhile,
> Then thanks the Doctor with a Smile.[5]

Thus, we read of the cure of "Mr. Owen, the Bookseller of Temple Bar, who now sees with the greatest Perfection, without having suffered the least Uneasiness." We also read that the Chevalier is to give "at the Rooms a Lecture on his new Manner of restoring Sight." It is probable that this "new Manner" was the extraction of the lens for cataract rather than couching, invented and first performed on a live patient by Charles de Saint Yves in 1707, but which method did not appear in an English translation until 1741.[6] However slow the Chevalier's uptake of the new operation, he was the first to perform it in England. The same article also claims,

"Yesterday one received Sight, who was born Blind; another by Means of an artificial Pupil of a new Invention," and we might want to ask whether the Chevalier's child born blind and made to see could tell a dog from a cat after the operation, or whether he used William Cheselden's method of opening the pupil.[7] However, all the article gives us for evidence is the poem.

The question that this compendious article begs, as was the case with Sir William Read, is whether the Chevalier's greatest skill might be as an operator or as a self-promoter. But there can be little doubt that if the Chevalier could not cure people successfully, then he would have had nothing to promote to the "Concourse of People [who came] for his Aid." There can be little argument about the Chevalier's skill, since people came to him in their thousands, from popes to kings to paupers, to be operated on for cataract as well as a number of other eye complaints, and he was de facto a specialist in eye surgery because, unlike William Read or William Cheselden, he did not attempt procedures on any other organs.

His son, the John Taylor who distinguished himself less grandiosely as "John Taylor, oculist of Hatton Garden," has been eclipsed by the debate over the Chevalier and his life reduced to an afterword in his father's *ODNB* entry. He is included there only because a scurrilous life of his father was published in his name, and because he is claimed to be oculist to George III from 1772 (a fact that is possibly not true since Baron Wenzel advertised his arrival in London in June 1777, calling himself "Oculist to his Britannick Majesty"),[8] and because he was the father of the fourth John Taylor, oculist to Kings George III and IV, who gets his own entry in the *ODNB* for giving up the family career to become a journalist and friend of the Romantic poets. But while the Chevalier was and still is open to the charge of being a mountebank, John Taylor, oculist of Hatton Garden, was the model of professional propriety. He set up business in a street of fine houses known for professional medical specialists, next door to Peter Billings, "Sole Professor of the Cure of Lunatics, experimentally, by a new and gentle Method,"[9] and patients came to him. Like the Chevalier, he was adept at advertising his skill and at least as profuse an advertiser.[10] But where the Chevalier made a career trying out and sometimes failing with new methods of operating, John Taylor, oculist of Hatton Garden, kept to the tried-and-tested method of couching cataracts and sought a regular income from an ingenious method of taxing parishes.

I shall not enter into the debate about an objective statement on the Chevalier's expertise but instead explore how both he and his son John Taylor, oculist of Hatton Garden, built their careers on the idea from William Cheselden that surgery should have a more important role in the armory of cures, and the idea from Peter Kennedy that narrow surgical specialism was necessary to raise success rates. The result of following this advice was remarkable: by the end of the century, eye care was being offered to the poor that was "free at the point of delivery" in an unprecedented cooperation between the careers of the Chevalier and his son.

A Professional Reputation?

In fact, working strictly from chronology, both of these ideas might be said to have originated from the Chevalier with a little help from his friends. The first time we hear from him is in 1727 with the publication of his *Account of the mechanism of the eye* by Henry Cross-Grove in Norwich. Its preface is a piece of self-advertisement asking for the Chevalier to be accepted as an expert in "the Profession of COUCHING" by local doctors whose old-fashioned practice is stubbornly generalist. At the same time, the preface calls for all properly trained surgeons to band together to bring "Home" the specialist operations that had become the "Distinguishing Excellency of Mountebanks."[11]

I mention the publisher of the *Account of the mechanism of the eye* since Henry Cross-Grove, also publisher of the *Norwich Gazette* since 1706,[12] may have been the progenitor of the Chevalier's orotund delivery and attention to self-publicity. It is a sad loss that copies for all but 1741 and 1742 of the *Norwich Gazette* cannot be located. However, in 1742, when the Chevalier made a stopover in Norwich on one of his surgical tours of the whole island of Great Britain, the accounts of his stay in "Cross-Grove's News," a column in the *Norwich Gazette* with the byline "H. Cross-Grove," are as florid as the Chevalier's would become as his career went from strength to strength. I quote the articles at length (although out of chronological sequence) to give evidence of the sort of language that the Chevalier would develop, as well as of the Chevalier's capability as an operator on eyes. It must also be remembered that the Chevalier was returning to his hometown so this is not a case of an itinerant oculist who "cuts and runs," covering up botched work with heavy bandages while he escapes to the next town.[13]

> Norwich, March 6. Agreeable to my last, JOHN TAYLOR, Esq; His Majesty's Oculist, arrived at Chapel-Field House; and not a Day has past since his Arrival here, without his Lodgings having been filled with People who have indeavoured [sic] his Assistance. Among those he has recovered, the following are the most remarkable, viz. Mr John Dove, of Weathering-Street near Debenham, who was born blind, recovered the Sight of one Eye by the Doctor 11 Years since at Ipswich, and now the other. Mr. John Lane of Broome, Mary Basey at St Martin's by the Palace, Mary Nobbs of St Michael's Coslaney, all which had been many years deprived of Sight: Mr. John Hudson, a Shoemaker, who has been upwards of 14 Years blind, and was recovered to Sight at the House of the Printer of this Paper, (in Presence of many Worthy gentlemen) so as to distinguish Objects immediately with great Perfection. On Wednesday the Doctor gave a Lecture at his House, in order to show the Nature of his many happy Discoveries in the Cure of these Diseases since he has been Abroad. A great Number of Persons of Learning and Distinction, as well Gentlemen and Ladies, were present on these Occasions. On Account of his extraordinary Success, he will not proceed to London till the latter End of next Week.
>
> JOHN TAYLOR, Esq; His Majesty's Oculist, Knight of the Order of Portugal, Doctor of Physick, &c. Since his Arrival here has given such eminent and convincing Proofs of his Superior Abilities to All who ever pretend to Science, and of the astonishing Certainty he has arrived at in it, that he has even struck Envy and Malice dumb. I was an Eye-Witness to his restoring to Sight Two Persons at my House on Thursday last, in the Presence of several Worthy Gentlemen; which Two Persons in a few Minutes had so perfect a Sight, as to distinguish Objects and one of them said that he saw the Doctor's Face as he performed the Operation. This I affirm for truth, on the

Faith of a Christian; and am so assured of the Certainty of my own Senses in the Case that even the Doctor himself can never make me believe that he imposed upon me doing it. And Yesterday several other Persons, whom he has brought to Sight in a most happy and wonderful Manner, since his Arrival here, called at my House, and informed me of their being by him restored to Sight, after their having been long blind: To all which Truths I give my Testimony; and must farther declare, that it is my real and sincere Opinion, that the *mean* Things which have been *more meanly* raised of him, was not owing so much to Ignorance, as to real Envy of the Merit of this Surprising Man, and the many great Honours conferred upon him Abroad.[14]

The following week, Cross-Grove named six more people the Chevalier had cured, and concluded the article with the greatest of hyperbole: "In a Word, He has the Applause of every one who beholds him; he being (in all Probability) the First Man in the World who ever Arrived to so consummate a Knowledge in his Science, and very possibly may be the Last who will be capable of putting in Practice so fine a Theory."[15] The next week Cross-Grove's article returns to reality: "But what is most remarkable, the Gentlemen of the Faculty who have been with him, as well as the chief Gentry of this Place, now agree with one Voice in his surprising Abilities in the Cure of the Distempers of the Eye."[16] This comment about the Faculty's—that is, the local doctors'—approbation vindicates the preface to the *Account of the mechanism of the eye,* which in turn suggests that Henry Cross-Grove might have had a hand in that work too. Granted Cross-Grove would have made money out of advertising the Chevalier's 1742 visit to Norwich, and almost certainly made money out of the Chevalier's lectures, but at bottom this meant that his faith in the Chevalier's belief that it was possible to be a specialist surgeon had—literally—paid off. Cross-Grove died in 1744, but his creation, the Chevalier, built his career on the sort of advertising campaign that he learned from his Norwich mentor.

As chapters 4 and 5 demonstrated, the Chevalier was not the first eye specialist who made use of an advertising campaign. Furthermore, as I surmised at the end of chapter 4, it is possible that the young Chevalier followed William Read's example to become an itinerant specialist eye surgeon. Taylor was born in 1703, and Read is recorded as touring East Anglia in 1712, when the Chevalier was nine years old.[17] He became an apothecary's assistant in London in 1722 and studied anatomy with William Cheselden at St. Thomas's Hospital. By 1727 he was practicing in Norwich, where he wrote *Account of the mechanism of the eye* as a manifesto for a surgeon specializing in couching operations. The date of the publication, 1727, coincides with William Cheselden's couching of the "young Gentleman,"[18] so there can be no surprise that the Chevalier dedicated his book to Cheselden as his "General." However, in the same preface the Chevalier calls himself a specialist eye surgeon: "I declare before I enter upon the Work, that I have no other View in it than to satisfy the World that I am no *Empirick* (as I have been vilely and maliciously represented to be) in my Profession of COUCHING; but that I know as much about the Nature and Structure of the EYE, as is requir'd of any one who pretends to the Operation."[19]

In damning empiricks (operators who performed a single operation who were not trained as doctors), this statement also departs from everything in which William Cheselden believed. According to Cheselden's *Anatomy*, the surgeon's "Intelligent Hand" could perform every operation with a minimum of theoretical knowledge about the function of the organ being operated on. And the Chevalier knew this as he wrote:

> The Reason why this Nice and necessary Operation is so rarely performed by Gentlemen regularly bred to the Profession of Surgery, I take to be this; That it having been a long Time the Distinguishing Excellency of several of our famous Mountebanks, the regular Surgeons, by undertaking it, are under the dreadful Apprehension of being rank'd with itinerant Operators, commonly known as Quacks: The Fault is absolutely their own; for did they not join with the Empiricks . . . to oppress every young Fellow who dares to attempt a Thing which is not the general Profession of the whole Fraternity . . . how ineffectual would all the little Malice and Calumny of these contemptible *Wretches* be towards ruining the reputation of a regular Surgeon![20]

The implication is that surgeons' belief in general practice makes them as bad practitioners as untrained empiricks. And the Chevalier goes on: "And how easie it would be for us, (for 'tis We only who can do it) by making a Collection of the injudicious and barbarous Practices of those illiterate murdering *Rascals,* so to destroy their Reputations . . . that in a few Years we might be able to take this and some other Branches of our Profession Home to ourselves, the Original Proprietors, without any Manner of Danger of the foregoing Imputation."[21] This sentence, which ends the preface, is a battle cry for the profession of specialist surgeon, and the Chevalier is the general of his new model army. But it was not a battle cry that would rouse many, if any, general surgeons to his cause. As in the advertisements in the *Norwich Gazette* of 1742, quoted above, the Chevalier was popular with the people he cured, and he certainly did cure many blind people by restricting himself to the operations he was good at. But he built his success upon the very mode of practice that would associate him with the empiricks, the "itinerant Operators, commonly known as Quacks."

After this we hear little until 1735, since the Chevalier toured Britain, Ireland, and Europe, making his reputation. His autobiography, *The History of the Travels and Adventures of the Chevalier John Taylor, Opthalmiater,*[22] gives an itinerary for his travels, which, while inaccurate, is worth quoting as it gives us some idea of how busy he was:

I set out from my native country, and began my travels in the year	1727
I was in my progress through every town in all *England,* without exception, to the end of the year	1728
I was in *Edinburgh,* and in my progress through all *Scotland,* to the end of the year	1729
I was in *Dublin,* and in my progress through every town in *Ireland* without exception, to the end of the two following years	1730 1731
I returned to *Dublin,* and parted thence in *September,* 1731, and crossed the water to *North Wales,* and continued in that till *March,*	1732
I returned to *London* that month, and made another progress though all *England,* to the latter end of	1733
Returned to *London,* and there continued till *March*	1734

> In this month I went to *Paris,* and after a few months be-   1735
> ing there, I went all through *France,* every town of any
> consideration, without exception; and thence thro'
> all *Holland,* and every town, without exception; and
> all this with such amazing rapidity, that I returned to
> *London* in *November.*

A letter published in May 1735 from Amsterdam suggests the performances in Norwich were repeated throughout Europe: "The famous Dr. Taylor ... made several curious Operations upon blind People, in the Presence of most of our principal Physicians and Surgeons, and Multitudes of Persons of Distinction, who were all exceedingly pleased with the uncommon Dexterity of the Performance."[23] Finally, a long press release of 15 July 1735 tells of his return "from off his Progress, of near Eight Years thro' Great Britain, Ireland, France, Italy, Germany, Flanders, Swisserland and Holland, for a Continuance at his House in great Suffolk Street, Charing Cross." Although the advertisement does not use the title "Chevalier," it does refer to Taylor as "Doctor Taylor, Occulist to her Most Serene Highness the Archduchess, Member of several of the most celebrated Academies of Physicians, and Author of the New Treatise of the Diseases of the immediate Organ of Sight (a work that appears to Day in all the Neighbouring Languages)."[24]

I cannot locate the *New Treatise of the Diseases of the Immediate Organ of Sight* in English,[25] in which both this advertisement and the *Travels and Adventures* list are found, although a possible partial English translation did appear in 1742 under the title *An impartial inquiry into the seat of the immediate organ of sight: viz. whether the retina or choroïdes.*[26] However, the week following his return, the London *Daily Journal* printed what is claimed to be a letter "Published with Doctor Taylor's Treatise on the Organ of Sight ... by that learned Professor of Philosophy and Physick, Doctor Swinger, Dean of the University of Basil."[27] Presumably a prefatory recommendation to the *New Treatise,* Johann Rodolph Zwinger's letter was republished in 1742, in Latin, as part of *The Sentiments of the Professors of Physick in the Foreign Universities,*[28] a series of twenty-six such letters of recommendation from medical faculties all around Europe, which were published as an advertisement for a course of Lectures the Chevalier was giving in "*Great Queen-street, Lincoln's Inn fields.*"

Zwinger (1692–1777), who held the Basel University chair in logic for nine years, was from 1721 to 1724 the chair in anatomy and botany, and from 1725 chair in practical medicine and dean of the Faculty of Medicine. If the letter is real, and there is no reason to believe it is simply a fake, it was something to make the Chevalier justly proud:

> In this shining Part of Physick [Diseases of the Eye], John Taylor, Doctor of Physick, &c. has in our Judgment, infinitely surpassed the Studies and Endeavours of all others; nay, what is most incredible, that being very Young, yet has he left at a great Distance behind him all those who have preceded him, as well as his Cotemporaries [sic] in this Noble Science; and he has a long Time made evident to all the Universe, to the great Surprise of each Particular, not by any vain Ostentation, or Force of Language, but by various and daily Experiments, a happy Genius formed by Nature for this Sort of Study, an Industry surprising, an Application inconceivable, and in the Practice a Delicacy and Address not to be paralleled.[29]

But if such a paean was good for his career, it was hardly likely to make the Chevalier popular among his fellow practitioners. Likewise, the sort of caper he advertised between August and November of 1735, in which "twenty Persons labouring under twenty different Disorders of Sight" were examined by "the Gentlemen of the Faculty" for six days while being kept in the Chevalier's house and then cured on the seventh.[30] The *London Daily Post and General Advertiser* for 29 September informed its readers: "We are assured that a very great Number of Gentlemen of the first Quality, as well as the first of the Profession, intend to visit these Persons before he attempts their Cure, and to be Eye-Witnesses of his Success with them."[31]

But together, the lectures, Zwinger's recommendation, and the public demonstrations of cures ensured the Chevalier's presentation to the king. The *Daily Gazetteer* of 12 November includes the announcement: "Last Monday the celebrated Dr. Taylor was introduced to his Majesty at St. James's, and had the Honour to kiss his Majesty's Hand, in Consideration of his extraordinary Capacity and Service in the Science he professes . . . [and] Yesterday his Highness the Prince of Modena, and several other Persons of the first Quality, were to see several of his curious Operations of the Eye, at the Doctor's House in Suffolk-st."[32]

On 13 November, the *Grub-Street Journal* gently placed the satirical knife against his breast, repeating almost verbatim the report of kissing the king's hand, and the visit from the Prince of Modena from the *Daily Gazetteer:* "Yesterday the celebrated Dr. Taylor was presented to the King at St. James's, and had the honour to kiss his majesty's hand, in consideration of his extraordinary capacity in the science he profess'd, and this day about twelve, his Highness the Prince of Modena, with a great many persons of the quality, were at Dr. Taylor's house in Suffolk-street, to see several of his curious operations of the eye."[33] The alterations are slight but not unnoticeable. By removing "and Service" and altering the tense of the clause "in Consideration of his extraordinary Capacity and Service in the Science he professes," the *Grub-Street Journal* emphasizes the Chevalier's placing himself in the center of his own achievement, echoing the *Treatise on the diseases of the Chrystalline Humour,* which repeats over and over again the phrase "my new Operation." The *Treatise* was not, in fact, published until Christmas 1735, but, probably unbeknownst to the Chevalier, James Roberts, bookseller "near the *Oxford Arms* in *Warwick Lane,*" was involved in both projects. The Grub Street satirists had likely got hold of a prepublication copy, and they went to town on it. After the apparently innocuous reprint of the presentation to the king, there followed a slash-and-burn satire.

> We are inform'd that a dissertation which will shortly be publish'd, on Dr. Taylor's new method of removing a Cataract, is plainly demonstrated, that the common operation (or that practised by all others) can never be made without exposing the patient to the most violent pain, inflammation, and irrecoverable loss of sight, and very frequently with an abscess and total destruction of the figure of the globe; and sometimes, after having suffer'd many weeks of the most insupportable torture, to loss of life; and that on the contrary, by his new method, 'tis almost impossible to be disappointed of success not only in a certain state and species of this disease, (as is essentially necessary to have even a chance of success by the common operation) but, in every state and species of it, without exposing the patient to the

least pain or danger, or even the necessity of many days confinement.—
A very great variety of instances have appear'd since his arrival, and have
been often seen by a multitude of spectators, and agreed to be such by all,
even of the faculty, except two or three of those who would persuade the
public, that they are of the profession, and that they are expos'd to suffer
greatly (from their want of practice) by the success of such a useful and
important discovery: and by consequence, no method that envy may dis-
courage them to attempt to prevent the impressions of a truth of such importance, can have any great weight with those who have some use of sight,
whatever effect it may have on those who are perfectly blind.[34]

The scathing attack was followed by two named cases in which the new operation was successful, and another, where "Dr. Taylor made an artificial pupil in the eye of one William Arkenhart."[35] Only a careful word-by-word read-through of the longest middle paragraph (which is reprinted in full above) would unleash the satirical content. Only a careful reader would catch on that the paragraphs were not attributed to another newspaper as was usual in the "Domestic News" section of the *Grub-Street Journal*.

The Chevalier was a ripe target for the satire of the Grubs. Richard Russel and John Martyn had begun the journal in 1730 with the vowed intent of lampooning "all such reading as was never read,"[36] and the Chevalier's *Treatise on the diseases of the Chrystalline Humour* would never be read by many to learn how to perform the operation "except two or three of those who would persuade the public, that they are of the profession": it was an unabashed piece of self-aggrandizement and self-advertising, and thus might be thought to be the work of a dunce.

Although the *Grub-Street Journal* has long been associated with Alexander Pope as an extension of his poem *The Dunciad* (which attacked imposture, pedantry, and poor writing), Bertrand Goldgar has convincingly argued that there is no proof of a connection between journal and poet.[37] Nor might we expect Pope to be bothered to lampoon an oculist, whereas Martyn was a scientist, a Fellow of the Royal Society (a botanist) who had used the journal to attack rivals such as Richard Bradley, professor of botany at Cambridge, whose job he managed to finesse. Furthermore, as Goldgar has argued, both Russel and Martyn were nonjurors (Russel a minister, who lost his parish, and Martyn a layman, who in the end publicly renounced his belief to be eligible to take up the professorship of botany at Cambridge), and so neither felt any love for the Hanoverian monarch whose hand the Chevalier was so pleased to kiss. Furthermore, like many satirical magazines of their time and today, the writers were not so bent upon unmasking imposture, pedantry, and poor writing as entertaining people who shared their political point of view. Again, as Goldgar suggested, "the endless sniping at other periodicals, the manipulation of contemporary scandals and court cases for purposes of political innuendo—all this is . . . characteristic of the flavor of the Journal not simply in its infancy but throughout its life."[38]

For this reason, we should be very careful not simply to ascribe objectivity or truth to the satirist even when faced with the bombast of the Chevalier. After all, advertising his skill and patenting his method of operating was doing little more than the fourth and subsequent editions of Cheselden's *Anatomy*, right down to the operation to make a new pupil (and it is noteworthy that the Chevalier does not describe the shape of his). Furthermore, as the *Grub-Street Journal* moved to outright warfare, the battle was fought between the named "Dr. Taylor" and the byline "Peter Queer." The tactic of a journalist to hide behind a byline can but suggest that they are pretending to objectivity by concealing who they really are. We cannot be certain about whom the byline "Peter Queer" masked, but though the name would suggest that it might be the rival oculist Peter Kennedy, the fact of the Chevalier's breaking of the patented pupil operation would suggest that Peter Queer hid no lesser personage than William Cheselden.

Peter Queer's opening salvo at the Chevalier in *Grub-Street Journal* no. 310 covered nearly two columns, working by extensive quote and comment of what had already been published in no. 307. The method allowed a nearly complete reprint of the original article accompanied by a gloss for those who had not read the first version with careful attention. The method protected the *Grub-Street Journal* from a charge of libel since they could claim they had published the first article in praise of the Chevalier, and the reply was a response by an irate reader: it is introduced as an attack on "Mr. Bavius," the byline of Richard Russel, "turn'd trumpeter to the Prince of Puffers." The article makes out that couching is "thought one of the easiest operations relating to the eyes," such that there is no need for the Chevalier to invent a new operation.

So far the Chevalier had not entered the *Grub-Street Journal*'s paper war, but the Grubs were soon given a second gift when the Chevalier was presented to the queen, "and had the honour to present her with the first part of his Universal Treatise on the Eye . . . [which is] this morning published."[39] This time, *Grub-Street Journal* no. 313 of 25 December 1735 reprinted, verbatim and unattributed, two paragraphs that had been inserted the day before in the *London Daily Post and General Advertiser*,[40] both of which note that the Treatise "is prefix'd with a Letter to the physicians and surgeons of London."

It was in this letter, prefixed to the Chevalier's *Treatise on the diseases of the Chrystalline Humour,* dated 21 December 1735, that he first replied to the *Grub-Street Journal* and Peter Queer. Addressed as though to William Cheselden's failures with the operation, he chides the surgeon with the accusation that "little Attention has been given to this Branch of Knowledge, and . . . few have engaged in its Practice." He continues: "There is no Doubt that the Cause of this Ignorance arises from the great Nicety that attends its Study, and the little Success that has flow'd from its Practice."[41] If this was not enough to anger his addressee, the Chevalier then sings his own praises:

> If, therefore, from the following Sheets, it may appear I have apply'd myself in the latter with more Diligence to the former; or if the Success which I have met with in the latter may be every Day known, I question not, but these will be sufficient Motives to recommend this Piece to your Perusal; and of this I am the more persuaded, because I apprehend, you, who are particularly distinguish'd in the Learned World from your Superior Judgment in Physick, can't be well pleas'd with any Industry, that may be conducive to the improving this most useful, and perhaps only Part, which has been hitherto least known.[42]

The Chevalier also addressed what he had called in the *Account of the mechanism of the eye* "the dreadful Apprehension of being rank'd with itinerant Operators, commonly known as Quacks," stating that travel was important for his development as a specialist oculist since "it furnished me with an Opportunity of making my Remarks upon a greater Number of Subjects in a few Years, than the whole Series of my Life, in a settled Way, could possibly have afforded me." There is no doubt that traveling around Europe would bring him to more people with cataracts than if he remained in London and let the patients find him. And there can also be little doubt that, given the number of successful operations he claimed to have performed, "I have been furnish'd with those Lights which have enabled me to form a more certain and extensive Theory than my Predecessors could pretend to, or my Contemporaries can boast of." Nevertheless, his hope that "what I present you, will be read and examined, without the least Regard to any private Ends, but purely in the View of rendring [sic] Service to the Publick"[43] can but ring hollowly in a book dedicated to and presented publicly to the queen.

The core of the new procedure which gave the grounds for his self-aggrandizement, the letter tells his readers, would be presented in "the Account here given of the Manner of my removing these Disorders, that I am the first who have discover'd the Means to avoid that painful Delay of a Cataract's Maturity, and to remove the several Species of it with less Danger."[44] The method, which entailed the removal of the whole lens before the cataract "was ripe" (that is, had completely obscured vision), was revolutionary since it meant that the patient did not have to wait through years of deteriorating sight until they had become completely blind and could be couched. Furthermore, the Chevalier claimed that the same operation was indicated for people who had hitherto been thought inoperable: those suffering from a "Cataract which arises from a Blow received near the Eye,"[45] with the "shaking Cataract,"[46] with the "false Cataract,"[47] and in cases of Glaucoma.[48]

Whether the procedure can be called "new" or the Chevalier was "the first who have discover'd the Means" is open to doubt, though as noted above, Charles de St. Yves's *Treatise* in which a lens removal was described would not be translated into English until 1741. However, the work of Brisseau (1705 and 1709), Maître-Jean (1707), St-Yves and Jean-Louis Petit (in the 1710s), mentioned in the introduction, had at least laid the groundwork for the sort of lens-extraction operations that the Chevalier described. It may well be that the Chevalier had observed versions of his "new" operation in Paris and had improved on it, but it was just this fact that Peter Queer picked up on in his next salvo in the *Grub-Street Journal*.

In *Grub-Street Journal* no. 316 of 16 January 1736,[49] the Chevalier and Peter Queer covered nearly all of the front page. The letter to the Physicians and Surgeons was printed in full, followed by a suggestive disclaimer: "It is unusual for us to insert whole *Prefatory Letters;* but inasmuch as the following *Remarks* were actually order'd for the Press, before the above-recited *Letter* came to hand, we judged it most fair to insert them both. And we hereby give notice to PETER QUEER, that (if he intends we should print any more of his Papers on this subject) we expect he should make himself known to our Printer." Peter Queer's remarks are dated "Jan. 3, 1735–6," which makes nonsense of the first sentence, in particular since the *Treatise* was advertised as published on 23 December. But it does suggest that Peter Queer must have read the *Treatise* before the Chevalier had asked James Roberts to add the letter. Furthermore, the letter, which has been quoted extensively above, is of the species of bombast that was a staple of fun for the Grubs. And they had, as usual, made subtle alterations in the wording to make the Chevalier look more ridiculous. Thus, the final sentence of the letter, which should read:

> I shall beg leave to finish with this reflection, That whatever fate *attends* this work, I know no enemies amongst you, except those who sacrifice more to Mammon than Reason.

in the *Journal,* reads:

> I shall beg leave to finish with this reflection, That whatever fate *amends* this work, I know no enemies amongst you, except those who sacrifice more to Mammon than Reason.

In the event, Peter Queer makes but one amendment to the Chevalier's book, which is in the rendering of an account of Jean-Louis Petit's dissection and measurement of the weights of the different parts of the eye. Where the Chevalier has given the weight of the vitreous humor as "ten grains,"[50] Peter Queer notes it should have been "104 grains," although the total weight of the eye is given correctly. Nevertheless, Peter Queer makes big of the error, offering it as "a specimen of the Dr's care in the account (the errors whereof his skill in addition might have rectify'd) and how little is to be expected from his account of any thing."

There is no doubt that the Chevalier's *Treatise* makes the error in addition, but where Peter Queer claims he will "demonstrate . . . [that] it is Dr Petit's; to whom he is indebted for all that is valuable in his operation," no such demonstration was forthcoming, perhaps because to do so Peter Queer would have had to expose his name.

The Chevalier's reply, printed in the next issue of the *Grub-Street Journal*, begins with this very question of Peter Queer's identity: "Not having the honour of knowing that worthy Gentleman, who signs himself Peter Queer in your past Paper, I beg leave to take this method to return him thanks for his singular exactness, in his Examen of the treatise of the Cataract, I lately published."[51] In a moment of candor, the Chevalier notes the similarity of one of his operations and Petit's, thanks Peter Queer "for leaving me the right of invention of the other three," and then explains that he developed the fourth operation based on Petit's original since "his is not practicable, as I am persuaded the Gentleman knows."

A Reputable Professional?

We must rely on another moment of candor from Peter Kennedy to gain a more accurate contemporary account of the Chevalier's prowess in couching cataracts. Kennedy, it will be remembered, had not begun to voice his concerns about Cheselden's *Appendix* of 1730 until 1739 (four years after the *Grub-Street Journal* issues attacking the Chevalier), but in the *Supplement to Kennedy's Ophthalmographia*, in which Cheselden was brought to task, the Chevalier is the focus of Kennedy's argument. For Kennedy, Cheselden was in no position to criticize "*Occulist T-r.*"

> I must, nevertheless, at the same time say, that to judge right and truly well, such who pretend to make a proper Judgment of a Person's Knowledge in any particular Way, they ought to be more learned in that Way than those they pretend to judge of, or at least very near as much; otherwise they will

not only be very liable to the being *deceiv'd themselves,* but by such means also most ready to *impose on others.*[52]

On the other hand, Kennedy's assessment of the Chevalier was that he "*was a fine Hand, a clever Operator* . . . [although] at the same time. . . . he has *no Head.*"[53] In this criticism, though we discover that the real difference between the two operators is technique. Thus, Kennedy freely admits:

> My old acquaintance Mr. *Serjeant Amyand,* . . . has even told me as well as others that he must do Justice to this *Operator* [the Chevalier], (however defective otherwise) much to commend him for such his *Adroitness,* &c and particularly, (continues he) in the so steady manner of operating, as by that of resting his *Elbow,* &c. . . . as to the resting of his *Elbow,* in the Operation of the Cataract, I am fully convinced that it is *Quite wrong,* being of the opinion that the said *Elbow* ought to be *entirely free,* and *at full Liberty.*[54]

No reason is given for Kennedy's opinion on where the elbow should be, and it could be argued to be a case of personal practice. Nor does Kennedy agree with the Chevalier's practice of making an "Incision with his *Lancet,* before he introduces his *Needle,*" and although he suggests that the incision may allow the aqueous humor to be squeezed out, this is the procedure invented by Charles de St. Yves in 1707, who also invented a method of closing the wound with a sector,[55] which Kennedy calls "a golden Screw."[56]

Quack or Specialist?

Despite the attack on his integrity by the *Grub-Street Journal,* the Chevalier's career went from strength to strength with national advertisements for his *Treatise*[57] followed by a second progress through England and Scotland.[58] With such universal notice and the level of praise heaped upon him could but come detraction, and the long list of deprecating pamphlets, squibs, and implications of charlatanry first begun by George Coats in 1915[59] could be expanded almost indefinitely with the use of modern search technology. While it is important to note that there were a huge number of negative, or at least satirical, representations of the Chevalier

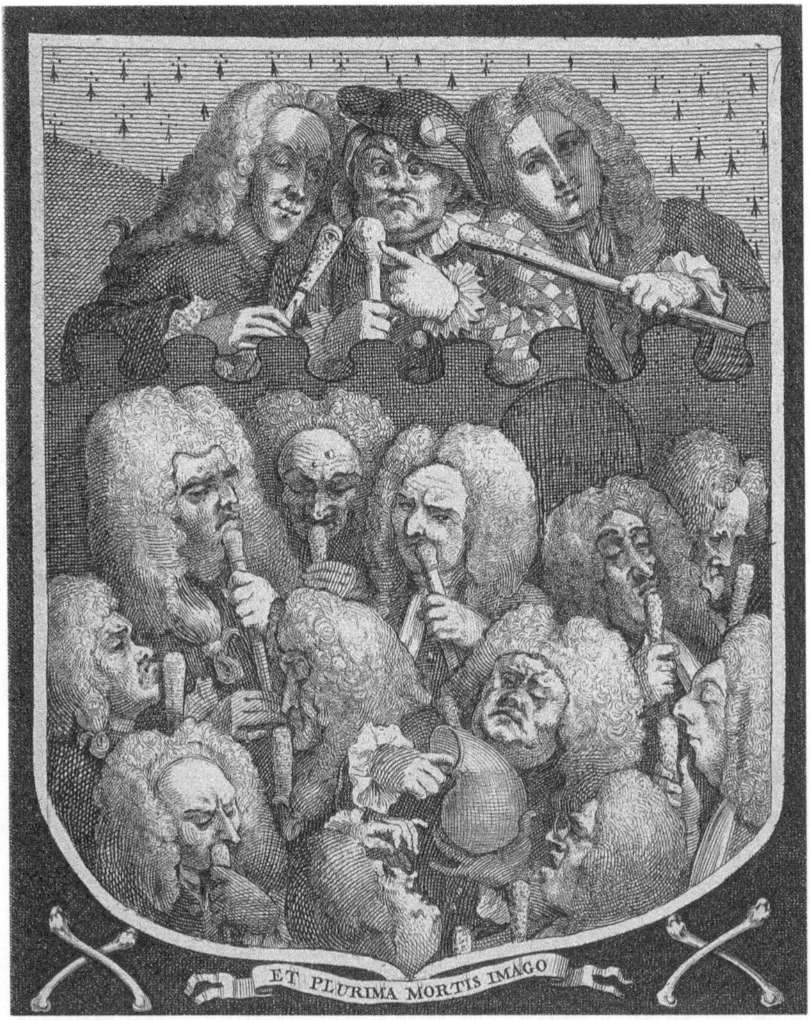

FIGURE 6. *The Company of Undertakers*, William Hogarth. (Wellcome Collection, CC BY)

to balance the articles of praise and that they began very early in his career,[60] there was only one that has really affected his historical reputation and cemented the associated between his name and the word "Quack": Hogarth's print *The Company of Undertakers* (see fig. 6).

Hogarth's etching, which dates to "March the 3d 1736," shows the Chevalier, Sally Mapp, a bonesetter, and Joshua Ward, purveyor of a "Pill and

Drop," presiding above twelve doctors (recognizable from their wigs and their pomander sticks, which they are smelling), who surround a urine jar into which one of them points. Fiona Haslam argues that the print was originally called *A Consultation of Physicians,* and argues that it "seems to encapsulate the commonly held attitude towards the medical profession that it was not always easy to distinguish the orthodox medical profession from the quack or charlatan and that, in fact, the dividing line between the two was rather ill-defined and the result of their ministrations similar."[61] This is a difficult argument to sustain when we consider that Hogarth was a governor of St. Bartholomew's Hospital and that between April and July 1736 he painted the famous staircase leading to the Great Hall with scenes that celebrated the work of legitimate doctors: *The Pool of Bethesda* and *The Good Samaritan.*[62]

The Company of Undertakers print actually dates from after the staircase, since "March the 3d 1736" is rather 3 March 1737, at which time there were a number of references to Hogarth's new print, called *Quacks in Consultation,* such as the *Daily Gazetteer* of Saturday, 5 March 1737, which advertised:

Just Publish'd

(Price Three Shillings)

A Print representing a Distrest POET. Also four Etchings of different Characters of Heads in Groups, viz. a Chorus of Singers, a pleas'd Audience at a Play, Scholars at a Lecture, and Quacks in Consultation. Price 6d each. To be either bound together with all Mr Hogarth's late engraved Works (except Harlot's Progress) or singly, at the Golden Head in Leicester-Fields, and Mr Bakewell's, Printseller, next the Horn-Tavern, Fleet-street.[63]

Thus, a much more likely reading of the print would point up the distinction (homophonous pun intended) between the workaday hospital doctors illustrated at the bottom of the shield, who sniff urine in order to make diagnoses for little reward, and the three successful specialists who have become known as "Quacks," who were all becoming known to ride in coaches and four.

The context of the Hogarth print, which cemented forever the association between the Chevalier, Mapp, and Ward, is important since it smears all three practitioners with the same brush. They were linked in the newspapers in August 1736, when a poem in praise of Mapp, at the expense of Ward and the Chevalier, was recorded in a number of regional papers:

> *To Mrs.* Mapp *the ingenious* Bone-Setter
> Of late, without the least *Pretence* to Skill,
> Ward's grown a famed Physician by a Pill;
> Yet he can but a doubtful Honour claim,
> While envious Death oft blasts his rising Fame:
> Next travell'd Taylor fills us with Surprize,
> Who pours new Light upon the blindest Eyes;
> Each *Journal* tells his *Circuit* thro' the Land;
> Each *Journal* tells the *Blessings* of his *Hand:*
> And lest some hireling Scribbler of the Town
> Injure his History, *he* writes his *own:*
> We read the *long Account* with Wonder o'er;
> But if he *less* had *wrote,* we'd believe him *more.*
> Let these O Mapp, thou Wonder of the Age,
> With dubious Arts endeavour to engage;
> While *you,* irregularly strict to Rules,
> Teach dull *Collegiate Pedants* they are *Fools;*
> By *Merit,* the sure Path to *Fame* pursue,
> For all who *see* thy Art, must *own* it *true.*[64]

The import of the first four lines of the poem is that whereas Ward's practice carried a risk, Mapp's did not. Ward's "Pill and Drop," based upon antimony, was poisonous in high dosage and was prescribed to be taken in tiny amounts. The invention was not Ward's own but derived from Pliny's *Natural History,* where the sulfide of antimony is recommended as an expectorant, cathartic, antipyretic, and emetic. Joshua Ward was another victim of the *Grub-Street Journal,* which, in November 1734, listed twelve named cases where the results of taking his "drop" for "chronical conditions" led to extremity and sometimes death.[65] Whether these patients exceeded the dosage can never be known, but nor can we simply label Ward as a "Quack" for not knowing that the medicine with which he made his fortune worked through sublethal poisoning.[66] Many modern medicines which are only slightly less fatal work the same way, such as chemotherapy for cancer. And a great number of people, such as Friedrich Wilhelm I, King of Prussia, claimed their cure from using Ward's "drop."[67] And neither must we forget that William Cheselden's skill at lithotomy came with a one in seven chance of dying of infection after the operation, or that James Jurin's soap treatment for the bladder stone killed Robert Walpole.

The Chevalier is attacked next in the poem for writing his own advertising material, an accusation also made in the *Grub-Street Journal* in late 1735, the import of which was that Sally Mapp, the bonesetter, must only reset a dislocated joint to be proved skillful and need not rely upon the press since people could see the results of her work.

What is important is that Mapp herself was not recorded in the newspapers before early August 1736, when, for example, the day of her wedding was announced, alongside "an extraordinary operation she perform'd in her Journey up to Town,"[68] which was [to be] recounted in the next day's newspaper.[69] The dates of their rise to public attention, one per year from 1734 to 1736, would suggest that from their first association, the three appear less as what Haslam has called a "trinity of Doctors" and more as a succession of celebrities who would come into and fall out of favor, in succession, as celebrities do.[70]

Thus, we should read Hogarth's print as a reaction to the incident which took place in October 1736, an incident which was so much what we would now call a "media event" that we should be very careful whether we believe it in every detail. A note in the *Gentleman's Magazine* for October 1736 reads:

Saturday, 6.

Mrs *Mapp* the bonesetter, with Dr *Taylor*, the Oculist, being at the Playhouse in *Lincoln's-Inn Fields*, to see a Comedy call'd the Husband's Relief, with the Female Bonesetter and Worm Doctor; it occasion'd a full House and the following:

Epigram

While *Mapp* to th'actors shew'd a kind regard,
On one Side *Taylor* sat, on th'other *Ward:*
Both *Ward* and *Taylor* thought it hurt their *Fame;*

Wonder'd how *Mapp* cou'd in good Humour be—
Zoons, crys the Manly Dame, it hurts not *me;*
Quacks without Art may either blind or kill;
But **Demonstration* shows mine's a *Skill.*

* This alludes to some Surprising Cures she perform'd before Sir *Hans Sloane* at the *Grecian* Coffee-house (where she comes once a Week from *Epsom* in her Chariot with four Horses) viz. a Man on *Wardour-street* whose Back had been broken 9 years, and stuck out 2 Inches; a Niece of Sir *Hans Sloane* in the like condition; and a Gentleman who went with one Shoe heel 6 Inches high, having been lame 20 Years, of his Hip and Knee; whom she set strait and brought his Leg down even with the other.

And the following was sung upon the Stage.
YOU Surgeons of *London* who puzzle your Pates,
To ride in your Coaches and purchase Estates,
Give over for Shame, for your Pride has a Fall,
And the Doctress of *Epsom* has out-done you all.
Derry Down &c.

What signifies Learning, or going to School,
When a Woman can do, without Reason or Rule,
What puts you to Nonplus, & baffles your Art;
For Pettycoat-Practice has now got a Start.

In Physick, as well as in Fashions, we find,
The newest has always its Run with Mankind:
Forgot is the Bustle 'bout *Taylor* and *Ward;*
Now *Mapp*'s all they Cry, her Fame's on Record.

Dame Nature has given her a Doctor's Degree,
She gets all the Patients, and pockets the Fee;
So if you don't instantly prove her a Cheat
She'll loll in her Chariot whilst you walk in the Street
Derry Down &c.

The report is full of mistakes as well as facts. The evening's entertainment advertised on 6 October to be acted at the Theatre Royal, Lincoln's Inn Fields on Thursday, 7 October was Charles Johnson's *The Wife's Relief, or The Husband's Cure,* with an after piece, "a Ballad Opera, The Honest

Yorkshire-Man."[71] There was no suggestion that Mrs. Mapp, the Chevalier, or Joshua Ward would attend.

However, the following day, Friday, 8 October, the *London Daily Post and General Advertiser* announced a performance on Saturday, 9 October of "The Wonder: A Woman Keeps a Secret" after which was to be played "A Pantomime Entertainment, call'd The CHYMICAL COUNTERFEITS: or Harlequin Worm-Doctor: . . . In which will be Introduc'd a new Scene of Action call'd Harlequin Female Bone-Setter. . . . The Female Bone Setter, by Harlequin. Bandage, Mr. Rosco; Callous, Mr. Ray; Vertebra, Mr Lyon; Dislocation, Mr Davis; South, an Innkeeper, by Mr Hewitt."[72]

There can be little doubt that it is to this pantomime that the *Gentleman's Magazine* was referring and in which the song was sung and from which the Epigram was derived. But whether Mrs. Mapp was there, or was accompanied by the Chevalier or Ward is not recorded before the event.

The following week, Saturday, 16 October 1736, the whole performance was repeated, and after this second performance the *Daily Journal* recorded there was chaos due to the popularity of Mrs. Mapp herself:

> On Saturday Evening there was such a Concourse of People at the Theatre Royal in Lincoln's-Inn Fields, to see the famous Mrs Mapp, that several Gentlemen and Ladies were obliged to return back for want of Room. She came there in her Coach and Four, and saw the Comedy called, *The Wife's Relief; or, the Husband's Cure*, with the Pantomime Entertainment, called *The Worm Doctor; or, Harlequin Female Bone-Setter*; which were performed to the Satisfaction of the whole Audience. The Confusion at going out was so great that several Gentlemen and Ladies had their Pockets picked, and many of the latter lost their Fans, &c. Mrs Mapp continues in Town till this Afternoon, when she returns again to Epsom to attend her Patients.[73]

We can probably be certain that the second performance was an advertisement for Mapp's practice, and the description of it demonstrates that she made herself part of the show. Thus, when we read that she was accompanied by the Chevalier in the *Ipswich Gazette* of Friday. 15–22 October[74] and the *Newcastle Courant*, of Saturday, 30 October,[75] we must be careful to ask whether it was really the Chevalier or rather an actor:

Last Saturday Night Mrs Mapp was at the Theatre Royal in Lincoln's-Inn Fields, and saw the Comedy called *The Wife's Relief; or the Husband's Cure,* with the Pantomime Entertainment called *The Worm Doctor,* in which was introduced, *Harlequin Female Bone-Setter:* there was in the Stage Box with her Dr Taylor the Oculist: In performing the Entertainment Mrs. *Love puppy* brought in under her Arm, wrapt up, a Dog to be *couched,* which Dr. *Pestle* (the chief Performer in the Entertainment) handled, and turned up his Eyes, to see if he had a *Gutta Serena;* upon which the whole House fell a clapping and hollowing, which held some Minutes; and Mrs Mapp shook her Hands and pointed at Dr. Taylor, which greatly added to the Mirth; upon which the Doctor retired a little, but returned, and stayed out the Performance with a great deal of good Humour; and when *Harlequin Female Bone-setter* appearred [sic] and performed her Operations, the House was again in Uproar, hollowing and clapping; but Mrs Mapp laugh'd with the rest and set out the whole Scene, and seemed highly delighted.

The story, mentioning the correct main piece for 16 October, suggests that at least this was a staged event. Thus, when we examine the moment in the account where "Mrs. Mapp shook her Hands and pointed at Dr. Taylor, which greatly added to the Mirth; upon which the Doctor retired a little, but returned, and stayed out the Performance with a great deal of good Humour," we would appear to be reading about part of the pantomime rather than the Chevalier's good humor at a joke made against him. It must also be noted that Joshua Ward was not recorded in this story, though he appeared in the Epigram from the *Gentleman's Magazine.*

We shall always remain uncertain as to whether or not the Chevalier was at either performance, and the same goes for Joshua Ward. Ward and Mapp appear to have been linked only after the second, when the *Daily Gazette* on Monday, 18 October, reported "Yesterday, she was elegantly entertain'd by Dr Ward in his house in Pall Mall."[76] Whether the Epigram, which links the Chevalier with Mapp and Ward, is real or the work of actors, we must read the Harlequin Female Bone-setter as part of just the sort of self-promotion in which the Chevalier would become more and more deeply engaged. Nevertheless, the Epigram, which was probably meant to raise the "Demonstration" of Mapp's "Skill" in the account of the cures she performed before Sir Hans Sloane at the Grecian Coffee House above those of her rivals, had the unwonted secondary effect of associating the Chevalier with Mapp and Ward as Quacks who will ultimately fail in their practice:

> YOU Surgeons of *London* who puzzle your Pates,
> To ride in your Coaches and purchase Estates,
> Give over for Shame, for your Pride has a Fall,
> And the Doctress of *Epsom* has out-done you all.

It might therefore be argued that fear of loss of reputation due to the Mapp performance led the Chevalier to leave England soon after he came to London in October 1736. While he was away he was represented in his own ballad opera called *The Operator*,[77] which was never publicly performed,[78] in the character of an oculist called Dr. Hurry. Whether the play was meant to be another salvo against him by the medical profession is not certain, since it is a lawyer who outwits him and steals one of his girlfriends. The play was "Printed for the Author." which suggests it might have been acted privately, perhaps by medical students, and had been well received. Some of the jokes are medical in-jokes, such as references to collyrium (an eyewash) that Hurry claims will cure any eye condition, William Salmon's *Pharmacopoeia* appears as Salmon's Drug Shop, as does a medical instrument for taking out eyes and putting them back the next day.

The play as a whole might be added to the Hogarthian legacy complaining that specialists (mountebanks, quacks, or empiricks) were paid more than establishment doctors, as well as part of the "noise and Bustle" of the doctors' attacks on the Chevalier which Peter Kennedy had noticed the year before but pointed in favor of the surgeons over the physicians.

Lecturer or Showman?

Either despite or because of the satirical attention, the Chevalier undertook another progress around Britain. The tour, begun in October 1736, resembled the Chevalier's earlier tours in all but one respect. Whereas earlier his operations were observed by other physicians,[79] now his operations were accompanied by lectures. An advertisement in the *Daily Advertiser* of 19 January 1743 announced a course of nine to run at his house in Great Queen Street:

> At Six this Evening Dr. John Taylor, Oculist to his Majesty, will begin his Course of Lectures on the Nature and Cure of the Diseases of the Eye, (and will be continued about the same House every Wednesday Evening till finish'd) at his House in Great Queen-Street, Lincoln's Inn Fields, in the Order he has for many Years given them in the Universities abroad, and of which he lately gave a general Account in a Lecture at Cambridge and Oxford. As the Doctor intends this Course to be free to the Gentlemen of the Faculty and Distinction, all such are hereby invited to be present.—This Day may be had at Mr. Cooper's in Pater-noster-Row, (which 'tis necessary each Person who attends these lectures should have with him) Syllabus Cursus Anatomiae Infirmitatum atque Operationum Globi Ocularis, & Partium contiguarum, D.D. Josepho Cervy, Regiae Majestatis Catholicae Praeclarisimo Medico Primario, Meritissimoque Praesidi, Proto-Medicatus Regnorum Hispanicae, &c, Didicatus a D.D. Joanne Taylor, M.D. Regisque Magnae Britanniae Medico Oculario, multique in Academiis celeberrimis Socio, Authore.[80]

The advertisement is interesting as it suggests that the Chevalier may well have learned from the Mapp affair and was developing his performance into something more theatrical. The rehearsal period would have been in the "Years [he had] given them in the Universities abroad," and the dress rehearsal in England the "general Account [given] in a Lecture at Cambridge and Oxford." To further guarantee the quality of his performance, the Chevalier offered complementary tickets to "the Gentlemen of the Faculty and Distinction." And making it a media event, there was merchandising of a souvenir brochure which "This Day may be had at Mr. Cooper's in Pater-noster-Row, (which 'tis necessary each Person who attends these lectures should have with him)." All this might be reading too much into the advertisement, which ends with a list of titles of each of the lectures that present a comprehensive study of diseases and operations on the eye, but it was just the sort of thing offered by other medical professionals.

We get an idea of what his performance might have been like in the spoof biography *The Life and Extraordinary History of the Chevalier John Taylor* published in 1761, supposedly by his son, John Taylor, oculist of Hatton Garden:[81]

> He lands at *Dublin*—is well received—gives a *Syllabus* lectures in Public *gratis*. Here he is followed by People of Fashion who invite him and caress him; for, being a little of the Knight Errant, which from our Doctor is inseparable, there was something whimsical and not disagreeable mixed with his Manner. His Style, though it sometimes bordered upon the Burlesque, yet his Deportment was so rapid and shining, one had not Time to reckon the Ridiculous, it was carried off in the Vortex of his Elocution, which made an Impression tho' singular indeed, yet not unpleasing; it puts one in Mind of the Poem, called, *The Splendid Shilling*.[82]

This passage, in a biography in which the incidents rush on, piling Pelion upon Ossa in accusations of Quixotic mule-headedness,[83] fornication,[84] sodomy,[85] religious irregularity[86] and political vacillation,[87] is probably a moment of clarity amid the satire. The reference to *The Splendid Shilling*, a poem by John Philips, gives us echoes of the Chevalier's orotund mock-Miltonic diction in the lectures:

> Not blacker Tube, nor of a shorter Size
> Smoaks Cambro-Britain (vers'd in Pedigree,
> Sprung from Cadwalader and Arthur, ancient Kings,
> Full famous in Romantick tale) when he
> O're many a craggy Hill, and fruitless Cliff,
> Upon a Cargo of fam'd Cestrian Cheese,
> High over-shadowing rides, with a design
> To vend his Wares, or at the Arvonian Mart,
> Or Maridunum, or the ancient Town
> Hight Morgannumia, or where Vaga's Stream
> Encircles Ariconium, fruitful Soil,
> Whence flow Nectareous Wines, that well may vye
> With Massic, Setian, or Renown'd Falern.[88]

The Life and Extraordinary History of the Chevalier John Taylor gives a sample lecture, labeled *The Mountebank's Speech,* which begins:

> The Nature of Good, my worthy Countrymen, is to communicate itself. Good is a communicative Thing. Good is not selfish, or solitary. Good is no Good, except it is diffused, Good, like a Dunghill, is good for nothing, till it is spread about; and for the Matter of that, no more is a Heap of Gold itself.
>
> This Remark, the Banker and the Husbandman will judge a good one. The Miser may perhaps put in his Exception; but my Lord *Bacon* and the Gold Finder will both tell him, that he lies. And, what is Gold; or even Dung itself, a much more useful Commodity? I say, what is either of them, or both of them, when they are compared to the Manure of the Mind? when they are compared to Knowledge, to saving Knowledge; such saving Knowledge in the greatest Good to Mortals? Gold, and Dung, rate Creatures of the Earth; Knowledge is the Child of Heaven.[89]

It was Joseph Addison who judged John Philips's poem *The Splendid Shilling* "the finest Burlesque Poem in the *British* Language."[90] It was also Joseph Addison who declared that a poet "ought in particular to be careful of not letting his subject debase his style, and betray him into meanness of expression," while failing to criticize Virgil for using the word "manure" in his second Georgic.[91] But if this satire, claimed by the Chevalier's grandson to be by Henry Jones, the bricklayer poet,[92] runs the gamut between subtlety, forthrightness, and the outright rude, it pales into insignificance when set beside the Chevalier's reply to it in his autobiography *The History of the Travels and Adventures of the Chevalier John Taylor, Ophthalmiater.*

It is necessary to quote at length from this remarkable book to give something of the effect of its extraordinary delivery. The preface begins innocently enough repeating the statements of the *Account of the mechanism of the eye* that ophthalmology is a specialism that must be addressed only after a general medical education since it is "a part of physic distinct and independent of every other, as well with regard to the theory as practice. That any great knowledge in the theory is never to be acquired but by a long and painful study, and the man must be born to the practice, *whoever hopes to excel.* To have any merit in the theory, he must be bred . . . to general practice; he must be acquainted with the laws of animal oeconomy, and capable of reasoning on the diseases, not of a part, but of the whole body; and for the practice, we all agree, that the works of the hand can never be improved but by the hand; and the difficulty must be in proportion to the delicacy of it."[93]

There follows a subtle and clever metaphor:

> To attend a painter, suppose, even for years together, to see all the various motions of his hand, will any man say, that he should do, because he saw it done? if here we admit of the impossibility, is it not, at least, equally impossible in the operations of the eye? if, in passing a pencil, a wrong colour is given, it may be removed, another is put in its place, and all again is well; but alas! it is not so with me; going almost the thickness of a hair beyond what I ought, may prove fatal; there is no calling back, no passing that way twice; the error once made, repentance is vain; must not then all men, who, for some envious or selfish view, call these things easy, abuse the judgment of thinking minds? must not all such believe, that men who report such idle tales, are strangers to the labour.[94]

The metaphor leads back to the arguments of the *Account of the mechanism of the eye* that poor practitioners blame the condition they are treating rather than their lack of skill. But then rather than move on to make another point, the Chevalier begins a long exposition of his technique that uses language, just as Henry Jones's satire declares, which is redolent of the burlesque language of *The Splendid Shilling*:

> For the truth of what I have related, I appeal to every honest and judicious man—To pass a needle immediately under a pellicle, finer than the finest cobweb, a pellicle that intimately incloses a body, whose surface is not plane but convex, and even that (when an operation is wanted) unequal and undetermined, without wounding or dividing the one of the other, to carry a needle immediately under, and about so small a circle as that to the pupil, whose diameter, on account of the different quantities of light, which enter the eye, in the progress of the operation cannot be determined. To attend this circle in all its changes, continuing the needle intimately round all its circumference, without wounding any part of it; and yet more, to pass the same needle immediately under, and carry it about another circle, before

you arrive at that of the pupil, a circle which cannot be seen (and much more delicate) and the sounding of which would be followed at least with an irrecoverable loss of sight—What almost incredible exactness must be required in the movement of the hand to succeed in such work as this! to make an opening of a determined length, in a certain part of so fine a pellicle, to force out of that opening various contents, which differ greatly in their composition—part solid—part fluid—This specifically heavier, that lighter, without enlarging the opening, or leaving any of the contents to hinder the perfection of sight; and what is yet more, placing them so well out of the way, where the light should pass, that they shall never be able to return to interrupt the progress to the immediate organ of sight—And above all, to pass a needle through parts in an unnatural state, so delicate, as those which compose the coloured part of the eye, dividing the insensible, avoiding the sensible, to make this opening of a determined diameter and figure—To pass through all the various parts in the way thither, wounding some, avoiding others, when the smallest error in either would destroy the eye, or render the attempt unsuccessful—If to all, we add the agitations of a thinking mind, when thus employed, knowing the difficulty, not forgetting the danger; can any say there are works yet done by the wit of man, that exceed such as these?[95]

Without more than a line space, the Chevalier follows his description of couching with an eye-watering series of invocations of the great and the good:

Oh! thou mighty—Oh! thou sovereign Pontiff—Oh! thou great luminary of the church; given to mankind, in the sense of so many nations, as a star to the Christian world—The great excellence of whose diadem is faith—Whose glory is the defence of virtue—who can believe, that you, *most holy father*, who art placed as the first inspector of the deeds of man, would proclaim to all the inhabitants of the earth, *as you have done,* your high approbation of my works, but by the voice of truth.

Oh! ye Imperial—Oh! ye Royal—Oh! ye great masters of empire—who have so far extended your benevolence, as to be witnesses of my labours—Behold me at your feet—To you, with all humility I now appear—Have ye not, oh! ye great powers, been graciously pleased to declare, under your hands and seals, the happy event of my enterprizes? How often have you condescended to behold the transports that affected the mind, when from before the dark eye, by my hands, the dismal veil was removed. The curtain drawn, and saw, by my labours, this beauteous little globe reassume its native power, and was again a lucid orb?—Who then can suppose, that you, the rulers of man—The protectors of virtue—the greatest lustre of whose diadem is justice, would point out, *as it were,* with the sceptre in hand, me alone amongst all mankind for these things, but from the strongest evidence that could be possibly desired for the support of truth?

Oh! ye Empresses—Oh! ye Queens! Great partners of the governors of the people of the earth—You, whose gentleness, whose goodness of heart, have so often engaged your awful presence on these occasions—What satisfaction have you expressed at seeing the blind, by me, enabled to behold again the marvels of heaven!—And finding them prostrate at your feet, expressing their joy at what they first saw—*Because,* 'twas you they first saw—The first object of their duty—The highest object of their duty—The highest in their wishes.—Have you not with your own gracious hands affirmed, that these things you have seen and where is the man so *daring,* and so *imperious,* as to call into question what you have said?

Oh! ye great people of *Rome,* once masters of the wiling world, governors of that great mistress of out terrestrial globe—Have you not, in the *sacred name of your people and senate,* declared with one voice, in praise of my works? and who will venture to say, that a body so illustrious, who for so many ages was revered as the rulers of all, could possibly err in their defence, of a cause like mine?

Oh! ye learned—Great in the knowledge of physic—Excellent in virtue—You, who are placed as at the head of human wisdom—Have you not told to mankind how highly you approve my deeds? Have you not, under your hands and seals, declared to the world how much you were pleased at my labours? Have you not often received me as a brother, and introduced me as a member of your bodies, with every mark of the most singular esteem: presenting me with *diplomas* to shew my authority, mixt in your praises for your motives, my knowledge in theory, my successes in practice, summing up all the most elevated reflections from the excellencies of my deeds; and promising, that my memory should to you be ever dear—Is it then possible to believe, that the most celebrated societies now existing, and bodies of men so eminent for learning and knowledge, would these things have done, *for me a stranger,* but from a consciousness of doing right?

It remains for me now only to add, that I flatter myself, that on due consideration of the motives that induced me to write, at this time, the story of my life, my readers will not blame me for having laid aside so often that gravity becoming the professor, and the physician, on the promise, when I speak or write as such I shall ever endeavour to appear—If then, in the following sheets, I may in this be said to have erred, I presume it will only be from my well educated brethren, and all such I hope to please hereafter in my own way—having many works already prepared from the press, which treat only on the objects of my profession.[96]

The apostrophe and hyperbole are perhaps what the Chevalier meant as "my own way," and the language is certainly personal and distinctive, eccentric and egocentric. However, we must not simply dismiss it as the work of a mountebank demanding to be taken seriously when he has nothing to offer. The invocations of the pope, emperors and kings, empresses and queens, the people of Rome and the academics of Europe, if taken at face value, are "royal seals of approval" given for excellent work in treating the highest echelons of society. It is as though the Chevalier had come top of a modern-day league table of surgeons, and so would presumably be any patient's choice.

The Importance of Itinerancy

And one more important point was made in the spoof biography *The Life and Extraordinary History of the Chevalier Taylor*. It was written at the height of *Tristram Shandy* mania and bears a resemblance to that novel's narrative strategy, beginning with an interlocking group of letters that appear to set the Chevalier and his son at odds with one another:

My Son,

If you should unguardedly have suffered your name at the head of a work, which must make us all contemptible, this must be printed in it as the best apology for yourself and father,

To the Printer.

My dear and only Son, having respectfully represented to me, that he has composed a Work, in titled *My Life and Adventures,* and required my Consent for its Publication, notwithstanding I am as yet a Stranger to the Composition, and consequently can be no longer of its Merit, I am so well persuaded, that my Son is every way incapable of saying ought of his Father, but what must redound to his Honour and Reputation; and so perfectly convinced of the Goodness of his Heart, that it does not seem possible I should err in my Judgment, by giving my Consent to the Publication of the said Work. And as I have long been employed in writing my own Life and Adventures, which will with all Expedition be published, 'twill be hereafter left with all due Attention to the Candid reader, whether the Life of the Father written by himself best deserves Approbation.

Oxford, Jan 10 1761.
The Chevalier Taylor, Ophthalmiator
Pontifical, Imperial, and Royal.

*** The above is a true copy of the letter my father sent me. All the answer I can make to the bills he sends about the town and country is, that I have maintained my mother these eight years, and do at this present time; and that, two years since I was concerned in his affairs, for which I have paid near 200*l*.

Hatton Garden, May 25, 1761.
As witness my hand, *John Taylor,* Oculist.[97]

However, the book is credible as a biography because of its Shandean subjects and because of the Shandean logic of these letters. On the one hand, the son, "John Taylor, oculist of Hatton Garden," is doing what his father bid him do in the first letter, by printing the second, and on the other, the son is getting revenge on his father, "John Taylor, Ophthalmiator, Pontifical, Imperial and Royal," for abandoning him and his mother. The fact that the two have the same name and overlong distinguishing titles was always meant to remind potential clients that the two worked in opposition to one another in the same trade, and in very different ways. Before this publication I can locate only one announcement which puts the two men in the same house, a press release in the *Public Advertiser* in 1758 which claims that the Chevalier "is expected every Hour in Town from Holland, at his Son's House in Hatton Garden."[98] And the inescapable logic of this is that if they did live close to one another, they encroached upon one another's business—so it was better for one to be itinerant, and the other static.

Indeed, though the *Public Advertiser* of 25 September 1761 announced that the Chevalier was back again in London for a month (at his son's house at No. 6 Hatton Garden), and advertises his practice and lectures, by Christmas 1761 the Chevalier had removed to Grevill Street, Hatton Garden, and by March 1762[99] he was out on the road again in Norwich.[100] The Chevalier spent the rest of 1762 on the road, and there is no suggestion that this was an escape from further vilification. He was already acknowledged as something very special, and people came to him in great numbers to be treated for problems with their eyes, which his grueling tour itinerary for 1762 demonstrates:

24 July:	Glocester
28 July:	Bristol
31 July:	Bath
3 August:	Bristol
6 August:	Wells
7 August:	Salisbury
11 August:	Winchester
14 August:	Portsmouth
17 August:	Chichester
18 August:	Lewes
21 August:	Rochester
24 August:	Canterbury
25 August:	Tunbridge
28 August:	Oxford
29 August:	Worcester

30 August: Birmingham
31 August: Newcastle under Line
1 September: Warrington and Liverpool
3 September: Wigan
4 September: Preston
15 September: Wigan
16 September: Liverpool
18 September: Manchester
20 September: Chester
22 September: Shrewsbury
23 September: Wolverhampton
24 September: Birmingham
27 September: Worcester
29 September: Glocester
30 September: Bristol
8 October: Wells
9 October: Sherborne
12 October: Exeter
18 October: Plymouth
23 October: Truro
26 October: Newport
28 October: Barnstaple
29 October: Tiverton
30 October: Exeter
2 November: Sherborne
3 November: Shaftesbury
4 November: Salisbury
5 November: Winchester
6 November: Portsmouth
10 November: Chichester
12 November: Lewes
14 November: Dover
18 November: Canterbury
20 November: Rochester
24 November: London for the winter.[101]

The parallel between the Chevalier's tour and that of a successful rock band in the 1970s is striking. It is as though he is promoting a successful album rather than suffering from a low point in his career. It might be best to understand the tour as his promoting his own success in his own specialism, but always he referred to it as part of a diverse medical profession:

> As has ever been the Chevalier's chief Study to deserve the good Opinion of the Publick, and above all his well educated Brethren of the Faculty: For the more effectually obtaining this desirable End, he intends hence forward, his Operations over, to leave the rest to their Care; this will be their Interest to acknowledge what they cannot but in their hearts believe, that the Art of restoring Sight is a Part of Physick distinct and independent of every other; and consequently for their Patients thus afflicted, will gladly call in his Aid. As the Cure of distempered Eyes is his peculiar Profession.[102]

Although he was never to learn that he did not need to expatiate infinitely on his own cleverness, he had become synonymous with his profession through his actions and not his words, as an epigram of the same year demonstrated:

> **To Dr Taylor**
> REpairer bright of IMpaired Sight,
> Best Oculist in Being,
> With gentle touch no longer couch—
> What *Briton*'s fond of seeing?—
> Whilst with their Tricks State Empiri-ricks
> Are *Blind* and *Screen*-Contrivers;
> What signifies an Eye or Eyes!
> Our *Seers* are but *Connivers*.[103]

And quite soon, even the medical profession embraced him:

> *From* Dr Erasmus Darwin, *an eminent physician at* Litchfield,
> *to* Dr Ash *of* Birmingham, *dated* Litchfield Oct, 21, 1763.
>
> Dear Sir,
> With this you'll receive that extraordinary, &c. the Chevalier Taylor, &c.—I think Mr Sharp has said it is three to one against being perfectly

restored to Sight in the Cases of the Cataract; here the Chevalier Taylor has couched four People by my Recommendation, one of whom was more than 70 Years old, and they all of them see perfectly. The Operations were all performed with great Judgment and Delicacy, the Patients seemed to endure very little Pain, and had scarce an Inflammation afterwards, &c.[104]

The Chevalier's career ended in success, probably in spite of himself, but the greater success was probably for the specialism of ophthalmic surgery itself, which he had firmly established in the minds of the people of Great Britain, if not in the minds of the medical profession.

Whether in the end it was because of his technique or because of his eccentric address to the world we shall never know. We might remember him for his diamond-encrusted pectoral cross, as some sort of eye-fixing Liberace, or as a hideously arrogant Tony Stark, who, like Iron Man, saved the nation's sight, or we might remember him in his self-appellation "Ophthalmiator, Pontifical, Imperial, Royal." Edward Young memorialized him in a poem which appears to describe his own operation for cataracts:

> Hail curious Occulist! to thee belongs
> To know what secret Springs of Vision move
> The Ball of Sight, what inward Cause retards
> Their native Force; what Operation clears
> A Clouded Speck, or bids the total Frame
> Resume the Lustre of the lucid Ray:—
> 'Tis thine to tell, how veil'd to gloomy Shade
> The darkling Eye retires, nor feels the Force
> Of solar Beam:—Anon a darting Gleam
> Shoots thro' the Glass, and gives the brighting Orb
> To visit Light:—I see the liquid Stream
> Flow, as the guiding Hand directs the Way,
> And bids it enter, where a total Gloom
> Had drawn dark Cover o'er the Seat of Sight;
> Whether in Choroid, or nervous Net,
> Fair Vision shines, thither the streaming Rays
> Converge their Force, and in due Order range
> Their colour'd Forms—Anon the Patient sees

A new Creation rising to the View,
In living Light!—There blows the flowery Mead
With sweets of every Bloom; there limpid Rill
Glides on soft Foot:—Here fair Pomona smiles
In Luxury of Charm; there Flora paints
Her vary-colour'd Train:—Here lunar Orb
Soft sheds her Silver Light, to cheer the Gloom
Of languid Night, 'till orient Sun reveals
A living Scene, with radient [sic] Lustre spread.—
    Go on, thou Favourite of Heaven, to bless
The darkling World with Light; give it to see
The Maker's Work, and teach the grateful Tongue
To sing his Praise, for what the Eye beholds,
To Rapture rais'd, fair Work of Power divine.—
While others court the Populace for Fame,
And every Merit which they cannot claim,—
Be thine the Task to beam in open Day,
And shine with Lustre of unborrow'd Ray.[105]

The poem has never been collected or reprinted, possibly because of its subject matter. The poet's importation of words such as "choroid" and "nervous Net" suggests he had heard the Chevalier's lectures in Bath before his operation. But whatever he thought about the ophthalmiator's self-presentation, Edward Young's joy at being able to see again and his delight that the Chevalier's talent had given him a new lease on life gives us a poignant reminder of how John "Chevalier" Taylor was accepted as a genius in his "profession of Couching."

7

FREE AND ACCESSIBLE EYE CARE FOR ALL

John Taylor, Oculist of Hatton Garden

However charismatic, however successful, no one can single-handedly found a medical specialism. Despite Sir William Read and the Chevalier Taylor narrowing the area of surgical intervention to hone their skill, the very fact of their traveling about the country (and Europe) to bring their dexterity to patients all but indelibly attached the epithet "itinerant" to anyone practicing as an oculist.[1] The word brought with it the further denigrating adjectives "mountebank" and "quack," something which twenty-first-century medical historians have barely been able to get beyond.[2] As has been demonstrated in chapters 3 and 5, this was probably because neither Read nor Cater's practice, nor the Chevalier's eccentric way of life and address, could be thought of as a solid foundation upon which a specialism might be built. But the Chevalier's son, his self-presentation, and fixed place of practice were exactly the sort of thing which was needed. Only ten years after John Taylor, oculist of Hatton Garden, began to practice we find this account of the benefits of medical specialism in the book designed to advertise the foundation of an eye hospital at No. 6 Hatton Garden: "It is less difficult to attain a superficial Knowledge of Disorders that affect the Body of Man in general, than a profound Knowledge of those which distress some Parts in particular, whereof the Eye is the Chief; complicated as it is."[3] If the Chevalier's life was characterized by showmanship and satirical attacks, the life of John Taylor, oculist of Hatton Garden, was so quiet and steady that at least two of his neighbors used his house at No. 6 as a fixed beacon to locate their businesses. Dr. Lowther, purveyor of various cures for nervous disorders, explained his address to potential buyers by telling them that "These medicines are sold in Parcels and Bottles of 6s. and 3s. each, at the Doctor's House, Number 14, between Mr. Taylor, Oculist, and the Golden Head, in Hatton Garden."[4] Mr. Warford, dancing master, likewise directed his clients to "the large genteel room, next Door to Mr Taylor's, Oculist in Hatton Garden."[5] What is perhaps most remarkable is that both of these advertisements were placed at the height of the fuss about the spoof *Life* of the Chevalier and his own *Travels and Adventures*, and both directions continued to be used for a number of years afterward. In the minds of the eighteenth-century consumer, John Taylor, oculist of Hatton Garden, was apparently unattached to his itinerant parent.

If the Chevalier's address was quirky, emotional, and at times ill-advised, his son's voice is all but absent. Where his father's querulous tone can be heard in every one of his press releases, and more and more in the forty publications he claimed, John Taylor, oculist of Hatton Garden, published nothing but a list of the names of many of the people whom he had treated as a summation of his career "in London only," two years before he retired from practice. It makes sixteen pages.[6] He also showed remarkable, even taciturn, restraint in his silence after the spurious *Life* of the Chevalier was attributed to him: a hiatus in his advertising between January and June 1761. Porter suspected silence suggested collusion,[7] but in a career that was marked by repeated dull advertisements and a complete lack of self-adulation, one might equally well argue that his silence was the best answer when any reply could only make things worse.

If the Chevalier's practice was tirelessly mobile, eagerly innovative, and began to slow down only in 1763, when he advertised that his success with a new operation was due to "a Resolution he has now taken, never henceforward to undertake any Person whatever, without giving his personal Attendance till each Patient is perfectly restored,"[8] John Taylor, oculist of Hatton Garden, traveled out of London for a protracted period only once, moved house twice in his life, and made only three recorded house calls out of London, twice to Grimesthorpe, Lincolnshire, the seat of Peregrine Bertie, the Duke of Ancaster,[9] and once to "Alexander Bence, Esq; Thorrenton Hall, near Saxmundham, in Suffolk," which left him so worried he might lose business that he published an advertisement when he returned.[10] Setting himself up in Hatton Garden was akin to being a modern Harley Street doctor, as Hatton Garden was home to a number of other more or less professional medical practitioners.

But this does not mean the career of John Taylor, oculist of Hatton Garden, is not worth remembering. The narrative of his struggle toward professional respectability demonstrates the same innovativeness and unstoppability as that demonstrated by his father. But instead of ceaselessly seeking glory in the moment, which led the Chevalier into debt everywhere he went,[11] John Taylor, oculist of Hatton Garden, sought and found a steady income and was possibly the first medical specialist to build up a regular practice paying a regular salary outside the public hospitals.

From Great Queen Street to Queen's Court and Back

John Taylor, oculist of Hatton Garden—Junior[12]—began to practice at the extraordinarily early age of nineteen, placing an advertisement in the *Daily Advertiser* of 30 November 1743 stating: "Whereas Dr. Taylor, Oculist to his Majesty, is at present in the Country; all who stand in Need of Attendance, are desired to apply to his Son, at the Doctor's House in Great Queen Street, Lincoln's Inn Fields, who will treat their respective ocular Disorders according to his Father's Methods, with the utmost Accuracy, till the Doctor's Return."[13] Porter suggests he was educated at the Collège du Plessis in Paris, from whence he returned to London in 1739 and studied under his father.[14] If he was born in 1724, this would mean that he finished his education at the age of fifteen and returned to London while his father was away on tour in Europe. Another advertisement in the *General Advertiser* of 18 March 1749 gives us a slightly different account:

> John Taylor, Oculist, Son of Dr. Taylor. Oculist to his Majesty, who attended his Father many Years in his Tour through most of the Principalities and Towns of Europe, and is thoroughly instructed in all his Father's curious Methods of Operation, and had practiced upwards of Six Years for himself,

with the most happy Success, continues to treat all Diseases of the Eyes and Eyelids, by the most safe and expeditious Methods, founded upon a regular Education in this Profession, and a lone Experience, at his House in Great Queen-street, Lincoln's Inn Fields, where Numbers of Poor attend daily, between Ten and Two, and are cured without Expence.[15]

The six years' practice fills the years 1743 to 1749, suggesting that Junior did not return to England in 1739, but traveled with the Chevalier in Europe for four years until he came to London in 1743, whence he was adept enough to perform eye surgery "with happy success." But the advertisement goes on to make two startling claims: that he had undergone "a regular Education in this Profession" and that the house in Great Queen Street was his.

Junior had not had a regular education in the profession of attending "ocular Disorders" since there was no regular education in medical specialisms. The Chevalier was educated by William Cheselden at St. Bartholomew's Hospital and in his *Account of the mechanism of the eye* claimed that he had a general medical education before he took up the "profession of Couching," so if either could be called a quack it is Junior and not the Chevalier. To ward off such an accusation, Junior, who did not write any books to preface with his ideas, used another advertisement in the *London Evening Post* of 1 November 1750 to explain that being a specialist in eye surgery was better than being a generalist:

> The numerous Defects and Diseases incident to the Eye, and its contiguous Parts, are so various in Kind, and of so tender a Nature, that they are more than sufficient to employ the whole Study and Attention of any one Person, be his Abilities ever so great, or his Knowledge ever so extensive. Hence it is, that Patients commonly meet with such bad Success, from their Application to Gentlemen whose Judgement and Skill in other Parts of the Human Body may indeed be unexceptionable, but whose Practice is too general to permit them to make any considerable Improvement in the knowledge on this one Organ; the Structure of which is so delicate, and its Parts so exquisitely fine and minute, that it will hardly bear any Mistakes in the treatment of its Diseases, since the first false Step in these Cases is always dangerous,

and very often of fatal Consequence. To obviate therefore this Difficulty, all Persons labouring under any ocular Disorders, may, with great Probability expect Relief, by applying in Time to

> Mr. John Taylor, Oculist in Great Queen-Street, Lincoln's Inn Fields;
> Whose Study from his Youth, and whose Practice since he came to Maturity, has for many Years been continued to the Diseases of the Eyes and Eyelids; from whom the Poor daily receive Advice and Medicines gratis.[16]

The statement is a development of his father's position in the *Account of the mechanism of the eye* and suggests that he believes that the treatment of ocular disorders was a specialism and required specialist training. However, in want of any such training being offered in the medical schools, as the advertisement of March 1749 explained, he had learned his profession of couching while traveling as some sort of unofficial apprentice to the Chevalier.[17] Junior also benefited from the change in title brought about by Cheselden's separation of the Company of Barbers and Surgeons, after which all surgeons have used the title "Mr.," and thus Junior did not need a physician's degree or to be called "Dr." in order to practice as a specialist eye surgeon. His self-presentation is the culmination of his father's teaching and Cheselden's politics: his status as eye specialist is de facto rather than de jure, but it was successful. Between 1748 and 1751, all his advertisements call him "oculist in Great Queen-street," and it would appear that he had bought his father out of the family home.

The relationship between father and son, which appears as Junior's advertisements progress, is a complex one. In the third advertisement placed for his practice, in the *Daily Advertiser* of 28 January 1744,[18] he no longer states that his father is "in the Country," but he still calls himself "John Taylor, Son of Dr. Taylor, Oculist to his Majesty." In the next, placed in the same newspaper at the end of March 1744, the slight changes in wording tell a completely different story: "Such Persons who unhappily labour under any Disorders of the Eyes, are desired to apply to John Taylor, Oculist, in Queen's Court, Great Queen-Street, Lincoln's Inn Fields."[19] Junior has moved his business out of his father's house and no longer refers to himself as his father's son. The same advertisement was repeated verbatim at least three more times[20] when, on 14 June 1744, the *London Evening Post* announced the Chevalier would be returning to "his House in Great Queen Street by the latter end of next Month."[21] The last advertisement the Chevalier had placed in a London newspaper was in July of the previous year,[22] and either Junior did not notice or believe the advertisement, or he was doing so well in his profession that he placed the same short advertisement in the *Daily Advertiser* a fortnight after his father's information.[23] Then he was silent for four months before he advertised that, "having lived for some years separate from his Father, in Queen's Court, Great Queen Street, Lincoln's Inn Fields, [he] continues to treat all curable Diseases of the Eyes."[24] The advertisement appears to be a shout of defiance at his absent father, but thereafter he was silent again for five months, when either his business thrived without advertising or he lived in fear of the collapse of his business when his father returned.

Still the Chevalier did not return to London, and Junior's advertising strategy began to use his absence as a selling point. In two advertisements in December 1744, the banner headline reads, "Dr. Taylor, Oculist to his Majesty," below which the sentence continues, "having long been absent from Town, and his Return quite uncertain, his Son, John Taylor, Oculist in Queen's Court, Great Queen Street, Lincoln's Inn Fields, still continues to his assistance in all Ocular Diseases, to whom all Poor People labouring under Disorders in the Eyes, applying between the Hours of Twelve and Two, may have proper Advice and Remedies, according to their respective Cases, gratis."[25] The tactic is to draw the reader's eye with his father's name and then to offer his own services in the Chevalier's absence. And it worked. For the first five months of 1745, the advertisement appeared at least seven times with the slightly altered wording of "being gone abroad" for "having been long absent from town."[26]

In May and June 1745, the Chevalier published a series of press releases in the *Dublin Journal*, listing cures and consultation times,[27] printing in full a letter of thanks from Charles Lucas, "the Irish Wilkes,"[28] and informing his correspondents of his "being requested home at London by the 25th of August next."[29] A month later,[30] Junior's advertisements were altered with his own name as the banner followed by half of his father's. I shall leave it to others to decide whatever might be said about the psychology of this change, but as a change in business strategy, it must have been spectacularly successful. While the Chevalier lingered in Ireland until the complete cessation of hostilities of the 1745 Jacobite Rebellion, Junior published the identical advertisement once in 1746[31] and then placed no further advertisements until October 1748, when his name dominated the longest description of his work to date.

The reason behind this show of grandeur is likely to have been that when the Chevalier finally returned from Ireland, in December 1747,[32] the two came to a working arrangement that suited them both. Either because it was the Chevalier's usual practice, or because he could not (or would not) compete with his son, he at once began an extensive tour of Britain,[33] from which he did not return to London until he advertised a lecture series from late October (the date of Junior's advertisement) to December 1748.[34] The Chevalier's lectures were held at the Exeter Exchange, and if he practiced at all, it was based around the course of lectures, at which: "On Tuesdays, the Nobility are invited, to see his Manner of restoring Sight—an extraordinary number of Persons with Defects of Sight will be assembled for that purpose To-morrow." Together, the advertisements suggest that he did demonstrations on the poor for "the Nobility," who were invited to watch, and he tells of one hundred cures but gives no consultation times. It appears that the Chevalier was making money from sales of tickets for the lectures of which there were to be no more than five hundred for each, and for which a subscription for the whole course was advertised at "one 3rd less Expence." The show—for show it must have been—fascinated his audience so much that the mimic Samuel Foote headlined in December 1748 with a skit called "An Oration in Praise of Sight" in his popular and long-running show "An Auction of Pictures."[35] Whether, as in 1743, the Chevalier's lecture course continued throughout December and January without further advertisements is uncertain. Foote's show began as the Chevalier's advertisements cease at the beginning of December, and no further mention is made of the "Oration in Praise of Sight" in Foote's advertisements after the end of January 1749.

Junior placed no advertisements in any London newspapers for the whole of 1747, which suggests that he was treating enough clients to obviate the need for publicity, and the large advertisement illustrated above, which is the only publicity I can locate for him in 1748, was printed just before his father came to London when his British tour ended and just before the course of lectures in London began. The very public nature of the Chevalier's business model, with his lectures being more important than his treating eyes, was in stark contrast to Junior's, which was what we would now consider thoroughly sober, serious, and professional. But it is a moot point whether Junior's private business model could have gotten off the ground without the popularity of the Chevalier raising public consciousness to the profession of ocular surgery to set it in motion.

Nevertheless, we can be sure that Junior's advertisement for 1744 and 1745 that hid his father's absence beneath the banner headline proclaiming the Chevalier's name, added to the advertisement for late 1745 and 1746 with his own name followed by the words "Son of" in the banner, led to the triumphant advertisement of 1748, which used his own name and profession as the whole banner and put his father's in brackets and in italics beneath. And Junior was successful, since the 1748 advertisement notes that he had moved back into Great Queen Street from Queen's Court. The Chevalier might be lording it in "His House next the Duke of Marlborough's, Pall Mall" from October to December 1748 while he gave his lectures, but by the end of January 1749 he had left England for the continent and did not return until 1755.

The question which still remains is whether the two oculists, father and son, fought tooth and nail or lived in symbiotic harmony. As suggested by the evidence presented above, the latter would appear more likely. Although the spurious *Life* of the Chevalier suggested itself to be the work of his son, and thus an act of revenge, the Chevalier's lectures at Exeter Exchange, for which tickets had to be bought in advance, were his main source of income, and his cures, limited to one hundred poor people who acted as guinea pigs, and who were cured for nothing, would not have impinged upon Junior's potential paying clientele. After all, treating eyes was not an ongoing process, once each eye had been treated, a client probably had no need to return. The only evidence that suggests that the Chevalier and Junior were at loggerheads is that although he first advertised that he was returning to London to "Queen's Street,"[36] when he finally arrived in London he moved into a house in the much more prestigious Pall Mall,[37] where Joshua Ward lived. Whether the house rental had been organized by Junior (and there is no evidence that it was, though it is not unlikely) as a sign that the Chevalier was one step up from him in their profession, we shall never know, unless any correspondence be discovered. But two years after his father's departure to the continent for another tour, Junior altered his business model once again, which also moved him to a higher status, or at least to Hatton Garden.

In Hatton Garden and Cures for All

Hatton Garden was a wide street of newly built houses. Far away from the vegetable smells of Covent Garden market that would have beset Great Queen Street, it was at the top of Holbourn [sic] Hill so was protected from the smell of the Fleet ditch, London's open sewer spanned by the nearby Holbourn Bridge. Opposite the church of St. Andrew's, Holborn, Hatton Garden was populated by a number of medical practitioners.[38] It must have been a reassuring place for middle-class people to go for treatment, but at the same time Junior did not exclude the poor, even in his press release telling of his move: "We are desired to acquaint the Publick, that, Mr. John Taylor, Oculist of Great Queen-street, Lincoln's Inn-Fields, is now removed to his House in Hatton Garden; where poor People labouring under any Disorders in their Eyes, or eye-lids, may apply for his Advice and Medicine (gratis) as usual."[39] The move heralded the only time in Junior's professional life that he ventured into the scale of publicity in which his father indulged, a campaign which would guarantee his popularity with the middle classes, and on the back of which he set up his practice with the poor.

Advertisements for Junior's cures were rare. In 1745, the first affidavit of a successful operation was made in a "voluntary and publick Declaration" by William Austin, "thirty-three years Clerk to the Sheepskin Market in Wood's Close, in the Parish of St James Clerkenwell."[40] Although this sort of statement had been used as a method of advertising by William Read and Mary Cater from the beginning of the century, Junior had never used it. Less than a month after the Chevalier left for the continent in

January 1749, John Jarret (or Jarratt), "Horse-Bridle Founder, in Hosier-Lane, Smithfield," made a similar public declaration about his cure by Junior, adding that "I laboured under a dangerous Distemper in my Eye, attended with the most racking Pain and Loss of Sight; wherefore I applied to the Surgeons of St. Bartholomew's Hospital, but was told my Disease was remediless, and rejected as incurable."[41] As if such self-promotion were beneath his dignity, the following month Junior published the advertisement stating that he had learned his trade from his father[42] and was once more silent until November 1750, when he published the press release that specialist eye surgeons are better than generalists.[43] So far in my argument I have suggested that no advertisements meant good trade, based in the logic that it would be a waste of money to place advertisements when the clients are coming in by word-of-mouth recommendation. But Austin's and Jarret's statements given voluntarily and presumably paid for by themselves were a form of word-of-mouth recommendation. Whether because of a drop-off in trade or because Junior was planning his move to the more salubrious, and more expensive, Hatton Garden, in April 1751, three reports of cures were published in quick succession. The first is a letter in quotation marks witnessing "by the Help of God, and the Assistance of Mr. Taylor, Occulist [sic] in Great Queen Street, Lincoln's Inn Fields, [James Dausit] is restored to Sight." It is marked from "Rumford in Essex" and signed by a chapel warden and two overseers of the poor.[44] The second is presented as a statement of fact: "Last week the Wife of Mr Dupleix, Peruke-maker in Quaker Street, Spittle-fields, was restor'd to sight by Mr Taylor, Oculist in Great Queen-street, Lincoln's Inn Fields."[45] A third followed with the identical wording but for the name of the cured, "the Son of Mr Selby, an eminent Linnen-draper in Smithfield."[46]

The cure of James Dausit is of a poor man and would have been paid for by the overseers of the poor in his parish of settlement, Romford in Essex, although we must assume he was working in London since he was treated by Junior. The cures of Mrs. Dupleix and the Son of Mr. Selby would presumably have been paid for by the relatives named in the advertisements. These two forms of payment would go to make Junior's stable income, but each was fraught with its own difficulties. The mechanism of payment of the first, by the doctor billing the parish of settlement, meant that witnesses from the parish had to be called to be present at the cure, return to their parish, and then bring the money back to the doctor, which could take a long time. The mechanism of getting the attention of those who could pay for their own cure was either to travel to them, as the Chevalier did, to advertise, or to hope that they would come of their own accord.

In June 1751, the problem of traveling to find patients rather than waiting for them to come to him beset Junior. We can read this in an advertisement in the *General Advertiser* that is filled with the annoyance of losing trade by going out of town: "Those Gentlemen, &c. who have enquired after Mr John Taylor, Oculist, in Great Queen-street, Lincoln's Inn Fields, in order to apply for his Assistance, are hereby informed that he is now returned from the Seat of Alexander Bence, Esq. in Thorrenton-Hall, near Saxmundham, in Suffolk, where he has been treating a Disorder in that Gentleman's Eyes, and may now be consulted in all ocular Diseases, at his House, as usual."[47] In October 1751, the advantages of having a fixed address in a recognizable street of doctors became apparent, and with his talent for business, Junior combined his two preferred forms of making income at one stroke: he would bring the middle-class blind to a specialist hospital and cure the poor from local parishes who prepaid for the service: and this was brought about with a careful advertising strategy.

The month after his move to Hatton Garden, Junior performed a double couching on an eight-year-old boy who had been blind from birth.[48] William Taylor of Ightham in Kent was the son of a farmer and was only the second case recorded in detail of a person who, though born blind, had been "made to see," since George Berkeley had thrown down his challenge to the medical profession to give a real case that would prove his theory that perception of depth was learned rather than perceived. Furthermore, it will be remembered that Peter Kennedy had mired William Cheselden's cure in controversy with his suggestion that the boy could not get about by himself even after the operation, so it could be argued that William Taylor was the first-ever blind person "made to see" within the Western tradition of empiricism and surgical procedure. Appropriately to the extraordinary importance of the cure, an etching was made of the boy's face by Thomas Worlidge, the English Rembrandt, which appeared early in 1752

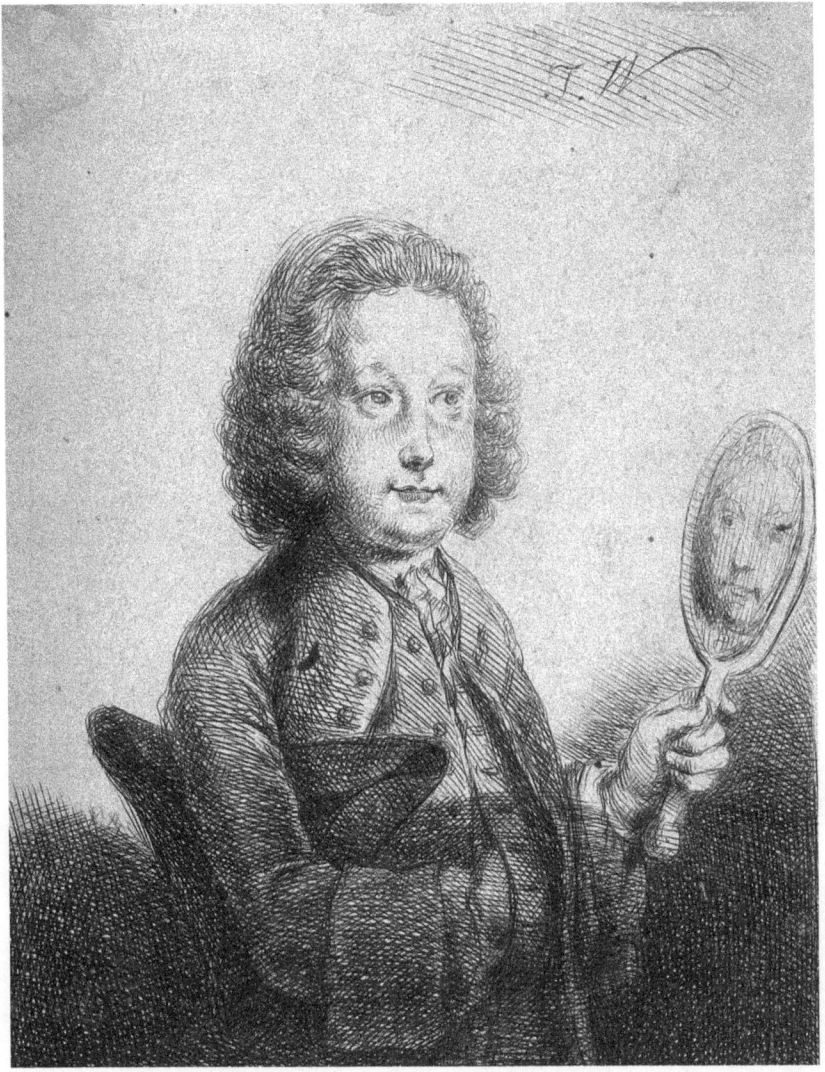

FIGURE 7. *William Taylor of Ightham, Kent,* Thomas Worlidge. (Wellcome Collection, CC BY)

(see fig. 7).[49] It is nowhere near the quality of Worlidge's usual representations but is worth reproducing as it is so rare.

In October 1752, William Oldys, an antiquarian who was a close friend of Junior,[50] wrote the incident up in a book which tells the story of the cure and gives details of the proposed hospital.[51] Where the Chevalier wrote his own story for himself, and in as many as forty books, Junior asked a friend with a track record in writing to do the honors, which was probably better for his reputation, at least at the time of writing.

Oldys's book, *Observations of the Cure of William Taylor, the Blind Boy of Ightham, in Kent,* and subtitled *Some Address to the Publick, for a Contribution towards the Foundation of an Hospital for the Blind, Already begun by noble Personages,* begins with the names of those "noble Personages" who were associated with the hospital project. Presented in the same way as the subscribers in a book, it is described as a "List of the Noblemen and eminent Persons who have permitted their Names to be mentioned for the Encouragement of this Treatise." Included are the Dukes of Ancaster, Grafton, and Leeds, Earls of Godolphin and Waldegrave, and William Windham of Fellbrigg Hall in Norfolk. These members of the aristocracy were associated with the project through medical connections: Ancaster was treated by Junior, and Godolphin employed Messenger Monsey, the dedicatee of the book, as his private physician.[52] Monsey still resided with Godolphin but was also physician to the Royal Hospital at Chelsea, the post which William Cheselden had held until April 1752. In 1739 Godolphin and Grafton were governors of the charity that set up the Foundling Hospital with Thomas Coram.[53] Windham was not only local to the Chevalier's home town of Ipswich but also had a blind daughter who became the character Helen in Elizabeth Sibthorpe Pinchard's *The Blind Child or Anecdotes of the Wyndham Family,*[54] a hugely successful children's book published by the Newbery family.

Following the list, the book prints three letters between Oldys and Monsey that confirm the treatise's strangeness. Oldys writes to Monsey as though he is asking a stranger for confirmation of Junior's character, when the two were close friends of Junior's who met regularly to drink and smoke together in his back kitchen.[55] The first letter from Oldys to Monsey is an opportunity to let it be known that Monsey had recommended patients to Junior, that Junior had treated the Duke of Ancaster, and that Monsey had seen William Taylor soon after the operation. Monsey's reply to Oldys duly confirms the facts of Junior's practice, gives a brief account of William Taylor's inverting things he sees, since the images on his retina have not been understood: "How the Mind turns it afterwards, is a Question of another Kind, and very hard to be resolved."⁵⁶ Surprisingly, Monsey also volunteers the information that "my worthy Friend Mr. *Chiselden* [sic], in his Life-time, gave this Man [Junior] all the Encouragement in his Power; and for good reason; because as he told me, he very well deserved it; which I think too, or else I had saved you, and myself the Trouble of this Answer."⁵⁷ In this we hear the irascible voice of Monsey, but it is a moot point whether Cheselden was well disposed to Junior or whether this is name-dropping; after all, Cheselden had died in April 1752, five months before Monsey's letter.

Both of these letters are dated "Sept. 20," and were probably composed at Junior's fireside. The third letter from Oldys to Monsey is not dated, is more formal, and claims that Monsey is out of town. It inverts the importance of the titles of the book and begins with the Hospital for the Blind, of which it states, "we know not to what extensive Benefit, the within proposed Foundation . . . may arrive." It also notes that Ancaster and Godolphin, "besides other noble and public-spirited Persons of Rank and Distinction, . . . have also signified their favourable Disposition, as well to establish and maintain the same, as to appropriate some reasonable Salary for the Encouragement of his Deserts who first offered this laudable Scheme thereof, and his Attendance upon the patients to be admitted therein."⁵⁸ The scheme might therefore appear to be for a hospital for treating the blind poor, and the hospital itself to be something like the Foundling Hospital, which offered free care for babies whose parents could not afford to bring them up. However, after the date of the two letters between Oldys and Monsey but before the publication of the *Observations* in March 1753, Junior advertised three cures and all of monied people: of "Mr Wood, an eminent Boat-builder at Rotherhithe";⁵⁹ of William Barton, the servant of Mr Faulks, Baker of Bloomsbury, who, "whitewashing his Master's Shop, some of the Lime fell into his right Eye";⁶⁰ and of "Mr DeEllens, a Swiss Gentleman, blind in both eyes, [who] was couched in the presence of Mr De Lafontaine, an eminent Surgeon in Meard's Court, Dean-street, Soho,"⁶¹ both of whom appear on the subscriber list. When the advertisements were finally placed for Oldys's *Observations*, they do not mention the hospital, but after noting William Taylor's "Strange Notion of Objects, upon his first Enjoyment of his New Sense," add that there are "Also some

Remarks Philosophical and Historical with the Author's Letter to the Doctor [Monsey] and the Doctor's Answer."[62]

In fact, Oldys's account of William Taylor's cure and of the hospital is neither a treatise on eye surgery,[63] nor an appeal for charity. It is a philosophical discussion of the importance of sight to human understanding and an argument for setting up a teaching hospital for training specialist eye surgeons to be run by John Taylor, oculist of Hatton Garden. "Under this Gentleman then," writes Oldys, "and such other Co-operators, as shall be appointed with competent Salaries, we may hence hope to see the beneficent *Foundation* here proposed, effectually pursued . . . will procure a Patent for the same, and elect such Governors to form the Plan, proportion the Expence, and provide such commodious Habitation, or settled Place of Abode, that, besides even those of better Rank, a Number of neglected and forlorn Patients also, . . . may know where to apply themselves, and meet the soundest Advice, most sovereign Medicines, and other Administrations."[64] Here, Oldys is advertising care for all, rich and poor, under one roof. But nor does he forget that hospitals have another function: education. Thus, Oldys argues that a specialist teaching hospital is necessary since "it is less difficult to attain a superficial Knowledge of the Disorders that affect the Body of Man in general, than a profound Knowledge of those which distress some Parts in particular, whereof the Eye is the Chief."[65] After quoting in full Junior's November 1750 advertisement about the benefits of specialist eye surgeons,[66] Oldys explains that the problem besetting specialism is that "the Transition of Studies and Experiments, from one ailing Part of the Body to another . . . is more engaging to the Curiosity of a Practitioner, thro' the Diversity of Objects and Operations, than the Constant and confined Attachment to any one Organ of Sense."[67] Furthermore, he points out, "there are fewer Patients, and more indigent Objects, there is less Prospect of Profit from professing to restore only one little Part, how useful and important soever, of the human Frame, than those usually meet with, who promise, and undertake to cure all Diseases, in every Part of every Body."[68]

While the Chevalier might travel to find patients, however wildly successful he might be, he did not set up a mechanism for training other eye surgeons. However well the Chevalier might finance his treatment of the poor with patents from the monarchs of every court in Europe, patients had to wait until he came to their town as there was no specialist center of excellence for them to turn to in their trouble. It will be remembered that early in the Chevalier's career, Henry Cross-Grove had advertised the cure of "Mr John Dove, of Weathering-Street near Debenham, who was born blind, recovered the Sight of one Eye by the Doctor 11 Years since at Ipswich, and now the other."[69]

William Taylor was a case in point. There were no oculists in Kent, the Chevalier was traveling in Europe, and so "he was recommended to the Care of the said Mr. *John Taylor, the Younger, at London.*"[70] Oldys handled the account of what William saw after the operation very well, and the detail was explored in chapter 1, which suggested that this is the most important and detailed discussion of a "blind person made to see" in the eighteenth century.[71] Here, it is only important to point out that this sort of affecting story of a real case of blindness cured is still used to advertise medical care: "one Evening, this young Patient of *Ightham,* then residing, for some time at Mr, *Taylor's* in *Hatton Garden,* stole to the Top of the House, and clamber'd out at the Window, along the leaden Gutter, without any Apprehension of Danger; but being discover'd, brought down, and asked, what induced him to hazard his Life, if by a Slip of his Foot, he had tumbled to the Ground? He reply'd that, *He only went thither to catch the Moon.*"[72] Nowhere does Oldys make any suggestion of the location for the "commodious Habitation" of the new eye hospital. But it must be borne in mind that by its very nature, a hospital for the blind would be nothing like the scale of the Foundling Hospital. Nor would there be a *Messiah* written for its foundation ceremony, though it did not go unrecorded by music; William Boyce, one of the leading London composers, set a lyric that was reproduced in Oldys's book.

Boyce, who is remembered largely for his songs for pleasure gardens, was organist of at least two churches in London, was "Master of the King's Music" from 1755, and, after the death of Handel, wrote for all the royal occasions. Of his writing for charities, the *ODNB* records: "For Mercer's Hospital in Dublin he composed the orchestral anthem 'Blessed is he that Considereth the Sick' (1741), which he later introduced at the festival of the sons of the clergy at St Paul's. He composed and conducted the funeral music for the burial of the philanthropist Captain Thomas Coram at the Foundling Hospital on 3 April 1751. For the benefit of the Leicester Infirmary he composed the ode *Lo! On the Thorny Bed of Care*, with words by Joseph Cradock, performed in St Martin's Church, Leicester, in September 1774."[73]

And to this we can now add that he wrote "While modest *Merit* does its Rays conceal" for the founding of the first hospital for the blind in England. Who the lyricist was is not known, although Boyce set words by Moses Mendez and Christopher Smart among others, the words might even be the work of Oldys himself. Nor do we know when the piece was performed or where, though the presence of David Garrick's name in the subscription list suggests that it might equally have been a theater as a church.[74] It is an accomplished piece of eighteenth-century occasional verse, and we get a real sense of Junior and how he was regarded by his contemporaries:

> While modest *Merit* does its Rays conceal,
> Let the just *Muse* draw the injurious Veil;
> 'Tis her's, fair *Truth*, distinguish'd to display,
> And place by *Vertue*, in its native Day.
> Then take rare *Oculist*, these artless Lays,
> As the *free* Tribute of *unpurchas'd* Praise.
> No longer timid, in *Retirement* pine,
> But claim the *Notice* that is justly *Thine*.
>
> Say, of the *Blessings* to Mankind decreed,
> From great *Hippocrates*, to the greater *Mead*,
> The sovereign *Secrets* of the Godlike Art,
> Which oft have warded *Fate's* approaching Dart;
> Can any with thy noble *Science* vie?
> Which guards that guiding Lamp of Life the Eye;
> Gives us the *heavenly Joys* of *Light* to know,
> For what is *Darkness*, but *infernal Woe!*
> And clear from Clouds, redeems the visual Ray,
> To bless the *Blind*, who wish in vain for *Day*.

Rare *Oculist!* couldn't thou restore aright
But intellectual, as Organic Sight;
Cou'd thy enlightning Needle but advance,
The Cataracts to remove, of Ignorance;
Unveil the Films, couch the distorted Eyes
Of squinting Envy, scolding Prejudice;
Art would, with Praise, and Wealth embroidered be,
And Worth, no more dwell with Obscurity;
Thy Cures, with Fame's best Quills, she should record
Thy Lights, thro' Men, should glorify their Lord,
Thy Skill, all Eyes, from deepest Darkness free;
Tho' none so *blind*, as those who *will not see*.[75]

The metaphor in the first verse of couching Modesty in order that the Muse might be truthful about Junior suggests that his lack of self-advertising was regarded as a virtue by those who knew him and his father. Added to this, the demand that he come out of retirement to claim his just notice was exactly what he was doing in his recent turn to advertising. It may be suggesting too much that an oculist is the greatest of the medical scientists, as the second verse argues, but to those who had been transformed from darkness to light, the operation that was Junior's staple may be claimed to have been like a "Godlike Art." Perhaps the most important metaphor of the three verses is, however, the last, that Junior should couch minds to enlighten people about the benefits of his hospital. Wherever it was.

I think it probable that we do not have to search long and far for the hospital for the blind, though we do have to be careful if we are to find it. I can locate no advertisements for a performance of the Boyce song for Junior's hospital, though his music was performed at many annual sermons for a number of other hospitals in London. This may have been due to animosity that arose between Junior and Boyce after he operated on Boyce's musical and political rival Thomas Arne[76] the month after Oldys's book was published. Furthermore, although the first advertisement for the cure of William Taylor tells us that the operation was performed on his father's dining table at Ightham, it also notes that "The . . . Lad is now at Mr Taylor's House in Hatton-Garden,"[77] where Oldys tells us that the first consultation took place. It is therefore not outside the bounds of possibility that Boyce felt tricked into writing the song, thinking it would be performed in St. Paul's at a large dedication ceremony, while the project was much more modest and the hospital no more than No. 6 Hatton Garden, Junior's own house. And the house still stands today (see fig. 8).

It may not look much, but an eye hospital treating only a few patients a week did not need to provide large wards for sick patients, since most were treated as day cases. As to training new eye surgeons, I can locate only one for certain as, typical of his family, Junior took on his son as an apprentice. John Taylor the fourth felt dragooned, believing himself more temperamentally suited to journalism, for which he left the profession of oculist after his father's death.[78] But his writing adds to the idea that No. 6 Hatton Garden might have been the first specialist eye hospital, since he records that he first lived in a house in Highgate (sometime after his birth in 1757) while his father still owned the Hatton Garden property.[79]

From the inception of the hospital, Junior's practice grew quickly, but in the long run it might be better to regard the "hospital" as more of a conceptual center than an entity restricted to a building. For a start, Junior became more confident in his technique and published a press release in May 1753 claiming that couching was safer than the "Operation said to be new" of removing the "Chrystalini" (that is, the hard part of the lens within the capsule), since "tho' it sometimes succeeds, yet where it fails, it destroys the Figure of the Eye, and leaves no hope of Recovery of Sight."[80] The purpose of the press statement was twofold: First, it attacked Samuel Sharp's paper read to the Royal Society on 12 April 1753,[81] which argued that extraction was a better method of curing cataracts. Second, he claims, against Sharp who attributes it to Jacques Daviel, that the extraction operation "was invented by my Father in the year 1735, and practised by him at Paris, and at that time approved on by Dr Petit," though the Chevalier had "long since laid it aside." In fact neither was correct since the extraction method was invented by Charles de Saint Yves in 1707, though it was perfected by Jean-Louis Petit, who possibly taught it to the Chevalier.

Attesting to the power of Junior and his specialist eye hospital, Sharp

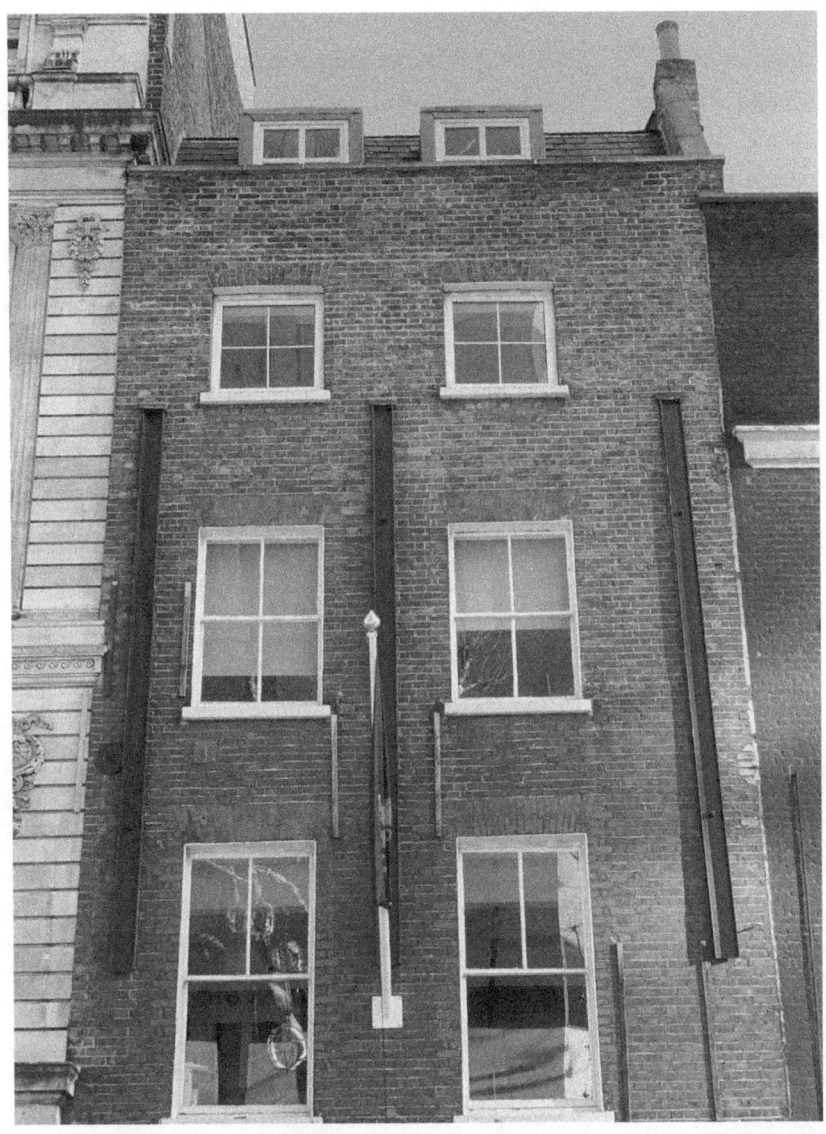

FIGURE 8. No. 6 Hatton Garden, probably the first eye hospital in Britain. Note the mansard windows from which William Taylor climbed to catch the moon.

read a second paper to the Royal Society on 22 November 1753, giving account of the eleven patients on whom he had operated.[82] Of these, only six operations could be called successful, all of the patients suffered from severe inflammation, and the account of the disasters in the other five patients hardly bears reading. Junior replied in matter-of-fact terms on 9 December that he had practised "his father's curious Methods of Operation . . . with the most happy Success, ever since 1743, in London, [and] treats all Diseases of the Eyes and Eyelids, as usual, at his House in Hatton Garden."[83] Even Sharp had conceded that the couching operation seldom led to inflammation and had a better than 50 percent success rate.

On the back of the news of the failure of Sharp's new operation, Junior advertised little between 1754 and 1756, but what advertisements were placed mark the beginning of a shift in his clientele toward children and the poor, which came to fruition in terms of making a stable income in 1758 and 1759.[84] In the meantime, his advertising became more regular and more repetitive. In 1757 he placed twelve advertisements, of which six were for "Business as usual," a form that was continued monthly until September 1758, when apparently previously unannounced, Junior published a list of the names of nine poor people whom he had cured since 1 August 1758.[85] The advertisement was repeated in October with a further nine names.[86] Each list was introduced with the words: "A List of . . . Patients recommended to Mr John Taylor, Oculist of Hatton Garden by the Churchwardens and Overseers of the several Parishes within the Bills of Mortality, since August 1, 1758." In these advertisements we find the first accounts of the success of Junior's scheme to finance cures for the poor of London, which was explained in *A Proposal to the Nobility, Clergy and Gentry, by Mr Taylor, Oculist,*[87] of which three paragraphs give the details of the scheme under which these eighteen people were cured.

> Although several very useful and extensive charities are already established, to the great good of the indigent and afflicted, and to the lasting praise of the generous benefactors; yet that many unhappy objects are still beyond the proper relief of any of those charities must be admitted without the least dispute. Nor is the imperfection of the several benevolent institutions in this metropolis for the purposes intended by them more glaring in any instance,

than in the great number of poor people we daily meet with, who are either totally blind, or else labour under such diseases of the eyes, as render them incapable of getting their bread: in which unhappy situation they must ever remain, unless relieved by the privately humane, who have now an opportunity, at a very trifling expense, of recommending them to a practitioner, whose study and practice are confined to the care of this one organ. . . .

In order therefore that such unhappy objects as labour under diseases of the eyes, may meet with all the relief the nature of their respective cases will admit of, MR TAYLOR makes this very reasonable proposal, that any person, subscribing two guineas a year, for medicines, operations, &c. shall be entitled to send as many patients to him as they shall think proper.

It is humbly presumed this very charitable undertaking will continue to meet with approbation from the humane and compassionate: to whom Mr. Taylor returns his grateful acknowledgements for the countenance they have already shewn to it.[88]

Who the "humane and compassionate" persons might be who would subscribe 2 guineas a year is not stated, but those who have "already shown . . . it" are addressed in a brief letter of thanks:

To the CHURCHWARDENS *and* OVERSEERS
of the POOR *within the* Bills *of* Mortality.

Gentlemen,
All poor objects under your care, afflicted with any kind of disorders in the eyes, I still continue to give assistance and relief to, without any expense, as they shall be directed under your hands to,

Gentlemen,
Your most humble Servant.
Hatton Garden.   John Taylor, Oculist.

A further note tells his readers that he has treated "one thousand seven hundred . . . and the greatest part so far relieved as to be able to get their bread."[89] The scheme therefore provided cure for eye problems that was free at the point of delivery to the poor blind, and the pay back to the benevolent donors was that the poor blind could return to work and would no longer have to live on charity. For example, an advertisement of 1767 tells us that Mr. Jackson of Cripplegate parish paid his 2 guineas "and at the same Time recommended John Ince, Shoe-maker, blind in both Eyes, whom Mr Taylor has restored to perfect Sight: What renders this Cure the more valuable, is, that Ince his Wife and Child are entirely dependent upon his Labour, who, with himself must have unavoidably fallen upon the Parish for Support, had it not been for this fortunate Recovery."[90]

If this makes him something of a saint, Junior was nevertheless ruthless about being paid for his work. In 1769 we hear of a defaulting parish brought back into the fold:

> A few days ago the parish of St. Matthew, Bethnal Green, ordered two guineas to be paid into the hands of Mr Taylor, oculist of Hatton Garden, as a subscription (towards the expense of medicines) for one year, for that gentleman's benevolent care of such of their poor who are, or may be, afflicted with disorders of the eyes. This parish, which was one of the first that subscribed, discontinued their subscription for two years, but others of their poor proving ill of these dangerous complaints, some of the principal gentlemen, and proper officers, taking it under consideration, most humanely determined, that their poor, so unhappily circumstanced, should have the benefit of the most skilful assistance, for the future; and therefore again avail themselves of Mr. Taylor's charitable institution, by renewing their subscription thereto, and ordering it to be paid annually.[91]

If this is draconian and falling something short of charity, it must be remembered that this was a very early scheme for providing a regular income for a specialist doctor, and in particular for one who charged only for his specialist services. And it was extremely successful. Advertisements in successive years mention he has cured, 300,[92] 400,[93] 500,[94] 600,[95] 700,[96] and, by 1770, 1,400 poor blind.[97] Another, in 1768, advertisements reported 1,200 poor blind cured and explained that a number of parishes, "amongst others Clerkenwell, Cripplegate, St Giles in the Fields, Shoreditch, Bermondsey, St Botolph Bishopsgate," are soon to be joined by St. Luke Middlesex, and all have "voluntarily agreed to pay the gentleman the annual sum of two guineas, not merely as a mark of gratitude for his past benevolence, but as a small incitement for his pursuing such charitable designs."[98] Three days later a similar advertisement which welcomed St Martin's in the Fields as a supporter, recorded that "The charitable Scheme of Mr Taylor, Oculist, in Hatton Garden, is on the Point of meeting with all the Success that such a laudable Institution deserves. This Design is for it's Object the curing, or relieving, gratis, the Indigent in general of this Metropolis and it's Environs, that may be afflicted with any Disorder of the Eyes."[99] London-wide accessibility for the poor was the second part of Junior's plan, begun in 1760,[100] which opened the scheme up to "persons and societies" other than parishes, one hundred in all, after which Junior would cure any poor person who came to him, deeming, one must suppose, that 200 guineas a year was an adequate remuneration for the public practice of an eye surgeon.

Free access at the point of delivery to medical care for the poor quickly became associated with two problems which Junior had to remedy. The first was that he had to remain, and to be known to remain, in London. Possibly due to his being mistaken for the Chevalier, a press release was necessary to quash the rumor "that Mr Taylor, Oculist, of Hatton Garden, has been travelling the country, and distributing Bills, within a Circuit of about twenty Miles round London, he thinks it necessary to acquaint the Public that he never goes out of Town on the Business of his profession, unless particularly sent for; and that the Extensiveness of his Practice in London (where it has met with the greatest success for these twenty Years past) not only prevents an Absence of this Nature, but renders the Step utterly unnecessary."[101] As a press release, this short piece does more than merely quash the rumor that he is often not at home; it tells us how Junior wanted his practice to be known. The practice is busy, successful, and confined to London.[102] Moreover, his son remarks in his own memoir that, when he was quite young, the family moved back to Hatton Garden from Highgate, where he was born, and if he does not give a date, it was probably after 1761, when the boy was four years old and might remember.[103]

The second problem was the idea that any poor person would be treated for free if they turned up at No. 6 Hatton Garden. In possibly the saddest press release I have ever read, we hear of one such blind man:

> Some little time since a parish in the country sent one of their poor, who was stone blind, up to town, for the charitable assistance of Mr. Taylor of Hatton-Garden. They were so parsimoniously inhuman not only to send him up without money, to keep him in London whilst under cure, but even to refuse allowing the unhappy wretch the comfort of riding in the wagon; but paid the driver some trifle for suffering him to be tied to the waggon, behind, like a dog; and he actually arrived in that situation. It is incredible what the poor creature suffered (as he says) in stumbling over stones, and other impediments, on the road.[104]

Here we must remember that Junior had always advertised to all classes of clients, as we can read in the quotes of his early advertisements above, which have been recorded here without excerpting them of their mention of treating the poor gratis. The original practice of offering free cures to the poor was another idea he had copied from William Read and the Chevalier; however, his father's use of the poor as guinea pigs for the cures that, when perfected, he would perform on the rich (as had happened at the Exeter Exchange show in 1748) is likely to have rankled with Junior and may well have been the impetus for the parish subscription. But his free-at-the-point-of-delivery practice among the poor was segregated from the paying clients. From 1761, Junior advertised that he practiced every morning "at his House in Hatton Garden; and on Mondays, Wednesdays and Fridays, from Three to Six, at his large Room between the Asylum and the Dog and Duck, St. George's Fields."[105] St. George's Fields was an area south of the River Thames owned by the City of London, and Junior would have reached it either by London Bridge, or the new Westminster Bridge (which had been completed in 1750). Although sometimes billed as a fashionable spa, the Dog and Duck is always depicted as being in decline,[106] and it was the nexus of the riots in favor of John Wilkes in 1768, the year after Junior ceased advertising his visits to the site, as well as the Gordon riots. Perhaps fortuitously, Thomas Boddington, James Ware, Samuel Bosanquet, and William Houlston set up the first School for the Indigent Blind, at the "notorious" Dog and Duck tavern, St. George's Fields, Southwark in 1799.

Another aspect of Junior's practice was preventative medical care for children affected in the eyes by "Small-Pox, Measles, and Colds from

Birth." Selling "a Certain Remedy" at half a guinea a bottle, Taylor moved into the tinctures, remedies, and nostrum market practiced by many of the other medical residents of Hatton Garden. How effective it was cannot be ascertained, but once again the marketing assured success, since it was claimed "to preserve the Eyes, if applied when they are first affected with those Diseases."[107] I can locate only one further advertisement for the remedy,[108] which, appearing twelve years later, would suggest that it needed no further marketing. There are twenty advertisements for children cured across his career, in which he claims a total of more than three thousand.[109]

Despite his success in making a career out of eye surgery, Junior's work was never innovative, but this was another aspect of his business strategy. In 1761, Junior gave a demonstration of the safety and efficacy of couching on Gilbert Dudley, who had been recommended for free treatment by the overseers of St. John Hackney, to Mr. Redhead, a surgeon "lately arrived from Antigua, with his Lady, who is afflicted with the same Disorder, and is now under Mr. Taylor's care."[110] Thus Junior couched a poor man to make a private fee, at the same time also explaining the procedure to another doctor and advertising his skill to future clients.

In 1763 he advertised couching John Parkes, a river pilot with cataracts, who came to him after "he was advised to make Application to the Gentlemen of the Faculty at one of the Publick Hospitals, which he consented to and there, underwent the Operation of extracting the Chrystalline, which instead of restoring him to Sight unfortunately occasioned the Eye to sink, (for a Disfigurement is ever the Case, where this dangerous Method of operating fails) past every Hope of Recovery." Parkes was so frightened at the thought of losing the other cataracted eye that he decided to "drop all farther Thoughts of Relief" until he consulted Junior, who "couched him, (an Operation, which perform'd by a Person of Judgment, where it does not succeed, still leaves the Eye in the same State it found it) and restored him to perfect Sight."[111]

Telling the same tale in a note added to the account of the cure of Sarah Fagan in April 1766, Junior advertised that he "can produce to any dubious persons, numberless instances of his success in the curing of cataracts, as will convince them of the great superiority of the operation of couching to that of extracting the chrystalline; the first being easy, safe, and, in most cases, sure; the other, dangerous and uncertain."[112]

From 1767 to the end of his practice in 1780, Junior advertised sixty-five more named cures, some of private people, some of children, and some recommendations by the overseers of the poor. He still used his advertisements strategically, flooding the newspapers with ten between June and October 1777 after the arrival in London of Baron Wenzel, who claimed to be oculist to his Britannick Majesty, and not advertising at all for longer and longer periods, until finally an advertisement in the *World and Fashionable Advertiser* read, under the heading "DIED": "Monday night, after a lingering illness, in his sixty-third year of his age, Mr. Taylor, Oculist of Hatton Garden."[113]

In Lieu of a Medical Model of "Disability"

The picture of eighteenth-century English medical practice in the treatment of eyes which has been mapped out is one of increasing specialism and its attendant features: a hospital, specialist training, and accessibility of care. Concomitantly, while treatment by physical intervention began to become more popular, practitioners reduced the types of procedures which they would attempt in order to increase the chance of success. This retrenchment might have been either because of, or even a cause of, an increase in patient expectation of, and understanding of, cure. And it would appear to have been because of the economic necessity of cure demonstrated by the offering of cures to the poor blind; though equally, it might have been because the sense of transitivity in the idea of "disabled" lingered throughout the century as we find in the often-used phrase "disabled from getting his bread."

From the earliest stages of the spread of surgery, complementary practice continued to be offered as an alternative to those who were frightened by the thought of "being cut" by surgeons.[114] At the same time, two further developments are noticeable. First, specialist practice required separate local and itinerant practitioners to reach the target group of patients: local practice in large cities, and itinerant practice to cover the rest of the nation. Second, specialist practice could benefit from two sources of income, a regular stipend from charitable work that is free at the point of delivery to poor patients, and another from the wealthy.

However, while cures that were more or less successful were offered, and practice appears to have improved in curing certain forms of blindness such as cataracts, there is no attendant sense of compulsory able-bodiedness demanded of their patients by the doctors arising from their medical intervention, nor from the patients' raised expectation of cure from their doctors. But nor, as the next part of the book demonstrates, does it appear that those who were not amenable to cure believed that there ought to be a cure for them, or that they had somehow been failed by or failed medical practice by their intractable condition.

PART III

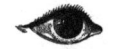

LIVES

8

THOMAS GILLS OF ST. EDMUNDS-BURY AND THE ITINERANT GIVER

In this third part of the book, we move from discussions of medical people to explore the lives of the blind people whom they could not treat. The dramatic shift is not intended to set up a binary opposition between "the doctors" and "the blind" but rather to offer examples of the farthest limit cases at either end of the spectrum of the people whose lives were vitally affected by vision and its failure. None of the blind people whose lives are considered in the next three chapters were amenable to cure, but their stories are no less important to an understanding of blindness in the eighteenth century. What we shall find is that their lives were never beset with obstacles that society put in their way, nor were they beset by some overarching idea of compulsory able-bodiedness. Rather, the lives of each suggests a journey toward a personal place of safety. Yet, neither of the three can be said to have run away from society; rather, their places of safety were constructed of a sense of economic independence and social responsibility. The purpose of these three chapters is therefore not just to tell the biographies of blind people to balance the discourse of the doctors but to confront the disease-treatment-cure paradigm that is so often foist upon the eighteenth century as the century of medicalization. Medicalization did not offer a universal panacea, and although the treatment for a number of blinding conditions was improved during the century, as now, some people were left out. They did not complain; they got on with their lives, and it is just how they did that with which the third part of this book will be concerned: in telling the stories of blind people who addressed their lives in a completely different way from "the sighted."

I have written elsewhere on Thomas Gills[1] of St. Edmunds-Bury in terms of his self-presentation through a number of rhyming catechisms written for children, where I argued that these publications "demonstrate how much a disabled man wanted to be independent, and established a complex relationship with the parish poor law for his income."[2] My argument suggested that Gills wrote for children in order to reach as wide as possible a buying public so as to give himself the best chance of making money within an "economy of makeshifts,"[3] typical of the poor at this time, but also that Gills wrote not simply with the "rhetoric of powerlessness" which would characterize begging but strategically to his individual and changing circumstances.[4]

In this chapter I want to return to Thomas Gills and his experience as a blind man based on the remarkable addition to his canon of eight pamphlets[5] that were gathered together in 1852 by "J.O.," an Edinburgh book collector.[6] Now to be found in the National Library of Scotland,[7] the group includes the two catechisms about which I have already written, *Instructions for children, in verse*, and *Advice to youth: or, instructions for young men and maids*,[8] with another, undated version of the first called *Practical catechism: or, instructions for children, in verse*. There is also a third catechism, printed in London and dated 1712, called *Questions and answers. In verse, upon the creation of the world, the fall of man, the flood, and several other passages out of the Old Testament*, which very much follows the style and approach of the other two, with its opening address, "The Author to the Reader," strategically placing it as worth buying since it will be of benefit to both, financially for the former and educationally for the latter:

> My Hands are Idle, but my Head
> Is still at Work to get my Bread,
> By Ways that none can justly blame,
> In One that's Poor and Blind and Lame:
> Now this of making Verse (tis true)
> And going out to Sell it too,
> Is all the Business I can do:
> And none I hope will think or say,
> But that it is an Honest Way;

Provided what I sell, in fine,
Be either Moral or Divine.

This short Extract of Holy Writ
Perhaps may yield some Benefit
To those who want the Means indeed,
More Large and Learned Books to read:
If so it does when you have bought it,
I Gain the End for which I wrote it.

The catechism ends with what might now be thought of as a typical sign-off for Gills: an advertisement for his next piece that continues the self-presentation of himself as an industrious blind man, while also introducing the next chance the buyer will have to purchase a poem from him.

And if the Public take it not amiss
But by their kind acceptance favour this,
It will encourage me, to use my Art,
Upon this theme to write a Second Part.

The other four pamphlets are completely different from the catechisms and comprise two poems on religious subjects and two secular. The first religious poem is an undated *Upon the Nativity of the Blessed Saviour,* and the second, *New-year's-gift: or, a poem on the circumcision of our Blessed Lord and Saviour Jesus Christ,* is dated 1712 and gives the name "R. Janeway" as the printer in London. The first of the secular poems is a sensational *Lamentation on the death of His Grace Duke Hamilton,*[9] which describes the effects of the fatal duel between James, Duke Hamilton, and Charles, Lord Mohun, in Hyde Park on 15 November 1712. Last and best of all is the irrepressibly cheery *The Blind man's case at London: or, a character of that city. Sent in a letter to his friend in the country,* printed in London in 1711, which describes the pell-mell of city life in a way that recalls Swift's *Description of a City Shower* and pleads with his benefactor to give him enough money to come home to St. Edmunds-Bury.[10]

Gills's self-presentation was one of advertising his situation, showing he was not incapable of "getting his bread," as he prefaced the catechism quoted above: "My Hands are Idle, but my Head/Is still at Work to get my

Bread." This chapter will not read the catechisms or the poem on the restoring and subsequent loss of his sight that I have explored before but will read only the recent additions to my knowledge of the Gills canon, giving some new biographical suggestions about him based on these pieces, and make some suggestions as to how he was ultimately treated by a charitable foundation which may have been the first in England to help a blind writer.

I shall argue that the four new poems extend the idea of Gills's strategic writing and allow us to understand his experience as a blind man interacting in a sighted world, with his poems and pamphlets acting not as pauper letters, which I argued formerly, but as commodities to be sold to those we should think of as "itinerant purchasers." For Thomas Gills was not an itinerant beggar, since, as we shall find, he took control of his situation as a blind man and attempted several different forms to please his buyers. What will emerge is a man who not only did his best to make as much money as he could out of an uncertain income stream, the "chance giver," but who was also no small fish caught up in the stream of circumstance but rather a boulder in the stream of life around which the waters parted. It is for this reason I would like to rename the "chance giver" as "itinerant giver," itinerant since Gills remained, or at least did his best to remain, in one place (his hometown, St. Edmunds-Bury) with the givers walking by him. In this way, I believe we should regard Gills as a shopkeeper trying out new lines on his regular customers, enticing them to come in and buy. But since Gills was not a bookseller with a book shop where he could wait in the relative peace and quiet until a customer entered, he needed to sell his wares out in the streets, and the quieter the street, the better it was for a blind man to do business. In this sense, I believe that St. Edmunds-Bury can be called his place of safety, and the readings I shall present of his poems will give some sense of what such a place of safety would be like for a blind man in the very early eighteenth century.

Biography

In my previous essay on Thomas Gills, I stated that nothing was known about him other than the brief addresses titled "The Author to the Reader" that opened each catechism and explored instead the reasons why his extant works were all published in London. I argued this was because "For Thomas Gills to make money out of his writing he did not fit with the economic model underpinning local publishers: he had to turn to London where publishers were becoming used to paying for copy."[11] This hypothesis was based on the idea that Gills's pamphlets were published, that is printed for sale in bookshops, and the payment for the printing was borne by a London bookseller. Underpinning this was another hypothesis that Gills was poor and, lacking a family to help him, indigent.

However, the "Argument" of Gills's *The Blind man's case at London* tells a different tale, explaining that: "THE Blind Man of Bury, by the Perswasions of His Printer and some other suppos'd Friends takes his Wife with him to London with an Intention to settle there." Of the twelve pamphlets, only *New-year's gift* bears the name of a printer, Richard Janeway. By 1710, this must be Richard Janeway Junior, since Janeway Senior, publisher and bookseller of "Queen's-Head-Court, in Pater Noster Square," had ceased work in 1691. Unlike his father, Janeway Junior was only ever a printer, working for, among others, the booksellers John Gwillim, near Sun Yard in Bishopsgate; Jonathan Robinson, at the Golden-Lion in St. Paul's Churchyard; T. Davis, in Red-Lion-Street, near Whitechapel; H. Walwyn, at the Three Legs in the Poultry, the corner of Old Jury; and S. Ballard, at the Blue Ball in Little Britain. He also printed books for the Company of Stationers, near Ludgate Street, such as William Salmon's *London Almanack*, for 1702, 1704, 1705, and 1706. He was succeeded in this in 1713 by "E. Janeway."

As Janeway was a printer who did not own a bookshop, he was not a publisher in the modern sense, that is, he did not pay authors for their work, pay for the printing, and then make his money out of selling books. Thus, we can be pretty certain that Thomas Gills had enough money to pay up front for the printing of his pamphlets and was in charge of his own distribution. This in turn suggests that he was not living within the "economy of makeshifts," an idea which is borne out by further internal evidence from *The Blind man's case*. For a start, Gills was not only married, as noted in the "Argument," he was in London "With little Deb and Nab my Wife,"[12] where Deb is presumably their daughter. During his stay in the city, Gills's disgust with their accommodation suggests he is unused to living three floors up, bedbugs, overly hot summers and cold winters, cracks in his walls, eating broth, a smoking chimney, being dirty, and having filthy furniture.

> In Summer thro' excessive Heat,
> We gap'd for Air and stew'd in Sweat;
> By Day with Clouds of Dust oppress'd,
> At Night by Buggs deprived of Rest;
> In Winter we abide so nigh
> The freezing Cold and Snowy Sky,
> And our exalted Habitation,
> So cleft for want of reparation,
> That now we Sweat not you'll suppose,
> Unless like Woodcocks at the Nose;
> We both blow Hot and Cold in troth,
> To warm our Nails and cool our Broth;
> A mess of this to heat the Carcass
> We get sometimes else tis a hard Case;
> But that which tries, and most provokes us,
> Our low-built treacherous Chimney smokes us,
> Afflicts our Eyes and almost chokes us.
> Our Linen looks like Skins of Witches,
> And we are Black'd like Bacon Flitches;
> Our Curtains, Valens, Cloths and Rug,
> That look'd so ruddy, fresh and smug,
> Are changed to sooty hue, and thus
> They mourn for good P.G. and us.[13]

This more middling-sort self-awareness is also suggested by Gills's fear that he should not remonstrate with passersby who have buffeted him in the street so badly that "Hat and Wig are both beat off."[14]

The Thomas Gills who dressed in "Hat and Wig" is probably the Thomas Gills, son of Henry, who was baptised on 14 May 1654, at St. Mary's Church, St. Edmunds-Bury, where he also married ffrancis Hawkins on 5 June 1675.[15] ffrancis "Nab" Hawkins may be the aunt or sister of the St. Edmunds-Bury clockmaker Mark Hawkins, which would give us something more of an idea of Gills's class. It is tempting to suggest that Thomas Gills was also in the clock- or watch-making trade, which was widespread in East Anglia in the seventeenth and eighteenth centuries, when there were a number of clock and watch makers with the name "Gill."[16] The close work involved would account for his early blindness, but whatever it was that finished off his sight, he must have been blind by 1707, when his first catechism was printed (by Janeway?). Exactly when Gills came to London at "His Printer's" advice cannot be certain, but he must have been in the city at least in the summer and winter of 1711 to make sense of *The Blind man's case* (that is, if it was printed before 11 March 1711, when the date would change to 1712, Old Style). The poem wishes that he could return to St. Edmunds-Bury, but he probably remained in London at least until after 15 November 1712, when the *Lamentation on the death of His Grace Duke Hamilton* was printed. Gills's death, recorded on 15 January 1715 in St. Mary's Church, St. Edmunds-Bury, suggests he finally did get home. It is unlikely that his body would have been transported there postmortem.

New-year's gift: or, a poem on the circumcision of our Blessed Lord and Saviour Jesus Christ

If I made a mistake in deducing that Gills was poor and indigent from the evidence of the catechisms, I believe that I was correct in my suggestion that the catechisms were not aimed at a particular religious group in order that they might sell to as wide as possible an audience.[17] The idea is confirmed by the choice of Richard Janeway as printer, whose background would appear to have been in the Dissenting tradition, but whose publications were legion. James and John Janeway were both associated with Puritanism, with the former being a Dissenting minister.[18] Richard Janeway Senior certainly published works by prominent Dissenters and their apologists such as Richard Baxter, Samuel Bold, and Increase Mather,[19] but he also had the common touch and a miscellaneous list reaching a much wider audience than Dissenters, which included the political and the sensational.[20] While Richard Janeway Junior's first two imprints were of works by John Bunyan,[21] and he is also named as the author's printer in anti-Quaker publications by, among others, Francis Bugg,[22] the evidence of those works on which his name can be found suggests he would print anything brought to him by authors, for example, A. J.'s *Account of the Portugueze language*,[23] and an anonymous satire, *The Celestial Envoy*.[24] Thus, it may well have been at Janeway's advice that Gills wrote his catechisms for a wide audience, and *The Blind man's case* tells us he took Janeway's advice to come to London, albeit he was not happy during his stay. This relationship between Gills and Janeway is also evident in Gills's preface to the poem on which Janeway put his name as printer, *A Poem upon the circumcision*:

> Good Reader,
> WHilst [sic] others who have Store of Coin,
> Blest by a kinder Fate than mine,
> Present their New-Year's Offerings,
> Of pretty Toys or costly Things
> To those whom they affect to prove
> Their gratitude, Respect, or Love,
> Poor I, whose Purse no Wealth contains,
> Present the fruit of my weak Brains,
> A Poem made for New Year's-Day,
> In which my humble Thoughts display
> How Christ first suffers Smart to ease us,
> And to the Holy Name of Jesus.
> I wish I could have handled it
> As does the Glorious Theme befit
> And that my Muse had here prepar'd
> An Offering worthy your Regard.
> But some perhaps who read my Verse
> Will say Bright Thoughts in me are Scarce.
> And I betray in every Line
> As great a Want of Wit as Coin:
> Well, granting this be so, yet still

The Theme I choose shows my Good-will;
And if what I have done can raise
One single Act of Love and Praise
In any soul to Jesus name,
I shall not wholly lose my Aim.
But, Gentlemen,
When I present this Gift to you,
I hope you'll give me something too;
For if I've no Return you know
I cann't content the Printer so.
What I expect from you is small
A Halfpeny or a Peny's all.
A Good New-Year, and many a one,
I wish you all, and so have done.

If the transactions herein described were simple gift giving, as the prefaces of the catechisms described, the poverty of Gills and the poverty of his poetry become forgivable and fulfilled in an act of charity. Gills gives poor poetry (that is, poetry written for children) and is rewarded not so much for the poetry as for his poverty, and the buyer becomes doubly blessed as giver of alms and their child as receiver of a useful lesson. But in this preface, Gills describes a secondary relationship in the transaction, with his printer, who must be "content[ed]" (that is, paid), and thus Gills must choose a theme important enough that the "Offering" is worthy of the buyer's regard so that both he and the printer have earned their pay. Thus, the work is no longer solely for the giver's children, and the sums Gills mentions, "A Halfpeny or a Peny," are large for the eight pages of flimsy paper and tiny type in which format the pamphlets are all printed. But the idea of the double work, for "the fruit of my weak Brains" and the printer's part in setting the words positions Gills in the economy of buying and selling typical of the middling sort of which he claims to be a member.

To forward the aim of writing something worthy enough for this market, the theme is Anglican in its language and directly interprets the words of the 1662 *Book of Common Prayer* collect for 1 January, the Feast of the

Circumcision: "ALMIGHTY God, who madest thy blessed Son to be circumcised, and obedient to the law for man: Grant us the true Circumcision of the Spirit; that, our hearts, and all our members, being mortified from all worldly and carnal lusts, we may in all things obey thy blessed will; through the same thy Son Jesus Christ our Lord. Amen." The date of the Feast is eight days after Christmas Eve, the traditional "octave" after birth when Jewish boys are circumcised. As the collect suggests, this is the first time the blood of Christ was shed, and thus this is the beginning of the process of the redemption of man, a demonstration that Christ was fully human and that he is obedient to biblical law.

Gills's words need little glossing as they act as an exegesis to the collect:

Besides his early Suff'ring Want and Cold,
The Spotless Lamb of God at Eight Days Old
Is Circumcis'd like other Males and thus
Begins betimes to smart and bleed for us:[25]

Must thou as soon as Born, begin
To bear the Shame and feel the Pain of Sin?
And with the Mis'ries of an Infant Life,
Endure the Bloody Circumcising Knife?
Thou, who behind the Veil of Infancy
Conceal'st that Infin'te Glorious Majesty[26]

To teach by this Obedient Act of thine
Exact Obedience to the Laws Divine
And that we never should offensive be
To others by our Singularity;
And that all those who will in thee have Part
Must Spiritually be Circumcis'd in Heart;[27]

Upon her Lap the Blessed Infant lyes,
She proper Medicines to the Wound applies,
And he declares his Pain in tears and Cries;
Yet inwardly he joys on this Occasion,
To have begun the Work of our Salvation.[28]

But there is one moment in the poem in which we come to understand Gills's self-awareness as a blind man: "Methinks I see the Foster-Father stand / With Bloody Knife held in his trembling hand[.]"[29]

Within the stricture of the collect, which demands that "our hearts, and all our members, being mortified from all worldly and carnal lusts, we may in all things obey thy blessed will," Gills's blindness, the mortification of his eyes, is something with which he must struggle to come to terms. The word of the collect "may," related to obeying God's will, is a word of hope and struggle against backsliding into self-pity. I would argue that it is the struggle against self-pity which urges Gills to remain economically viable in the difficult world of making money from work. Furthermore, naming Joseph "Foster-Father" of Jesus, something which I believe is unique to this poem, suggests the arbitrariness of Gills's blindness: it is not something God the Father would do to him, just as circumcision is not practiced among Christians. The image suggests that blindness is something which might happen accidentally to any of his itinerant purchasers and as such acts as a further lesson for them to get by heart.

Upon the Nativity of the Blessed Saviour

Upon the Nativity, a companion piece to *Upon the circumcision*, is undated and bears no place or publisher. The fact that it is eight pages long suggests that the copy in the National Library of Scotland is not lacking a title page, and the existence of the "Preface to the Charitable Reader" suggests it was to be sold separately. Likewise, Gills's preface emphasizes the work involved in writing as his only way "to get a Living these Hard Times,"[30] which in turn emphasizes the middling-sort nature of the economy in which he is working.

> Good Reader,
> This Subject is Divinity,
> And you perhaps may Censure me,
> That I presume to meddle here,

> With what's so much above my Sphere.
> But Gentlemen, consider pray,
> I'm Lame and Blind and see no Way
> But only this of making Rhimes,
> To get any Living these Hard Times.
> There's certainty tis better much
> To Publish serious thoughts and such
> As if the Good they do be small
> At least will cause no Harm at all:
> And if, like me, you will be Blind
> To all the Faults you here may Find,
> And lay a Penny out with me,
> I'll thank you for your Charity,
> Compose some other pious Lectures
> And pray for all my Benefactors.

The beginning of the preface thus takes up another important point, that as a layman Gills should not be writing religious materials. Robert Nelson, one of the founders of the Society for the Propagation of Christian Knowledge (SPCK), was equally worried by this when he wrote his *Companion to the Festivals and Fasts of the Church of England*,[31] and while Nelson was trying in effect to set national (and eventually international) standards for Anglican observance in order "to suppress the Dawnings of Enthusiasm"[32] he nevertheless took it upon himself to write his book, which he claims should have been the work of a convocation of ordained ministers. Nelson's argument for having the temerity to do it, made over many pages, is that it must simply be done and that any fear that he might be writing false doctrine must be discounted as "the same Fears may as well prevent Parents from instructing their Children, and Masters their Servants in these Duties that relate to themselves."[33] Gills, with his catechisms and these two longer religious poems, was possibly following Nelson's pattern, since we find in Nelson's *Festivals and Fasts* an exegetical catechism for each festival date followed by the collect for the day and a number of prayers. The difference between the two is their market, since though Nelson claims his was written by "a Man of Moderate Attainments [which nevertheless] may be serviceable to those that have lesser Degrees of Knowledge,"[34] he could only have been aiming a book of 554 pages at the wealthy. Gills's pamphlets make no claim for his scholarship of his writing other than claiming that "if the Good they do be small / At least will cause no Harm at all." If this is a comment on his being unordained but still writing on Divinity, it makes at the same time the same point that the giving of a halfpenny or penny for him to get his bread will not harm the pockets of itinerant purchasers.

This second religious poem is as charming as the first, and when it is remembered they were written for a niche market that included children and their parents, both rise above any charge of doggerel.

> Now when the Angels to Heaven were flown,
> To wait again before th'Almighty's Throne,
> The faithful Shepherds all by joint Consent
> With Eager Joy and Speed to Beth'lem went
> And ent'ring in the Stable they behold
> The Truth of every thing the Angel told[35]

> Invite him from the Manger to thy Breast
> And give thy Heart to be his Place of rest;[36]
> Th'Almighty King of Glory, God most High,
> Whom Angels Serve, Adore and Magnifie,
> Who sits enthroned above the Cherubims,
> Would in a Manger lay his blessed Limbs;
> Is Born amongst the Beasts as if design'd
> To be the Scorn out cast of Mankind.[37]

The link which can be made with Robert Nelson as a result of the discovery of these two poems suggests that Gills may have written similar works for the other dates in the Anglican calendar which are either lost or were not completed. If these two were the start of the whole cycle, with twenty-eight more festivals and eleven fasts to complete, Gills can but have thought himself facing a large task which in turn would have dignified the business of writing as a way of being economically independent for one who

Lame and Blind . . . [can] see no Way
But only this of making Rhimes
To get any Living these Hard Times.

Lamentation on the death of His Grace Duke Hamilton

The other two new poems, which might well have been written at the suggestion of a general printer like Richard Janeway, demonstrate that Gills tried other strategies to reach his target audience, the itinerant purchaser. The first, aimed at capturing their imagination and their pennies, exploits a sensational political event by giving an original angle on the duel fought between James Hamilton, 4th Duke of Hamilton, and Charles Mohun, 4th Baron Mohun in Hyde Park on 15 November 1712.

Jonathan Swift wrote up the duel in the *Examiner* as a political cause célèbre that demonstrated the Whigs' "return with fresh Vigour to their last Expedient of Murder."[38] He even went as far as comparing it to the recent assassination attempt on Robert Harley.[39] Swift's charge was a thinly veiled attack on the recently dismissed Whig John Churchill, Duke of Marlborough, as he suggested that General George Macartney, Mohun's second, was ordered by Churchill to call Hamilton out: "Their General [Churchill] set the Example of Party Duels, which was only to give them a Sanction (for Care was taken that his Person should not be exposed), and deputed that infamous Messenger of his Challenge, to be the general Bully of the Faction."

The facts of the duel lie somewhere between the three accounts of it in the *ODNB* entries for Hamilton, Mohun, and Macartney, but, briefly stated, the Tory Hamilton and the Whig Mohun had been wrangling over the Gawsworth estate of the Earl of Macclesfield for eleven years, and by 1712 the law awarded it to Hamilton. At the same time, and benefiting from the Tory ascendency, Hamilton was appointed ambassador to France, which the Whigs claimed would allow him to treat with the Pretender over the royal succession. Over whichever issue it was Hamilton and Mohun argued at the chambers of a lawyer, Olebar, both had been great duelists in their time and a challenge was issued for 15 November in Hyde Park. Both were killed; Macartney was accused of murder by Hamilton's second (his illegitimate son) and fled to the Netherlands, to return to England only after the Whig ascendency in the Hanoverian succession, when he was tried and acquitted.

Gills's poem on the event was probably intended to take advantage of the "sightseers [who] flocked to Hyde Park to carry away as macabre souvenirs fragments of the tree where the duke had died."[40] While this is a completely new direction from Gills's religious verse, it is neither sensational nor sentimental, even though it is written, in part, in the duchess's voice. While the choice of subject position allows reference to sighs and tears, the tone is a reminder that although a duke, Hamilton was also a man with a wife and family:

> With what deep Sighs, what Tears shall I deplore?
> His Death, Alas! My Lord is now no more;
> The dear lov'd Partner of my Joys and Bed,
> My better Part my Life my All is Dead;[41]

Nevertheless, Gills's choice of narrator lets us into his own politics, and there can be no doubt he takes the Tory side in the issue since he describes the illustrious duke in terms of his recent political appointment:

> To make the League of Friendship firm between
> The Gallic King and our Heroic Queen;
> To manage our Affairs and to Advance,
> The British Glory in the Court of France:[42]

It could be argued that these lines are more of a reflection of the political views of his readers than of his own, but the occasional turns to the personal, such as the line "His servants lost a good and generous Master,"[43] suggest that Gills may have been trying to account for all tastes. At the same time, the theme is also an admonition to the gaping sightseers:

> May none henceforth from City or from Court
> To that unlucky Hide-Park Ring resort;
> Let them for ever leave the hated Round,
> And come no more on that detested Ground;
> Let them no more with gaudy Pomp and Pride,
> About the Rails with Joy and Pleasure Ride;[44]

While the words "City" and "Court" might be references to political parties, such a stern reproach might equally be argued to be catering for yet another part of Gills's readership of itinerant purchasers. If so, theirs is the final message as the poem ends in "A Moral reflection":

> Reader, behold on this Occasion,
> The sad Effects of Pride and Passion;
> By which it seems Duke Hamilton,
> And Charles Lord Mohun were hurry'd on;
> . . . .
> Tis what they falsely Honour Call,
> To cherish that they hazard all,
> Their's no true Honour but proceeds,
> From noble Great and Vertues Deeds
> Yet self-Love blinds some Persons so,
> That all to them Respect must show,
> Whether they merit it or no.
> These for the least Affronting Action
> Cry D— me, I'le have Satisfaction;
> And one Reflecting hasty Word,
> Must be corrected by the Sword.[45]

Exactly where and when the poem was sold is a matter for conjecture, but it is not out of the question to argue that it was sold at one of the Hyde Park gates as something of a less bloody souvenir of the event. Whatever we might think of this, it demonstrates Gills's determination to take advantage of the market for occasional verse. The final new poem suggests Gills had become something of a common sight during his stay in London as he addresses his audience telling them of his desire to get home to St. Edmunds-Bury.

The Blind man's case at London or, a character of that city

Dated from London in 1711, *The Blind man's case* is rather like Swift's "Description of a City Shower," which first appeared in the *Tatler* in October

1710.[46] Whether Swift was once again the source or model for Gills's poem cannot be certain, but where Swift uses description to satirize the moral state of London, as Brendan O'Hehir suggests ("London is 'devoted'—set apart for destruction—for reasons suggested in Swift's poem. The city's corruption is betokened in the omens of rain—the stink of sewage [5–6], the throbbing of corns and toothache [9–10], the splenetic 'Dulman' enacting the eponymy of his race [11–12]—but still more radically in the behavior of the citizens caught in the downpour. Hypocrisy, or false seeming is the essence of their natures"),[47] Gills's London is simply to be escaped. The sojourn has been a mistaken enterprise, the food is not fresh but is nevertheless expensive, the accommodation inconvenient and unpleasant, the streets are teeming and noisy, everything the family owns is dirtied by contact with the city, the half-crowns his printer and his friends have promised for his verses have turned out to be halfpennies, and all he wants is to be home in St. Edmunds-Bury. By extension, Gills suggests that London contaminates all who live there, whereas St. Edmunds-Bury is his place of safety.

To be sure, busy streets can be terrifying for blind people, but the secondhand description Gills gives, detailed to him by his daughter looking at the scrum from their third-floor window, never fails to be as visual as it is entertaining. The final plea for help to return home is thereby carefully set up, and no reader, however much they love London, could fail to understand that the city was no place for this blind poet and hopefully after finishing the poem would be well enough disposed toward him for his description of their fair city to help him on his way out of it. As the poem exists only in two known printed copies, it is worth quoting in full, since it gives a fascinating account of being blind in a busy city.[48]

The Argument:
THE Blind Man of Bury, by the Perswasions of His Printer and some other suppos'd Friends takes his Wife with him to London with an Intention to settle there, where they meet with so many Inconveniences, and so great Difficulties and Charges as soon disgusted with the Place, made them repent their Rashness, and think of returning to their Native Home as soon as they should be able; they Winter'd at London in a very hard Season, and

with no Extraordinary Accommodation, at which time he sends the following Letter to his good Friend and Benefactor at Bury.

The Blind Man's Case
Oppress'd with Cares fatigued with Labours
Encompass'd round with unknown Neighbors;
By foes malign'd, by Friends neglected,
By none esteem'd, by few affected;
With foggy Ale and Bitter Beer,
With Bread and Flesh extremely dear,
With Potent Cheese, and frowy Butter,
In Dirt, and Stink and Noise, and Clutter;
In Ruinous Room Three Story High,
Up close dark Staircase here I live,
With little Deb and Nab my Wife,
Who share in these Fatigues of Life:
Sometimes to please herself (no doubt)
At Garret Window Deb looks out
And from that elevated Station
Casts down her Eyes with Admiration,
To see in miry Streets below
What different Throngs pass to and fro
As Lawyers, Ministers, and Laymen,
Chair-bearers, Hackney-Men and Dray-Men,
Black Chimney-sweepers, Brawny Porters,
Powder'd Beaux, Brave as Courtiers;
Fine Misses, primm'd with Paint and Patches,
And tatter'd Girls that sell Card Matches;
Starv'd Ragged Boys with Dirty Faces
Cry Two-A-Peny Long Thread Laces:
Some Folks deck'd richly to Excess,
And some in such a wretched Dress,
As scarcely covers nakedness;
Some Womens Necks with Pearls and Lockets
Some Yok'd between Two Tubs like Buckets;

Some Heads with Lace and Ribbons dress'd,
And some with heavy Loads oppress'd;
Milk-Wives with flat-Crown'd Caps and Biggins
Bear on their Heads huge Pails like Piggins,
Milk Dirt Hairs Straws, together Swigging;
Some few Complexions fresh and clear,
And numerous dowdy Ones are here;
Old wither'd Wives with Necks Flea-bitten,
And Maids that look as if Beshitten;
Low, Crooked, Forms and Homely features,
And many Blind and Crippl'd Creatures;
Some with their Arms quite shrunk and small,
And others have no Arms at all;
Some have but One and some no Legs,
But move upon Two Wooden Pegs;
Such is the mingled Medley Throng,
That hourly pass the Streets along;
Here goes a Furious Scolding Scab,
And there a Nasty Drunken Drab,
Who from the Brandy Shop new come,
With Draggled Tail goes Reeling Home,
Brimful of Kindness and Geneve,
She cries [to all] she meets Lord Save ye.
And as the Eye at these fine Sights
Is strangely ravish'd with Delights
Just so the various Noise is here
Affect, Regale, and Charm the Ear.
The Lame, the Blind, and hungry Poor,
With loud complaints some Alms implore
The many inarticulate Cries
Here strikes the Stranger with Surprize,
Who stares to hear them Bawl and Yell,
But knows not what they Say or Sell;
Here base Reviling, Cursing, Swearing,
And Imprecations great the Hearing;

With rumbling Carts, and rattling Coaches,
That crash by their too near Approaches;
And when Drays, Carts, and Coaches meet
Too thick and barricade the Street,
What Railing, Raving, Noise, and Rout!
What Horrid Curses fly about!
The Coaches thump, the weak Wheels crack,
Hold, D[amn] me, pull your Horses back,
A P[lag]ue, confound you, can't you see;
The Devil take that Dog for me;
Z[oun]ds, what does that damn'd Whore's bird mean?
Rot ye, I could have drove between:
Pox take ye, you Sir, keep your Reins out,
G—d damn your Blood I'll beat your Brains out;
With such rude Billingsgate-like Greetings
They treat at their unruly Meetings;
Besides the Quarrels, Brawls and Bustle,
When tugged Rakes and Bullies justle;
Nor can the Night afford us Peace,
Or make the Noise and Tumults cease;
Disturbing Clamours, frightful Cries,
From Accidental Mischiefs rise:
Mad Drunkards often meet and fight,
While Women Murder, Shriek outright.
The Watchman when he walks his Rounds
Tones his deep Voice in dismal Sounds,
Past Twelve a'Clock with hideous Yelling,
Bounce goes the door of every Dwelling;
At break of Day the Stony Ways
Are torn by jumbling jingling Drays,
That carry Drink as clear as strong,
Which jolted squirts thro' bor'd Clay-bung;
They bring it early lest their Ale
In two Day's time should grow too Stale.
    But Sir, whilst thus my Muse abroad does Roam,

The Jade forgets our case at Home
In Summer thro' excessive Heat,
We gap'd for Air and stew'd in Sweat;
By Day with Clouds of Dust oppress'd,
At Night by Buggs deprived of Rest;
In Winter we abide so nigh
The freezing Cold and Snowy Sky,
And our exalted Habitation,
So cleft for want of reparation,
That now we Sweat not you'll suppose,
Unless like Woodcocks at the Nose;
We both blow Hot and Cold in troth,
To warm our Nails and cool our Broth;
A mess of this to heat the Carcass
We get sometimes else tis a hard Case;
But that which tries, and most provokes us,
Our low-built treacherous Chimney smokes us,
Afflicts our Eyes and almost chokes us.
Our Linen looks like Skins of Witches,
And we are Black'd like Bacon Flitches;
Our Curtains, Valens, Cloths and Rug,
That look'd so ruddy, fresh and smug,
Are changed to sooty hue, and thus
They mourn for good P.G. and us.
And when the Wind from the South blows high,
About the Room Black Atoms fly
So thick, that Windows, Chairs, and Tables,
Are cover'd o'er with filthy Sables.
Amidst this Stifle, Stink, and Smother,
We cough and weep with one another;
Sometimes we fret, sometimes we pray,
And sometimes we know not what to say;
And sometimes we think to keep our Temper,
It will not be so nunc and semper:
Now we encourage then condole,

Ourselves in this vile smoky hole;
Sometime we laugh, and break a Jest on't,
The Market's Bad, let's make the best on't.
Thus, sometimes Sad and sometimes Merry,
We often wish ourselves at Bury.
   O how I long, Sir, to repair,
And breathe again my Native Air,
To walk securely up and down
The cleanly Streets of that sweet Town;
And certainly if wishes were
But Horses we should soon be there
And so perhaps in Time we may,
But till I'm able we must stay;
When I am once again I am fix'd there,
If I be drawn to live elsewhere,
May I be still Despised and Poor,
And never, never settle more.
Besides all this, it has of late
Freez'd here, and snow'd at such a rate,
I dare but seldom step Abroad,
So slipp'ry is my unseen Road
That going Out or coming Home,
Up flies my Heels and down comes Tom;
And this confinement keeps me poor,
And quite exhausts my Copper Store;
From here as well as from other Towns
I take more Half-pence than Halfcrowns.
And when I walk the Streets along,
There's such a Concourse, such a Throng,
I meet with many a Counter-buff
And durst not speak for fear they huff;
Tho' Hat and Wig are both beat off,
And some Relent while others Scoff
Thus, Sir, in wretched Poetry,
For which I beg you'll pardon me,

I've truly told you our Condition,
And humbly offer my Petition,
That you would please, &c.
And thus with pray'rs, and wishes fervent,
I am your very humble Servant,
             Thomas Gills

Making Money for the Blind Man of St. Edmunds-Bury

There are no new publications attributed to Gills after 1712. As he died in St. Edmunds-Bury in January 1715 (which might be 1716 in the O.S. calendar), his life ended with up to four years of apparent inactivity, something which his prefaces to his readers would suggest was not typical of him. He might have become unable to work or might have claimed himself unable to work and so was living off the parish poor law. This latter might have been the result of his deliberately making himself indigent, but whether his indigence was real or not, it would have required his resettlement in the parish of his birth or marriage, St. Mary's in St. Edmunds-Bury, something *The Blind man's case* tells us he wanted. However, such a strategy, calculated or not, is also not typical of the ebullient character who presents himself in the poems. Another possibility is that he had never been in the habit of putting his name to his works and continued to write the sort of pamphlets we know until his death. This is again unlikely if I am correct in my surmise that he was responsible for his own distribution, a marketing strategy which would require that he was a well-known face at or near events or churches selling his writings. Whatever it was that happened, if we work from the pattern of his extant publications, we can imagine another and more interesting turn of events.

Gills wrote three different catechisms for children, the first of which is known in more than one version:

1. *Instructions for children, in verse*, which appeared with that title and under his own name in two editions of 1707 and 1709.[49] Another version of the same catechism bears the title *Practical catechism: or, instructions for chil-*

dren, in verse and gives his name as "Thomas Gill" but is undated.[50] Finally there are two further versions of the same catechism with additions called *Useful and delightful instructions, by way of dialogue between the master & his scholar. Containing the duty of children.* Neither carries Gills's name, and they were "printed and sold by J. Downing of Bartholomew Close, near West-Smithfield" in 1712 and 1716.[51]

2. *Advice to youth: or, instructions for young men and maids,* which appeared under the name of Thomas Gill in 1708. The title page on the British Library copy has an MS addition of the date 1 March 1708/9, which has led cataloguers to suggest there were two editions or versions of the poem, which I cannot verify.[52]

3. *Questions and answers. In verse, upon the creation of the world, the fall of man, the flood, and several other passages out of the Old Testament,* which appeared under the name Thomas Gill in 1712.[53]

Where a place of publication is given, all editions and versions are printed in London except for the *Practical catechism* and *Questions and answers.* This allows that *Practical catechism* and *Questions and answers* may have been printed elsewhere, and it may have survived long after Gills died. An advertisement for an unattributed work called *The Weekly Exercise: Or, Plain and Easie Instructions for Youth* appeared in Ned Ward's *Honesty in Distress: but Reliev'd by No Party,* published in 1721(?), printed by Thomas Baily and William Thompson, who worked between Stamford, Lincolnshire, and St. Edmunds-Bury. No copy has been located, but the work may be yet another version of one of Gills's catechisms.

The long explanatory subtitle of *The Weekly Exercise* certainly follows the Anglican subject matter of Gills's other works: *Shewing First, The many Obligations Men are under to serve God. And, Secondly, How they may do it in the best Manner: Particularly, How they of the Church of England ought to behave themselves, whose Service and Prayers are herein fully Explain'd, and prov'd to be warrantable and Orthodox, by Quotations and Cases from Scripture, and the Examples of the Apostles themselves, and Rendered easie and intelligible to the meanest Capacities.* Furthermore, *The Weekly Exercise* is advertised to be sold at "Price Two-Pence, or 12s. a Hundred to those that are Charitably disposed to give them away," the same pricing structure of J. Downing's "Second Edition Enlarged" of Gills's catechism, printed in London in 1716.

Building narratives upon this evidence, it is possible that *Practical catechism* and *Questions and answers* may also have been published in St. Edmunds-Bury on Gills's return and financed his family for the last three or four years of his life. Another possibility is that J. Downing, who published a large number of works for the SPCK, bought *Instructions for Youth* from Gills for a fixed sum and financed their journey home, whence he wrote other works to sell there, for example, *Upon the Recovery of his Sight, and the Second Loss thereof,* whose date of 1710 is tentative and *Upon the Nativity of the Blessed Saviour,* which is also undated.

I shall go no further with my speculations, having learned the lesson from my first mistaken interpretation of Gills as a poor man when I had access to only half of his extant oeuvre. However, it might be argued that the man who could write *The Blind man's case at London* had a sense of humor, was devout, and faced his situation as a blind man with a family with fortitude. More importantly, his continued output of poems and his sadness at selling them at low prices suggests Gills was a man who was not daunted by his altered position in society and who had no sense of entitlement to parish handouts. If he did work out a deal with Downing for the reprinting of his *Instructions for children* in order that he could return to his place of safety, he gives us a fine example of how a middling-sort blind man understood himself as existing within the dignity of work and who spent his recompense the way he wanted to, far from the madding crowd, similarly, though in a different way, to John Maxwell and Priscilla Pointon.

9

JOHN MAXWELL

The Beauty of Gardens

We know very little about John Maxwell, "being blind," other than that he loved gardens and wrote much about them. For example:

> When, at the first, good Heav'n created Man,
> And, while he kept his native Purity,
> He needs must much enjoy those Delights
> Such as this Prospect gives.
> Heav'n plac'd him in a Garden; for such Scenes
> Well suit with Innocence; and is a Means
> Of height'ning Piety: As Musick in
> The Church enflames our Love, and charms us into Duty.
> Reflect my Soul, and take a full Survey
> Of all the Wonders that are here display'd;
> Extend thy Faculties, let Memory rise,
> And trace each beauteous Blossom as it blows;
> Then call up Understanding to apply
> Each Circumstance, accruing from the Whole:
> And, whilst I gaze upon those Miracles,
> Be thou, my Will, determined in this Choice,
> Steady t'obey that Power, which wrought 'em all;
> Which is so plainly seen in various Ways,
> I find it in the Odours of this Morn.[1]

For a blind poet to write of "this Prospect" and "Wonders that are here display'd . . . whilst I gaze upon those Miracles" is strange, though perhaps his use of visual expressions is explicable in terms of his having become blind late in life, more particularly since he tells himself to "Reflect my Soul ... [and] let Memory rise." There is no contemporary biography and little biographical information about this writer local to York, hitherto unknown to modern scholarship, and thus we do not know whether he could see until he was a young man or whether he was "born blind." But what we read in this extract from his poem *The reflection* is that Maxwell calls on other sensory information than the visual to enhance the effects of his metaphors. The garden's "Means / Of height'ning Piety: [is] As Musick in / The Church [which] enflames our Love, and charms us into Duty." God, "that Power, which wrought 'em all," is "seen in various Ways," and Maxwell himself *sees* God "in the Odours of this Morn."

Sighted poets' metaphors largely center on visual effects, and we might remember Alexander Pope's use of complementary colors in *Windsor Forest* to explore how in politics, "tho' all things differ, all agree."

> Here in full Light the russet Plains extend;
> There wrapt in Clouds the blueish Hills ascend:
> Ev'n the wild Heath displays her purple Dies,
> And 'midst the Desert fruitful Fields arise,
> That crown'd with tufted Trees and springing Corn,
> Like Verdant Isles the sable Waste adorn.[2]

However, even Pope struggled to write about sound, never took on the subject of music with the same easy brevity as Maxwell, and when he did, offered oddly silent similes and metaphors. In *An Essay on Criticism* he uses the word three times. He first imbues poets and composers with a mystical mastery of the "nameless graces" but says nothing about the power of music itself:

> Music resembles poetry, in each
> Are nameless graces which no methods teach,
> And which a master-hand alone can reach.[3]

Pope then tells us that music can "swell the Soul to rage, or kindle soft Desire," in a reference to Dryden's *Alexander's Feast: or the Power of Musique. An Ode for St Cecilia's Day:*[4]

> ... as Some to Church repair,
> Not for the Doctrine, but the Musick there.⁵

renders music merely pleasurable, while the third

> The Pow'r of Musick all our Hearts allow;
> And what Timotheus was, is Dryden now.⁶

Pope's own attempt to write for St. Cecilia, patron saint of music, was little better than these brief references to music in the *Essay on Criticism*, albeit that it was actually set to music by Maurice Greene and translated into Latin by Christopher Smart⁷ and Joseph Reeves.⁸ In 1961, Earl Wasserman relegated it to "the class of the respectable poor,"⁹ and it is hard to disagree when faced with lyrics which require some translation by music or language to give up their beauty:

> When the full organ joins the tuneful quire,
> Th'immortal pow'rs incline their ear;
> Born on the swelling notes our souls aspire,
> Whole solemn airs improve the sacred fire;
> And Angels lean from heav'n to hear!¹⁰

Perhaps the best brief poetic account of music before Maxwell belongs, surprisingly, to Elkanah Settle, who was so proud of the following couplet that he repeated it at least four times in four marriage poems, all called *Thalia Triumphans* and dedicated separately to David Mitchel, Lord Cobham, Richard Morgan, and John Buissiere:

> Love is itself but Musick more refined,
> Two well-tuned Hearts in one soft Consort join'd.¹¹

Alexander Pope rarely wrote about smells, other than a brief mention with reference to flowers or fruit and to lions having a better sense of smell than humans. And where other poets reference the sense, it is usually as a metaphor reminding readers that smells (and people) do not linger long. Thus, in Dryden's *Eleonora*, the life of the eponymous heroine is likened to a short-lived fragrance:

> As precious Gums are not for lasting Fire,
> They but perfume the Temple, and expire.

> So soon was she exhaled, and vanish'd hence;
> A short sweet Odour, of a vast Expence.[12]

On the other hand, Samuel Garth's *Dispensary* points out that not all smells are good: "So when Perfumes their fragrant Scent gave o'er, / Nought can their odour, like a Jakes, restore."[13]

The blind John Milton used the sense poetically only in a combination with the desire for food brought on by smell, and when the Tempter shows Eve the tree laden with apples, it is their odor that entices him to sin. He says:

> Till on a day roaving the field, I chanc'd
> A goodly Tree farr distant to behold
> Loaden with fruit of fairest colours mixt,
> Ruddie and Gold: I nearer drew to gaze;
> When from the boughes a savorie odour blow'n,
> Grateful to appetite, more pleas'd my sense
> Then smell of sweetest Fenel, or the Teats
> Of Ewe or Goat dropping with Milk at Eevn,
> Unsuckt of Lamb or Kid, that tend thir play.[14]

The scene is one which might have been written by a sighted poet since, like Pope's *Windsor Forest*, it paints the central motif with colors, this time, red and gold, and thus does not coax the reader to consider the poet's blindness as do Maxwell's color-free lines. But this is not to argue that Maxwell was unaware of the poetic conventions of his time; instead, I would suggest that he knew them and developed them according to his own perception of the world: a perception in which we might find a sense of his experience of being blind.

As we shall discover, Maxwell was well aware of a great deal of the literature of his time, and in *The reflection*, an early poem, we find a conscious quotation of Stephen Duck. In "The Thresher's Labour," Duck writes:

> Soon as the Harvest hath laid bare the Plains,
> And Barns well fill'd reward the Farmer's Pains;
> What Corn each Sheaf will yield, intent to hear,
> And guess from thence the Profits of the Year;

Or else impending Ruin to prevent,
By paying, timely, threat'ning Landlord's Rent,
He calls his Threshers forth:[15]

Maxwell, for his part, provides the farming year prequel in a fragment that might have come from a poem titled "The Reaper's Labour":

See! yon rich Valley, cover'd o'er with Corn,
Just ready for the healthy Reaper's Hand;
How does the Owner smile, to see his treasure!
And calls the Labourers forth:[16]

In his poem, Maxwell combines Duck's unfiltered experience of country life with the religious purpose of Milton (as well as his blank verse) and writes word pictures that owe more to other poetry than to vision:

See, that fair Meadow, richly clad with Flow'rs
Of different Kinds; wonderful both in Colours
And in Smell!
How does the sweet Variety at once,
Delight my Senses, and transport my Mind
While she contemplates the Hand that made 'em.[17]

The colors of the flowers are not named, individuated, or set in complementary pairs as in Pope's poem, such that the "sweet Variety" might equally delight the sense of smell which stops the half line, as the eye commanded to "See, that fair Meadow." I would even go as far as to argue that Maxwell has given his reader a complementary pair of color and smell as he did in "the Odours of this Morn" above. Furthermore, his mind's female sex might remind the reader of Aristotle's *De anima* rather than a companion on a walk, as we imagine her operation as the immortal part of the poet contemplating the divine in his solitary ramble.

Maxwell often makes this type of sudden shift away from the visual into more rarified knowledge, as though he is masking with learning his lack of ability to write about something he doesn't know:

Then mark those Insects, with their gawdy Wings,
Bask in its Beams, and feeding on their Sweets:

> There flies the Bee with her collected Store.
> Say, Infidel, how does she find her Home
> When at this Distance,
> Over such crooked Paths and Tracts of Ground?
> Reason she's none, and yet she travels on
> As tho' she understood:
> Does not this plainly show a Power Divine?[18]

It is difficult to work out whether Maxwell is writing here about butterflies with "gawdy Wings" of unnamed colors or the iridescence of bees' wings, and his turn to the discussion about how bees find their way back to the hive as part of the argument for the existence of God from design is a turn to information about something that he is certain of because he can learn it, whereas he can never see a bee or a butterfly.

It is not difficult to understand why Maxwell's next sudden shift in this poem is brought about by a sound: "Hark! from yon neighbouring Church a Sound for Death!"[19] The sound of a death knell ringing out over the fields of his walk which animates the reflection on death, sin, and redemption of the rest of the poem was used again by Thomas Gray in his *An Elegy wrote in a Country Churchyard* published eight years later. The knell, rung at the moment of death, nine for a man and six for a woman, has passed out of custom, so we can now only imagine the emotional effect caused by the interruption of the peace of a quiet country day by the sound of the bell rung at an unexpected time. The *memento mori* was a staple of eighteenth-century didactic poetry, so the similarities of language between Gray and Maxwell are hardly a sign of plagiarism:

> Sweet Meditation! see, how unobserved,
> I've reach'd this Church-Yard, here's a Field for thought!
> Now let the Ambitious come, and view this Scene,
> And tell me if it will not cure his Pride,
> When he reflects upon the mingled Mass,
> Which here lies wrap'd beneath those Beds of Turf.[20]

But what makes the meditation so significant, and Maxwell's poem particularly useful for this study, is that he refers consciously to his blindness in a way which gives us an understanding of how he understood himself. After hearing the knell, Maxwell gives a description of temptation and resistance of sin as a reminder of the free will all people have before they die:

> Perhaps a strong Temptation they shall find,
> So closely wove with Nature, it may be,
> Dear as their Eyes; which, to prevent, and cure,
> Heav'n will dispence another and another
> Tryal, equally as sharp:
> These may be Sufferings more than Martyr's Flames.
> Heav'n help all such, and yield them special Aid!
> And let them for their Comfort, be assur'd,
> That They are dear to Heav'n, and it is gracious,
> By thus impow'ring them to give to Heav'n
> Ev'n all their Faith, and Love and their Obedience,
> Which Heav'n will much reward; for Heav'n delights
> In Bounty.[21]

The idea that temptation is "more than Martyr's Flames" because it is a desire for the very thing that those tempted want the most is conventional enough. However, Maxwell's use of the phrase "Dear as their Eyes," which makes the value of sight a simile for the strength of temptation, turns the idea back on itself when written by a blind writer. Maxwell has no eyes, but the line suggests he knows how useful they might be. On one level, the line tells the sighted reader not to take sight for granted, but on another he might be setting himself up as a "blind seer," someone who does not sin, from whom his readers might learn. However, he continues the poem with a description of those who do not give in to sin in a visual metaphor:

> These shine like Stars of the first Magnitude,
> And are distinguish'd from the rest of Men,
> As holy Martyrs in their Time of Sufferings.
> O! how my Soul wou'd joy in such a Friend
> Whose Actions flow from Virtues pleasing Stream;
> That fears as much to act the smallest Sin,
> When Privacy has drawn a Veil around,
> As if expos'd in public Theatres.[22]

These lines halt any interpretation of himself as a virtuous man who is not tempted since he has no eyes, and instead we learn from them that Maxwell's blindness makes him feel that he is always being watched. Sight is a sense that he has learned can put him in contact with things he cannot touch, and so he knows that although the world he can reach out and touch is empty of people, there might still be someone looking in on his most private moments, and although he might believe from the evidence of touch that he is alone, he could as easily be onstage in a theater watched by an audience. Blindness does not allow him to live at ease in a world made certain because he can touch it; there might always be an eye seeking him out.

Maxwell explains the idea further as he turns his thoughts in on himself:

> And Now I will examine my own Heart,
> By asking it this Question: Can we not then
> Be sure of nothing which our Senses do
> Not prove? I'm satisfied we may; and this
> To me will prove it. Do I believe
> The Story of our *Royal Martyr*'s Death?
> As sure as I believe I view this Monument:
> And not to do so wou'd indeed be Folly;
> And yet I never saw one Circumstance
> Relating to his Sufferings; nor any who
> Was Witness of that Cruelty.
> Can we not then as readily believe
> The Hist'ry of our blest Redeemer's Death,
> And give our firm Assent to all those Truths.[23]

The first question attacks atheist empiricist materialism and answers it with the extraordinary insouciance of a blind man. He has the same certainty of the truth of the story of the Royal Martyr's death[24] as he has of the existence of the Monument to it that he cannot see. By the same method, he can therefore be as certain of the history of Christ and believe in the son of God. Rather than exhort the primacy of touch as a sure way to prove the material existence of objects in the world which can lead to atheism, Maxwell argues the idealist position that every experience is, at bottom, a mental state, but at the same time puts belief in God on the same level as believing in the existence of material objects. And it is before God whom he acts as though on stage in a theater, albeit in his most private moments.

Conversely, this also means that a life led piously and in constant mindfulness of the gifts of heaven brings heaven down to earth, although it might be in the imagination of the blind poet. Thus, where *The reflection* begins with a long description of an earthly garden which incites piety, it ends with a longer description of heaven as a garden, the reward for a pious life lived under the eye of God.

> Supposing then a pleasant Space or Ground,
> (Larger than what Imagination forms)
> Adorn'd with Hills, still rising as they spread,
> Where not the smallest Barrenness appears,
> But clad in every-green, and deck'd with Flowers,
> And Trees of ev'ry kind:
> Fair and Luxuriant All, as Nature e'er
> Produc'd, in every different Quarter of the World:
> Where Winter's never seen,
> But a perpetual Spring does ever bloom;
> Where the Sun always shines, but never burns:
> Where no rough Winds are heard, or Tempest comes;
> But All's serene, and blest with gentle Gales.
> That breath Aromatic Ordours [sic] all around,
> Whose blest Inhabitants are pleasing all;
> Having as those whom Blood or Friendship joyns.[25]

Heaven is a place peopled by the virtuous, who observe one another to balance each other's virtue. And this is a recurring theme in Maxwell's writing, since it is so like the world in which he lived as a blind man who saw by smell and sound.

In this way, Maxwell is a very useful example for our understanding of the self-presence of a blind person in the eighteenth century. The religious poet writes of a colourless world built up out of words that reference one another as the heavenly garden references the earthly. Thus, where Milton could use the colors "Ruddie and Gold" when writing with memory of apples, Maxwell describes a fruit tree to his sighted reader in a very different way:

> Now mark those Trees, and their delicious Fruit,
> With blushing Cheeks that ripen in the Sun;
> And listen to the sweet harmonious Sound
> Of all that variety of Birds,
> Which hop from Bough to Bough with painted Wings
> Warbling forth their sweet melodious Songs.[26]

No color is named since Maxwell does not know what red or gold is, but he does know what a blush is, and he knows he can apply the term to the skin of an apple, learned, perhaps, from Elizabeth Singer Rowe's *Tasso*: "Depending on the loaded branch are seen / The gold, the blushing Apple, and the green."[27] All this would suggest that John Maxwell was well educated, and he does mention his love of books: "Books are like Friends that serve us in out Need: / He has a mighty Blessing that enjoys 'em."[28]

But there is a question that hangs over his situation which leads from his education: Was he from the laboring class like Stephen Duck, from the middling sort like Thomas Gills, or from the aristocracy, which is possible since one "Lord Maxwell" subscribed to this poem? The answer to the question, which can be drawn from the few biographical details extant, gives us a fascinating insight into another blind person who refused to give in to his impairment and successfully made a living for himself.

Biography

We can be certain that Thomas Gent of York published eight pieces by "John Maxwell, being Blind" between 1740 and 1761, six of which carried long subscription lists. The first, *The faithful pair: or, virtue in Distress. A tragedy* (1740), is a short play in which Hiraxis guiltily desires Olinda, the daughter of the usurped king Archon but is foiled by his brother Marcellus, whose love is reciprocated by Olinda, and the two end up happily married as king and queen. There is a MS note on the front cover of the British Library copy: "Received 2D [2nd?] February 1739 five shillings for his majesties duty of this from [?], . . . containing 5 half sheets for the use of Mr Ea s_bardic . . . ," which suggests that it was a proof copy, and the fact that it carries no subscription list therefore might be explained as a printing anomaly. The names of the play's characters Olinda and her father, Archon, can be found respectively in Dryden's *Secret Love or The Maiden Queen*[29] and *Albion and Albanius, an opera*,[30] the latter being also used in Plutarch's *Lives*. The second, which we have already explored, is *The reflection, a poem* (1743) and carries a list of 263 subscribers. The third piece is another short play, *The royal captive* (1745), and given the date, the title might perhaps set bells ringing about Maxwell making a political point. The play carried a similar length list of 260 subscribers and features Mandana, the mother of Cyrus the Great, who is mentioned in Herodotus's *Histories* and Xenophon's *Cyropedia*. Mandana is also mentioned by Dryden in the epistle dedicatory to *Aureng-Zebe*.[31] In the fourth piece, Maxwell changed genre to write *The conversation, or, the lady's tale. A novel* (1747), which brought him 245 subscribers. The eponymous conversation occurs in a garden between Sulpitia and Rosalitta, the former of whose names occurs as half of a pair of female friends, Sulpitia and Lentulus, in Lady Mary Chudleigh's *Essays upon several subjects in prose and verse*, in the essay "Of Love."[32] Sulpitia is also named in the epistle dedicatory of Dryden's *An Evening's Love, or the Mock Astrologer*.[33] The title of the novel may also be derived from Madeleine de Scudery's *Conversations upon several subjects*.[34]

The fifth publication, *A new tragedy call'd the loves of Prince Emilius and Lovisa* (1755), another short play which concerns the pain of the loves of the highborn, appeared after a hiatus of seven rather than the usual two years. The only known copy in the Huntington Library bears a MS note on the title page stating it is "Collated and Perfect," although there is no subscription list, which usually comes at the end. This suggests that *The faithful pair* might also originally have had no subscribers, or it might be that the Huntington copy was stripped of its subscription list before binding, and perhaps even made up out of more than one original. Once again we can find the names of Maxwell's characters in other texts.

Billeront appears in Mary Pix's *The Inhumane Cardinal, or Innocence Betray'd, a novel*,[35] and Emilius might have been copied from either Dryden's translation of *Juvenal*[36] or Sir Robert Howard's play *The Vestal Virgin, or The Roman ladies*.[37] The sixth of Maxwell's pieces, which gained 264 subscribers, appeared the usual two years after the previous and is something like a prose version of *The reflection*; it also occurs in a garden. *The polite assembly, or, the Charms of Solitude Display'd* (1757) is more than a monologue, and others speak, including Arpasia, whose name might be copied from Scudery's, *Artamenes, or, The Grand Cyrus an excellent new romance*,[38] her *Conversations upon several subjects*,[39] or Nicholas Rowe's *Tamerlane*.[40] The *polite assembly* also contains a hymn by John Norris. There is only a single copy known of the follow-up to *The polite assembly*, which is called *A continuation of a book, lately publish'd; call'd, the polite assembly; or, the charms of solitude display'd* (1759). It garnered 249 subscribers, featured Arpasia in a garden once more, and quotes at length Edward Young's *Centaur not fabulous*, concerning Epicurus's thoughts about gardens, from a chapter called "On Pleasure."[41] The last extant work, *A new tragedy cali'd* [sic] *The distressed virgin* (1761), appeared after the "usual" time but collected the fewest subscribers at 219. It is specifically anti-Epicurean and begins with an argument for the existence of God by design. Also, as "usual," the names of two of its main characters, Archilas and Cleona, may have been copied from Nathaniel Lee's *Mithridates, King of Pontus*,[42] the former of which also featured an epilogue by Dryden, while Cleona is mentioned in the preface to *The Life of Cleomenes* by Dryden. The play also refers to the outbreak of cattle plague, similar to that which had been affecting Yorkshire herds of cattle for the past twenty years.

This brief survey of Maxwell's known output demonstrates the breadth of his reading. It might be reduced if we consider him to have had access to an edition of the *Dramatick Works of John Dryden*;[43] however, we must not forget the other references to Nathaniel Lee, Nicholas Rowe, Robert Howard, John Norris, Mary Chudleigh, Mary Pix, and Madeleine de Scudery, or the contemporary reference to Edward Young. In *The reflection*, Maxwell explains that he learned to "taste those Pleasures *Reading* doth afford"[44] from his mother, who may have owned copies of the books cited.

It is possible that the gap in publication between 1747 and 1755 was due to the loss of all copies, which quite probably were not printed in excess of the subscription list. The single known copy of *A continuation* in the library of York Minster is matched by the loss of almost all numbers of the early York newspapers: no one in York appears to have collected ephemera. Furthermore, we can learn little from the names of the subscribers. Some subscribed for all six, some for five, four, three, two, and some for just one. There are 812 separate names in total, including Thomas Herring, the archbishop of York, and his brother William. There is a Mr. John Barker, a Toyman from Coney Street, who subscribed to just *The polite assembly*, and Mr. John Camidge, organist of High-Petergate, who subscribed to the last three publications. Lady Fagg, wife of Sir Robert Fagg, who was married in the Minster, subscribed to all six. In the records of St. John Ousegate, 113 of the subscribers are mentioned, and given that there are forty-five churches in York, it would appear that further research might turn up records for most of the other subscribers as locals to the city.

Searches of the records of the parishes reveal a concentration of "Maxwells" as well as "Maxfields" christened and buried at All Saints Church, North Street, between 1658 and 1706, but then no more. This may have been because the family died out, as is recorded by the christenings and deaths of William, Thomas, John, Elizabeth, Isabell, Katherine, and Benjamin, all of whom died in childhood and are listed as son or daughter of John Maxwell. One Elizabeth Maxwell, wife of John Maxwell, and presumably their mother, died in 1701. After this date there are no more Maxwells in the parish register except for one Jane Maxwell ("a young woman"), who was buried there in 1706. The demise of the family is confirmed by the St. John Ousegate parish register, which duplicates the records of the burials at All Saints, North Street of Catherine [sic], and Benjamin daughter and son of John Maxwell, and Elizabeth, "Wife of John Maxwell, Cordwinder." The register also adds, "A male stillborn of Jno. Maxwell's" in 1697 and "John Maxwell, Cordwinder," who was buried in 1704 also at All Saints, North Street, although the records do not appear in that register. One last record notes the burial of "Grace, the daughter of William Cooper of Wakefield (Servant at John Maxwell's)," who was buried in 1695.

All these burials are probably too early to be in the nuclear family of John Maxwell the writer, but what is useful for us to know is that the two versions of the name "Maxwell" and "Maxfield" are a local confusion. We find in other parish registers that Stephen Maxwell, who married Anne Archer in 1719 at Holy Trinity, Goodramgate, appears in the parish register for St. Cuthbert's, Peasholm, as a churchwarden named "Stephen Maxfield" [sic] in 1723 and signs off the purchase of new pews in 1724 in the same register and on the next page as "Stephen Maxwell." Stephen and Anne Maxwell's daughter Elizabeth was christened in 1722 at St. Cuthbert's, Peasholm.[45]

Other Maxfield and Maxwell parish records include the death of "Isabell Maxfield (dau. of Matthew Maxfield Joyner)" in 1716 at St. Saviour's, and the marriages of John Maxwell and Mary Marshall in 1702, John Pickard and Mary Maxwell in 1707, and Thomas Maxwell and Jude Cousins in 1710 at Holy Trinity Micklegate.

If these are, as they may well be, fragmentary records of John Maxwell the writer's extended family, then we get a picture of professional people who might keep a servant and who were educated enough to become church functionaries. They also help us to understand the two apparently incontrovertible facts we have about the life of John Maxwell the writer. The first is the granting to "John Maxfield" on 23 October 1727 of £2 per year from the Dorothy Wilson Trust. The second is the making "by patrimony" of "John Maxwell, son of Benjamin Maxwell, carpenter," a freeman of the city of York in 1749.

The Dorothy Wilson Trust was one of the first charities which helped blind people. Set up after Wilson's death in 1717, it ran concurrently with a number of other charitable organizations including a hospital for ten old women at Fossebridge, and a school for twenty boys in the parish of St. Denys, which moved to the village of Nun Monkton. The arm of the charity which gave to blind people is not mentioned in a contemporary history by Francis Drake that mentions Dorothy Wilson's Hospital,[46] but it is mentioned briefly a century later in Baines's *History, Directory and Gazetteer of the County of York*, where we read: "The yearly sum of 2l. Each is supplied to three blind people."[47] The records of the charity demonstrate that the level of need was assessed by seven trustees, who voted on the blind people who applied for help.[48] The Minute Book of the Trust notes that Hannah Hick, who held the income stream before Maxwell, and Jony

Relph, who held another, were both voted for by a majority, but no vote is recorded for "John Maxfield." This might suggest Maxwell's greater need[49] or that the trust's secretary was of the same social position, or that members of the trust were well known to him. Drake notes an anomaly in the trust deed: "The lands are vested in seven trustees, citizens of *York*, but there is a remarkable clause in this settlement, *that if any one of these should be made an alderman of this city, he should cease to be trustee.*"[50] The clause suggests that trustees were intended by Dorothy Wilson to be ordinary citizens, which the occupations of the other Maxwells and Maxfields would suggest they were.

We can be almost certain that it was John Maxwell the writer who was created freeman in 1749, since the occupation of all other freemen is given as well as their fathers', and no occupation is given for John Maxwell (nor is he listed as a gentleman), which suggests he was thought not to work.[51] To have been created freeman of the city of York "by patrimony," his father must also have been a freeman of the city, and the granting of the status freeman, which was necessary for a man to vote, was available at the age of twenty-one. Since Maxwell was granted money by the Dorothy Wilson Trust in 1727 and began publishing in 1740, it is likely he was much older than twenty-one when he was made freeman.

These two pieces of information together suggest that, being blind, he was not thought competent to vote or use the other advantages of the status of freeman. However, it might be that being in receipt of a charitable donation excluded him. Since he was eventually made freeman, albeit when he was older than usual, we might conclude that he had become a local celebrity after the publication of at least four of his eight extant works which had been subscribed to by other freemen of York. In turn this would suggest that the subscriptions had made and continued to make him independent and that he was living as a blind writer, financing himself through his own work. There is even a suspicion in the Minute Books that Maxwell ceased to receive money from the Dorothy Wilson Trust at the time he became a freeman unless a fourth stream of finance was started, taken up by Thomas Wilson in 1753, when John Maxwell was still very much alive.[52] The long subscription list for a blind writer to become independent of charity was a model that would be used by Thomas

Blacklock in the subscription set up for him in 1756 by Joseph Spence, and by Priscilla Pointon in 1770 and 1794.

Religion

Perhaps the most difficult thing for a researcher to come to terms with is not finding the most basic facts about one's subject in the archives. However, the lack of a birth record must be set against the creation of John Maxwell freeman of York with neither an occupation nor the title of gentleman, which strongly suggests that he was born in York itself, son of Benjamin, a carpenter, even though neither of their births, marriages, or deaths were recorded in any of the city parish records.

As this is the time of Archbishop Herring's visitation (1743), which gave the names of more than five thousand Catholics in Yorkshire, it is tempting to argue that the Maxwell family were Roman Catholic. The suggestion is borne out by the inclusion of the name of Lady Haggerston, as subscriber to *A continuation* (1759) and *The distressed virgin* (1761). Married in 1758 to Sir William Haggerston-Constable of Everingham in the East Riding of Yorkshire, Lady Haggerston was formerly Lady Winifrede Maxwell, the granddaughter of the 5th Earl of Nithsdale and 9th Baron Herries, a Catholic Jacobite whose wife (another Winifrede Maxwell) famously helped her husband escape from the Tower of London after the 1715 rebellion on the eve of his execution, to return to France and the exiled court, where she was nurse to the Old Pretender. Herring's visitation notes that Everingham was still "a strong Roman Catholic centre" with six out of twenty-seven families being Catholic.[53] The hub of the village is Everingham Hall, built by John Carr for William Haggerston-Constable between 1757 and 1764, which now features a huge Roman Catholic chapel dating from the nineteenth century. However, there is a small abandoned chapel sixty meters east of the parish Church of St. Everilda, of classical design, which might have served the Haggerston-Constable family and the six Catholic families from the village during the eighteenth century. It would not be out of the question to argue that John Maxwell was related to Winifrede and that the garden he describes in each of his works is based

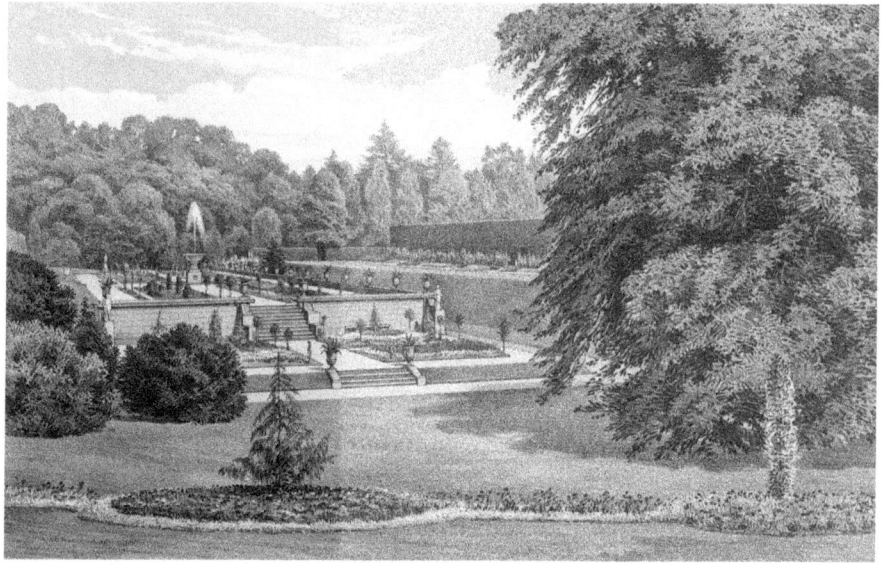

FIGURE 9. Terregles Garden, Dumfries. (National Library of Scotland, CC BY 4.0)

on the estate at Everingham Hall, or even at Terregles, near Dumfries, the seat of the Barony of Nithsdale, where as the brother of Winifrede he would have grown up (see fig. 9).

Whether or not he was the son of a carpenter, or the member of an aristocratic family, as a Catholic he might perhaps have developed his pious beliefs and written about them in terms of gardens from Richard Challoner's *Garden of the Soul*,[54] which lays out the duties of a catholic in a "Manual of Spiritual Exercises and Instructions for Christians who (living in the world) aspire to Devotion." The book was intended to help its reader to grow into what became known as a "'Garden of the Soul Catholic' as a spiritual type, devout but restrained."[55] However, its exhortations (for example, "At first waking in the morning . . . [t]ake great care not to let the devil run away with your first thoughts; for very much depends upon giving them to God, who is your first beginning, and last end, and therefore expects from you the first fruits of the day)[56] may as easily be from a Church of England divine such as Thomas Seaton, whose *The devotional Life render'd familiar, easy, and pleasant, in several hymns upon the most common occasions of human life* offers similar advice for the same moment:

"When first Awake in the Morning, let your thoughts be devout, and fix'd upon God, expressing your hearty Thanks for his protecting you the past night."[57]

Another reason why John Maxwell's name might not have appeared in any parish registers of York was that he came from a family which dissented for some other reason than Roman Catholicism. A number of names appear in the subscription lists: Calvert and Hotham were Independents; Wombwell, Baptist; Nelson and Coates, Wesleyan Methodists. Following this argument, we might ally John Maxwell's horticulturally based spiritual rumination with Johann Arndt and *The Garden of Paradise, or Holy Prayers and Exercises*,[58] which had recently been translated into English. Arndt's form of pietism resounds throughout Maxwell's works, but like that of Challoner or Seaton, may simply be the understanding of all believers what it was to be a good Christian despite the detail of worship and belief. Furthermore, it must be remembered that Archbishop Herring was a subscriber too, and the vast majority of subscribers appear to be conformists to the Anglican Church. Therefore, rather than speculate upon who was the Royal Martyr mentioned in *The reflection*, Charles or James, we might look instead at the way Maxwell's account of pious Christianity, with God watching him in all his actions as though he is in a theater, gives us an idea of his self-presence. And this is best tracked in dialogues and conversations that occur in gardens, or in dreams of gardens.

The faithful pair

When we first meet Olinda, the heroine, who is besieged by Hiraxis the king but who is in love with and faithful to his brother Marcellus, she is reading in "A Grove" from where she expatiates on sight and blindness:

> Knowledge! thou mighty much-desired Bliss!
> Delightful Source, from whence true Pleasures flow!
> By Thee we plainly view those Faculties
> The Soul possesses; the rich Gift of Heav'n,
> When it vouchsaf'd to breathe into us Life.[59]

It is "knowledge" by which we "plainly view" rather than the senses themselves giving us information as though we are machines. Through "knowledge" gained from language we interpret the "rich Gift of Heav'n" and "Bliss" using our understanding. On one level this is the philosophers' message from Plato's Cave: that what we experience needs to be interpreted for us to understand it. On another, it is a blind man writing about his lack of eyes in the self-consciously constructed language of heroic lines in blank verse: language which draws our attention to the fact of language bringing forth the information.

Maxwell develops the idea in a conversation between Olinda and her father, Archon, who is in prison. A concrete representation of a blind man, Archon can see nothing in his confinement but uses the idea of sight to explain to Olinda that virtuous acts on earth, however painful to perform, will be rewarded in heaven with a cornucopia of "Beauties":

> . . . and when we sacrifice
> What is most dear rather than disobey, then most
> We please; and larger our Performances of Goodness,
> Greater the Reward; and that so great, we
> Cannot comprehend it; let us but take a View
> Of what is present: How lovely is each Part of
> This Creation! How various are its Beauties! And
> What do some with Innocence enjoy, even in this
> Fall'n State! Then how much greater had not Man
> Transgress'd? Then can we think that in Variety Heav'n
> Will be barren? No: The Difference is so wide,
> It will bear Comparison; let this suffice
> To make us persevere.[60]

For Archon, nothing is "present" to his "view" except his memory of the world, which brings to him its "various . . . Beauties." This means he can make judgments with similar certainty about the greater "Variety" of the world to come, which he also cannot see, but of which he also has knowledge. Again, this is a standard Christian interpretation of the fallen world and the perfection of heaven as a reward for virtue, but encased in the language of blindness, together with the strange shift from heroic pentameter to heroic hexameter in which Archon speaks,[61] it appears to be a deliberate attempt to make language as the carrier of knowledge "visible" to the reader in the process of reading. For Maxwell, the world on earth and the world in heaven both come to him with equal certainty through the medium of language.

Language and the meaning of words becomes the subject of a discussion of sexual and virtuous love between Hiraxis and his brother Marcellus, which leads us to the reason the play is called a tragedy, though it is not strictly so since at the end the lovers are reunited when the king dies of rage at his unfulfilled desire for Olinda. In the argument with his brother, we hear Hiraxis claim that desire should lead to physical fulfilment:

> Now let me hear your Sentiments of what you call
> A virtuous Passion. I ne'er experienced any, but what
> Serv'd to gratify each Sense with most Delight, and to
> Make room to entertain another, and another yet
> More new.[62]

Marcellus replies that this is "Just so the Brutes enjoy," to which Hiraxis asks, "Does not each Fair afford us as much Love as any of your Virtuous Ones can do?" So Marcellus explains that the life of the mind is more important than the senses when understanding the single word "Love":

> How often is that sacred Word abus'd?
> Nothing's more common than to say, We love;
> When 'tis most sure 't shou'd bear a fouler Name.
> Our Love when pure, dwells chiefly in the Mind,
> And finds a many Pleasures that's unknown
> To Persons you describe.
> A virtuous Love can easily forgo
> All gross Enjoyment rather than destroy
> The Peace of what it loves. All that is spoke
> Of Friendship may in it be found with this
> Peculiar Happiness annext,
> That all we do administers Delight;
> And may, perhaps, be a Resemblance
> Of Love divine.[63]

Once again, the superficial message of the verse is conventional enough: love that is enflamed by sensuous interaction leads to fornication, but Christian spiritual love does not require a physical outlet. However, the same passage understood in terms of the blind writer who cannot see anything transforms the idea that "Love when pure, dwells chiefly in the Mind" into something truly tragic. Everything "dwells" in Maxwell's mind, nothing of any "Fair" comes to his eyes from the sensuous world, and he is trapped within his body trying to come to terms with the failure of a sense he knows exists. Later in the play, Olinda reads lines written by Marcellus giving an extended metaphor of virtue as a garden which explores the idea further:

> Virtue the choicest Blessing we can boast;
> Virtue as lovely as the blushing Morn,
> All soft and fair as Winds that gently fan
> The opening Buds whose balmy Sweets distill
> In fragrant Odours,
> Shedding their healthy Influence around!
> Happy's the Breast possess'd of such a Treasure;
> A Treasure far beyond the gaudy Riches
> Of the fading World.
> A Treasure everlasting and divine:
> For Virtue's ever merciful and kind.
> Virtue is all forgiving; its only Care
> Is to do good to all as Angels are.
> Happy indeed's the Mind that is this bless'd
> With solid Virtue. Virtue has a Charm,
> To make us bear Misfortune as we ought:
> To make us even look on Death with Pleasure.
> . . . .
> As when we hope to meet a Friend from far,
> Which we are satisfied some time will come.
> But when we know not when he does arrive,
> We wonder at the long expected Guest;
> Then mingle with the Dust, and are at Rest?[64]

The first six lines make Maxwell's typical invocation of the breezes, sounds, and smells of a garden; we find him in sensuous reverie brought on by the things to which he has access. The same lines tell us of the knowledge he can derive from what he can know: if there is a breeze bringing the smell to him, then there are buds making the smell, though he cannot see them. But this process of deriving knowledge, which is the blind man making sense of where he is from the information he has of it, takes him away from the moment of experiencing the garden further into his mind fixating on the process itself. Maxwell does not rest, lazily watching the garden in the morning; his mind turns inward as the process of making knowledge from experience continues relentlessly. Deprived of the "Treasure" of seeing the garden, he makes permanent knowledge about it, as though the thought of the garden brings unasked the memory of other things he knows, crowding him with thoughts of angels, mercy, and kindness in an effort to push away the pain of being blind. The memory of virtue which began in the innocence of the garden becomes in the reverie the harbinger of death: it "makes us bear Misfortune as we ought: To make us even look on Death with Pleasure." For Marcellus in the play, it is the loss of Olinda (although they both live in the same palace); for Maxwell, it is the loss of his sight (which perhaps accounts for Marcellus not "seeing" Olinda). The loss of the beloved person or sense becomes, through the relentless process of making knowledge out of experience, death. As Marcellus's finds pleasure in the thought of death since he is without Olinda, so Maxwell's life without sight is a living death, and we are left to wonder whether there was a real-life Olinda for the writer. This is borne out when the Olinda of the play "rewrites" the lines quoted above immediately after reading them, with an emphasis on the visual:

> How beauteous is the Face of this fair Morn!
> O! how my wearied Soul longs to enjoy
> Her wonted Happiness in rural Pleasures!
> How poor are gilded Roofs, with all the
> Grandeur that a Court can find, to those
> Sweet Scenes of Evening Sun, gilding the
> Mountain-Tops, and the fair Moon, with all

> Her Sister-Train of glitt'ring Stars, which
> Dress the Face of Heaven.[65]

In these lines Olinda is not recording what she is experiencing but transforming the golden roofs of the palace in the morning into a rural evening scene. In effect she is reversing the process that Maxwell uses to describe his experiences: she brings her knowledge gained from vision to change what her sight shows her. At once this confirms that Maxwell has some understanding of how sight works to bring visual information to the seer, but the overwhelming note of sadness gives us a sense of how he felt about being blind. The song which Olinda next commands her servant Delia to sing suggests that his sadness derives from feeling that he can never win a real-life Olinda:

> Ye fellow Swains, who sport and toil
> From early Dawn to Shade pursue,
> With pity view the cruel Spoil,
> And triumph o'er a Heart as true,
> As e'er at Paphos Off'rings made:
> And fly with Care the cruel Maid.
>
> Shun all those Shades, where at high Day
> She leads her fleecy Flocks to feed:
> Nor dart a random Glance that way,
> Or vainly hope you may succeed:
> And sure 'tis vain for every Art
> Of Love, I've try'd to touch her Heart.[66]

The offerings made at Paphos in the first verse recall Ovid's story of Pygmalion, in which an ivory statue of a beautiful woman is brought to life through prayers to Venus. Linking the story with Maxwell's predicament, in the translation by Dryden, we read that Pygmalion made the ivory statue as he,

> ... loathing their lascivious Life,
> Abhorr'd all Womankind, but most a Wife:
> So single chose to live and shunned to wed,
> Was pleas'd to want a Consort of his Bed.[67]

Pygmalion's fear of sexually active women, at war with his sexual desire, becomes doubly problematic for a blind man who cannot know what his wife is doing even when she is in front of him, as was famously made comedy in Mary Pix's play *The Deceiver Deceiv'd,* in which a blind man's wife makes love before his face.[68] In Dryden's Ovid, we learn that the statue made flesh is at least faithful until the birth of their first son, Paphos, since Venus

> So bless'd the Bed, such Fruitfulness convey'd,
> That e'er ten Months had sharpen'd either Horn,
> To crown their Bliss, a love'y Boy was born;
> *Paphos* his Name, who grown to Manhood, wall'd
> The City *Paphos,* from the Founder call'd.[69]

The statue wife does not have time to sharpen Pygmalion's cuckold's horns, a trait which is transferred to their son, who can wall around a city to protect it in like manner.

The second verse of Delia's song reminds married people that neither are their spouses necessarily faithful. The "random Glance" recalls Loveless from Vanbrugh's *The Relapse,* who falls in love with Berintha at the theater and tells her that his love began with their eyes meeting:

> When 'twas my Chance to see you at the Play,
> A randome Glance you threw, at first alarm'd me,
> I cou'd not turn my Eyes from whence the danger came:
> I gaz'd upon you 'till you shot again,
> And then my Fears came on me.
> My Heart began to pant, my limbs to tremble,
> My Blood grew thin, my Pulse beat quick,
> My Eyes grew hot and dim, and all the frame of Nature Shook with
>   Apprehension.[70]

Loveless, whose fidelity is being tried by his wife, Amanda, in the sequel to Colley Cibber's *Love's Last Shift,* is a reformed rake who has relapsed and fallen in love, hook, line, and sinker "at first sight" and failed the test. But falling in love that way is something Maxwell cannot do. And thus, in his own play, Maxwell becomes something of his own creation, Marcellus, looking for his Olinda, blindly fumbling around the same palace where both live. And in this way also we can understand Maxwell's sense of himself as something less than a man: he is alone in a world he cannot trust and only to be loved by someone who is blind to his blindness.

If this is the worst of self-pity, Maxwell's tragedy and the tragedy of the play is transformed when Marcellus and Olinda meet unexpectedly just at the point when Hiraxis has vowed to kill her father, Archon, sworn revenge on Olinda's lover (not knowing it is his own brother), and to rape her because she will not marry him. The faithful pair are happy to be reunited but are watched secretly by Hiraxis, who breaks into their scene of recognition and joy, commanding his brother to give Olinda up. Marcellus swears he will do anything for his king except give up his love, Olinda reminds Hiraxis that she has sworn fidelity to Marcellus before God, and Hiraxis dies suddenly of a heart attack. If there is something comic in the scene, it must be balanced by the similar scene of secret observation from Pix's *Deceiver Deceiv'd,* which was meant as comedy. Melito Bondi is a senator of Venice who feigns blindness to avoid being president of Dalmatia. His pretense is the basis of the comedy, and in a scene where his wife meets and kisses her first lover, Count Andrea, in front of him, he can say nothing to stop them. But this is just not funny for a blind man. Bondi's aside, "Oh, the Garden, the Devil!,"[71] brings us directly to Maxwell's own obsession with gardens, and so it is no surprise that the play finishes with a poem about a garden with no devil in it.

The description of the garden reads very much like an ideal retreat for blind person, always full of fruit, warm and with neighbors, a priest and most importantly a friend or two:

> Whose honest Hearts participate our Woe,
> And share our Joys. For, should Affliction rise,
> To vent our Sorrows in a friendly Breast,
> Eases the Load: And if our Lives are crown'd
> By smiling Joy, to share the Pleasure with
> A gen'rous Friend, doth add a Lustre to
> The mighty Bliss:[72]

The desire for this garden and its description is the burden of most of Maxwell's other works: *The reflection* we have explored, *The conversation*, *The polite assembly*, and *A continuation of . . . the polite assembly*, all develop the idea with Sulpitia and Arpasia as the friend who takes the place of Olinda. So much so that Maxwell appears to be calling out for the institutions for the blind which would be founded forty years after he died.

If Christian virtue in all its variations is the marketing strategy, the pain of being blind is the product Maxwell is selling, a pain which the buying of his book will alleviate. Thus, he avoids pity because the subscribers have all been given something for their money, and it is no longer charity.

10

PRISCILLA POINTON GETS MARRIED

No modern collection of eighteenth-century poetry is complete without Priscilla Pointon's "Address to a Bachelor, On a Delicate Occasion," a poem which describes a blind woman's dilemma when caught short needing to go to the toilet while visiting the house of a friend in all-male company.[1] The poem was published in her 1770 collection *Poems on Several Occasions*[2] and demonstrates an irascible side of her character that must be set against her more reflective side, represented by the much less well-known "Consolatary [sic] Ode" on her blindness.[3] This doubleness is expressed further in the little contemporary biographical information we have about Pointon that comes from the evidence of the poems, the long subscription list, and from the author of the preface of her *Poems on Several Occasions*.

I have written elsewhere on the subject of what we may or may not include as biographical information with relation to Pointon and argued that the subscription list of 1,577 names demonstrates that PP, as she called herself, made a "grand tour" of the theaters and public houses of the Midlands of England, where she recited her verses before an audience whom she then thanked in an "Extempore Address" in the finished collection.[4] The ability to perform and compose on the hoof suggests PP's extrovert character, and her "Address to a Bachelor, On a Delicate Occasion" appears to be less a sad tale of an unpleasant joke at the expense of a blind woman's modesty, as Simon Dickie reads it,[5] than revenge on the bachelor of the title and his friend Chatfree, who have come down in history as two of the nastiest men in eighteenth-century Chester.

PP's reflective side is based on telling the simple facts of her situation, and one version of the poem on her blindness is even called "Consolatory Reflections":

> My rip'ning joys, by stern misfortune cross'd,
> Thus blasted seem'd, and I to pleasure lost:
> And to myself I many times have said,
> Now all intrinsic satisfaction's fled;
> Of various comforts, what a curious store,
> By me, must now alas! be view'd no more!
> So simple and so ignorant was I,
> A truth so flagrant let me not deny.[6]

Exactly how repeating the fact that she will never again receive pleasure from seeing things can be a consolation is explained in the rest of the poem in which she claims devoutly if rather tritely: "Yea, though he slay me, in my God I'll trust, / Who's infinitely wise, and good, and just."[7] Stronger are the lines on her resignation to her situation when she draws a parallel between Eve's seeing, desiring, and being "wretchedly enthrall'd" by the "transient, vain and trifling" "External object," the apple, from which she concludes, perhaps with some pause: "Wherefore, in some respects, (if well we mind) / Tis an advantage, truly, to be blind."[8] If Eve had been blind, she would not have fallen into temptation.

In the main, PP's work expresses both sides of the doubleness of her character together, as in a poem to a friend:

> But how I do, will strait prepare to tell—
> Know then, my friend, sometimes I gay appear,
> Sometimes, as usual, Prissy's low, my dear;
> Each place does spirits much avail,
> I'm under deck, or else top-gallant sail.
> You'll smile at this, and think my humour strange,
> Because alas! thus subject I'm to change:
> Pardon in me this wonderful defect;
> Tho' mutable, I seem in some respect,
> Yet know, dear madam, I will ever be
> Your's to command—and much oblig'd P.P.[9]

When we search her writing for an understanding of herself as a blind woman, therefore, we must navigate a careful course between these two poles, avoiding reading her as either a Pollyanna or an Eeyore. I choose two such obviously one-dimensional fictional characters to remind us that PP was a real person faced with a real dilemma: how to care for herself financially as a blind woman who presumably did not expect to enter the marriage market but whose family could not or would not help her after her parents' death.

PP addressed only two members of her immediate family in her poems, her brother, Ned, in the 1770 collection and, in her second collection that was published in 1794, her sister, Maria. Ned became a ship's surgeon,[10] so must have been away from Britain for much of the time and is not mentioned in the second collection. Maria, married to a farmer, refused two invitations to come to Chester, one of which was to PP's wedding.[11] Behind the three children, and perhaps accounting for much of their behavior, is "Mamma," whom PP never addressed directly, but whose presence looms like a malignant ghost in the otherwise jovial 1770 poem to her brother on her arrival in Chester. "Mamma" comes across as something rather sinister: something of an Aunt Read to PP's Jane Eyre. However, PP's own lines on her "Mamma" are freighted with very unfilial thoughts that suggest the old woman was a valetudinarian:

> But first my duty to Mamma must give—
> May Heaven grant her health and long to live;
> When to this transient world she bids adieu,
> Crown her with joy that's ever, ever new![12]

It might be thought that this reading is going a bit far, but I would argue, and will argue below, that PP is always direct in the moment of writing and does not hide her emotions. Wishing her mother "long to live" in one line is all well and good, but wishing her joy in death equally suggests Mamma's ghoulish character, or at least PP's thought that her mother's devoutness hid her away from the "giddy world" which she really wanted to experience, and did experience while on her tour of the Midlands of England. How PP managed to escape from her "convent" of a family home to travel so widely to collect subscriptions cannot be imagined, but much of her enthusiasm in her early verse is likely due to newly tasted freedom, as she writes to her brother, Ned:

> Thou best of brothers, and thou truest friend,
> Forbear to chide the simple strain I send;
> My infant Muse, say now, dear Ned, you'll spare,
> For scarce three months I've known myself this Fair.
> To such a stranger sure you'll candour shew,
> Tho' rustic now—she may improve, you know—[13]

This verse epistle, sent from Chester, where the Pointon family had relations,[14] tells us she had been away from Lichfield for three months and suggests that she is finding a new language free of former criticism, perhaps from her mother, who, if the example of the "Consolatory Reflections" is to be believed, allowed her to write only religious poetry. If this verse epistle was for the private consumption of her brother, the second to him, on his appointment to the navy, is stilted and appears to have been written to be read out in front of their martinet of a parent:

> Though, Brother, you in busy life now are,
> Let Heav'n alone be your peculiar care;
> Then to your wish, propitious Fate, my dear,
> May grant you health, and friends that are sincere.[15]

There is little of sibling affection in a single line of the poem, and it is noticeable that she no longer asks him to spare her criticism as though another unnamed but expected listener can brook nothing but perfection. But free from Lichfield, and presumably her mother, the way she regards herself in terms of poetry is as a natural genius whose muse poured forth grateful verse in a proto-romantic vein, as she speaks extempore "On Gratitude":

> Superior Bards, no doubt, wou'd better fit;
> Let then their sheets with lofty language swell,
> In mine, simplicity be seen to dwell:
> Nor need I blush to own I nothing know,
> But what from Nature does spontaneous flow:

> Nature 'tis true, from every art is free,
> Yet by the Candid oft admir'd we see.[16]

For a blind poet, her writing would necessarily be a spontaneous overflow as she could not review the lines she had spoken other than by hearing them again and again, read by her amanuensis, a process which precludes minor alterations. As Jess Domanico points out, "A brief overview of Poynton's canon of poetry might suggest that she does not, in fact, read her own narrative through the act of composition, but instead simply replies to friends and acquaintances or responds to their wish for her to recite her work."[17] This would certainly account for the fact that most of her poems are in the form of verse epistles, first noted by Bill Overton.[18] Her method of composition also accounts for repeated words and phrases such as "simple" to describe herself or her work,[19] "the Nine [muses],"[20] and the overreliance on reference to other blind poets such as Milton and Homer.[21]

Adding together the ideas of her forgetting to write to friends, her writing as "spontaneous overflow," its occasional nature in her verse epistles, and her repetition of herself, we can begin to draw together some account of how PP understood her self-presence in her poems as a woman who lived fully in the moment, without thought of people or places not in her immediate vicinity.

Thus, the poem to the bachelor, "On a Delicate Occasion," might have been funny in its context of utterance, but in the published collection that gentleman would have found himself described in a very poor light. As would Lister Dighton's goddaughter Lucy Mason, who is described as poor company:

> Know first of all, to L.D.'s house I came,
> And who I ask'd for there, I need not name;
> The hour-glass near twice its course had run,
> Before the nymph, to welcome me, did come;
> And when, at length, she did on me attend,
> All hopes of pleasure disappear'd, my friend;—
> So flat her converse, and so grave her air,
> Instead of nineteen, ninety did appear;
> Wednesday and Thursday, with her stupid past.[22]

Other victims of PP's pen who might not have been happy to read of themselves are "a Young tradesman, Who complained that he had secretly languished for a Lady of Distinction ... without the least hope of a favourable return";[23] PP's accuser in "The Author, one evening, in company with some gentlemen, repeated a Poem of her own composition; when one of them was so cruel to tell her, her boasted Muse was borrowed, without being able to give the least account from whom or where: she being something chagrin'd at his unjust censure, in less than an hour sent him the following lines";[24] the infantilised "Master Jemmy ——, in his 32nd Year. An Extempore Epistle";[25] and even one named victim, Francis Grapel, "a young Gentleman, who, after a long correspondence with the Author, in poetic strain, voluntarily offer'd (when she publish'd) to return all those lines she had so obligingly favour'd him with: and he coming to see her a few months after she had begun her subscription, earnestly requested him to perform his promise, to which he shewed some reluctance; but after a short pause, he sneeringly reply'd, That in a few days she might depend upon him sending back all her empty Verse, as he was then pleas'd to phrase it";[26] an unnamed doctor, "a young Surgeon who had repeatedly broke his promise to the Author";[27] and finally, "a Bachelor who daily visited the Author before he went House-keeping."[28]

To include one attack on a close friend who had perhaps wounded her greatly might be excused, but eight in a collection of no more than one hundred pages suggests that PP might be labeled vindictive. The idea might be countered with the evidence of so many others of her poems which demonstrate a loving and caring nature, such as those giving "advice to a gay Bachelor, upon the Marriage State,"[29] and the heartrending pair of poems on the deaths of William Barker, who was "cast away, in crossing the River Weaver, a day or two before he was to have been married to an amiable young lady,"[30] and his sweetheart Anne Gaman,[31] who appears to have died of a broken heart. Similar such testimony to her kind nature is PP's ability to maintain the long-term and long-distance, if intermittent, friendship with Maria Lloyd, as well as with James Pickering, who would become her husband in 1780, twelve years after she met him in Chester.

One might suggest that the revenge and the friendship poems demonstrated the "top gallant" and "under deck" sides of her character. But all these explanations avoid the empirical fact of her blindness and the effect it might well have had on her sense of language in its spoken and written forms. The two types of poem might well exist side by side due to the fact that PP had no conception of the power of printed words to draw out the effect of the spoken moment of anger, sadness, or happiness. She could not conceive how printed words allowed a momentary situation to linger and bring old memories to life, she had no experience of how other people who were not present at an occasion might recognise the person she chided for saying or doing something stupid, and she did not understand how her most private feelings would become open to her mother when the book was in print no matter how much she hid them when they were in her carefully chosen amanuensis's hand.

To which it might be replied, how could she? For PP, poetry was extempore; it lasted in the moment of her speaking its words, as briefly as the emotions of anger, sadness, and happiness they expressed. And though she might repeat a few words or clenches between her verses that did not matter because words for PP were only spoken, as it were, into the wind and blown away like the few seconds of anger, sadness, and happiness they expressed.

Thus, rather than reading PP as vindictive or victim, Pollyanna or Eeyore, we might understand her as a blind woman doing what she could do, composing poetry, and in the event making enough money to buy a house in Saughall, some five miles outside Chester. But only after the disaster of publication, after which it would appear that her Mamma read the collection and shut her up in a convent. If that is what happened, and it is granted that PP did not understand the power and permanence of words.

This idea of PP is supported by the evidence her poems give about her courtship of and by James Pickering and their ultimate marriage at least twelve years after they met, which reads like the combination of both love affairs in Shakespeare's *Much Ado about Nothing* in all its twists and turns.

James Pickering

We know four facts about James Pickering: his name is in the subscription list of the 1770 collection, two advertisements in Chester newspapers mention his name,[32] the second being the announcement of his marriage to PP, and their marriage license.[33] And if we read the four facts alongside the poems addressed to James Pickering, and in the order in which they are printed across the two volumes, we get a picture of a tempestuous courtship between PP and James Pickering that required two deaths to lead eventually to a happy and fruitful marriage. At the same time, the poems give us some understanding of the experience of a blind woman who wrestled with the fact that her lack of sight excluded her from marriage.

The group of poems to James Pickering in the 1770 collection might be called the "courting" poems, and those in the 1794 collection the "marriage" poems. While only one in the earlier collection is indubitably directed to him, "An Invitation to J.P., written Extempore,"[34] his status as addressee of the others can be convincingly argued from circumstantial evidence. In the 1794 collection there are two poems addressed to "J.P." in the form of valentines. The first, "Valentine, On a Leap Year,"[35] addresses her husband, whom she calls "Strephon":

> Ev'ry grace will I study, my mind for to dress,
> That the hour Hymen join'd us he may ever bless.
> His converse I'll wisely prefer, Sir, to all;
> And scorn all those cheats the world pleasure does call:
> Abroad for amusement I seldom will roam,
> Thrice happy the pair, that are pleas'd best at home.[36]

The second, "To Mr J.P. On Drawing him Four Years Successively for a Valentine" recalls the poem in the 1770 collection "A Valentine, Extempore; On Drawing a young Gentleman three times successively.'" Thus, it is out of the question to argue that all the poems which use the word "Valentine" in the title are addressed to James Pickering as are the 1770 poems which also address "Strephon": "A Pastoral Piece," and "The following Advice to a gay Bachelor, upon the Marriage State."[37]

Likewise, since the poem in the 1770 collection which addresses "J.P." in the title is an invitation, it is also likely that the male "friend" in the title of another invitation, "The following Invitation, Extempore. To a Friend," is James Pickering. The courtship poems which add to the description of James Pickering but are less certain ascriptions are "Mr. Trueworth" in the "Address to a Bachelor," and the much less complimentary: "To Master Jemmy ———, in his 32nd Year. An Extempore Epistle," which describes a man tied to his mother's apron strings. But in this poem, I shall argue, we find further reason why PP waited twelve years before she married him.

I use the expression "further reason" as there are no grounds to believe that PP ever regarded marriage as a prospect. The first poem to James Pickering declares that although on Valentine's Day it is an ancient courting custom for women to address themselves to men: "Mine is but Friendship, others may be love."[38] On one level, PP's attitude derives directly from the strong vein of writing against submitting themselves to men in marriage that marks much of eighteenth-century women's verse:

> But once wed, we find it to our cost,
> That in the wife the goddess soon is lost:
> No more you sigh, no more in transport view,
> For strait we're mortals, and mere husbands you.[39]

But at the same time PP recognizes both that while she can love, she cannot believe those who claim to love her:

> With me, ye Pow'rs! let friendship ever reign,
> I ask no more, nor let me ask in vain:
> For shou'd I love, and meet with no return,
> How wou'd my bosom, like to *Sappho*, burn!
> Pity on me, perhaps they might bestow,
> But pity cannot ease the pangs of woe.[40]

These lines do not resound with self-pity and weakness of resolve but rather begin to give us something of the experience of a blind woman who has met more often with the pity of others than with their friendship, let alone their love.

Thus, in her valentines PP offers friendship and not love to James Pickering with the aim of avoiding the pain of unrequited love, and at the same time the withdrawal from love means she can continue to wield her poetic pen. In effect the poems create a space for her as a blind "seer" who can write commentaries on the people around her, and on men in particular, with whom she will interact as an equal:

Nay, dare to tell us in provoking strain,
That over woman, man was born to reign;
Him to obey shou'd be her chiefest care:
Adieu—P.P. such dire thoughts can't bear.[41]

Disguised beneath the bravado of the surface of the poem is the fear of a blind woman that she might never be able to participate in the sexual world because of her blindness. This is not an aspect of the cultural model of disability since it is a simple fact of blindness that you cannot see when a person loves you. If you are a sighted reader, remember that a blind person cannot see the tiny gestures and facial expressions of love that convince, but only hear the blandishments that words might belie. In the two poles of bravado and fear, we are introduced to the action of her "wonderful defect" in her changeable complex moods from "under deck" to "top gallant," a confession which could only be made to a woman friend. But this was a confession which was made in private to a woman friend. When it became public in printed words, such candor was extraordinary and probably the unique selling point of the 1770 collection.

Giving herself the authority to comment on men accounts for her preference for writing to male addressees, as it does her tendency to chide them, which we saw above in the two poems to men whom she thought had been rude to her. Likewise, she scolds her host in "Address to a Bachelor, who sneered:

... Dear Miss, make free;
Let me conduct you—don't be nice—
Or if a bason is your choice,
To fetch you one I'll instant fly.[42]

In this poem, once again, we might also understand PP's boisterous retelling of the incident as both a scold and as a disguise for her fear that as a blind woman she cannot look after herself even in a most basic function as going to the toilet. An unspoken implication of her host's offer to take her to the privy or bring her a "bason" is that she might at least offer herself sexually: as her forwardness of character and her preference for all-male company might suggest.[43] The implication is confirmed by the appellation of her host's friend "Chatfree," a character from Eliza Haywood's 1751 novel *The Adventures of Miss Betsy Thoughtless*. Chatfree is a stock, comic, theater villain who first appears in a scene in which Betsy, like PP, finds herself a lone woman in all-male company. In the novel, Mr. Goodman reproves Betsy in no uncertain terms, telling her that she "ought to have left the abbey as soon as divine service was ended;—that for a person of her sex, age, and appearance, to walk in a place where there were always a great concourse of young sparks, who come for no other purpose than to make remarks upon the ladies, could not but be looked on as very odd by all who saw her."[44]

Betsy's response to Goodman is to blush "not through a conscious shame of imagining what she had done deserved the least rebuke, but because her spirit, yet unbroke, could not bear controul."[45] PP's response to the sneering of her host and "Chatfree" is to accept the offer of help to the privy by James Pickering, who fulfils the role of "Trueworth," the hero of *Betsy Thoughtless*, whom she marries in the last chapter: "To go with me, Miss, don't refuse, / Your loss this freedom will excuse."[46] Where Mr. Goodman is reproving, Trueworth, who is called "all that could make us truly happy"[47] in Haywood's novel, lives up to this description in PP's poem. He understands her predicament and offers her practical and lighthearted help to "lose" her urine without losing face.

While I would not suggest that PP lived her life through the lens of romantic comedy, the final paragraph of Haywood's novel is telling: "Thus were the virtues of our heroine, (those follies that had defaced them being fully corrected) at length rewarded with a happiness, retarded only till she had render'd herself wholly worthy of receiving it."[48] For PP, the defacement of her virtue was not correctable; it was her blindness. And it was this that she sold in her verses: her readers "simply" had to accept her for what she was. As would her own Mr. Trueworth.

The placing of the next poem in the collection, "To Master Jemmy ——, in his 32nd Year. An Extempore Epistle," which I believe also to be addressed to James Pickering,[49] offers a more fully rounded picture of the man whom she would marry: for how many men are really thoroughgoing Trueworths? Nor does the addressee of the poem in the least resemble the eponymous hero of Haywood's last novel, *The History of Jemmy and Jenny*

Jessamy, of 1753. Where Jemmy Jessamy's casual sexuality is expected of his unmarried state, PP's "Jemmy ——" is described as childish, delighted by childish toys, and still living with his mother. To be sure, PP's line, "Nay, a whistle I'll buy you, and a hobby-horse too," can at a pinch be read as metaphors for sexual peccadilloes, as can her suggestion that "boys like apes, mischievous will be,"[50] but I doubt that the woman who wrote that, after marriage, "strait we're mortals, and mere husbands you" could ever agree with Lady Speck's explanation to Jenny Jessamy that she must accept Jemmy's sexual infidelity before marriage: "If criminal in no greater matters than a transient amour, . . . I think you might forgive him without putting him to the penance even of a blush by your reproaches.—In good truth we women have nothing to do with the men's affairs in this point before marriage:—and as I now begin to believe, in spite of all I have heard to the contrary, that he addresses no other woman than yourself upon honourable terms, these are but venial transgressions, which you ought to overlook until you have made him your own."[51]

Instead we are presented on the surface with an affectionate chiding of "Jemmy," who has failed to remember to return a book PP lent him. The effect is something like Virginia Woolf's scolding of E. M. Forster for spending too much time rowing his mother and aunt around the Serpentine, concerned that he has his mind on the wrong thing. So, unsurprisingly, there is another and perhaps not unexpected meaning to the poem, that Jemmy is spending far too much time looking for his mother's approval:

> To bring it yourself I darn't ask you to do,
> As I fear to offend your Mamma, it is true; . . .
> Then quickly reply, if this is your case;
> If it is, child, sincerely I wish you more grace.[52]

Mrs. Pickering's name is not included on the subscription list, and it is not out of the realm of possibility that she told her son that PP was not a fit wife, perhaps because she was blind or perhaps because she purposefully made a spectacle of herself performing on her "grand tour" and was too "forward." Following this interpretation of these lines, we can find a reason she chose the reduction "Jemmy ——" for James Pickering. While there may be no resemblance between the two Jemmys, there is, as underlies most comedy, a serious shared message in both PP and Haywood. Haywood outlines her message midway through the novel:

> According to all the observations which reason and a long experience has enabled me to make, happiness is a thing which ought to be totally erased out of the vocabulary of sublunary enjoyments;—the human heart is liable to so many passions, and the events of fortune so uncertain and precarious, that life is little more than a continued series of anxieties and suspence:— what we pursue as the ultimate of our desires, the summum bonum of all our wishes, fleets before us, dances in the wind, seems at sometimes ready to meet our grasp, at others soaring quite out of our reach; or, when attain'd, deceives our expectations, baffles our high-raised hopes, and shews the fancy'd heaven a mere vapour.[53]

I think we can read this disappointment in the whole poem about James Pickering as childish, and especially in PP's words, "I wish you more grace." She knows that she cannot hope to win the battle with James Pickering's mother for his attention, and that even if she does, she worries the marriage might not be quite what she could hope.

If the poem "To Master Jemmy ——, in his 32nd Year. An Extempore Epistle" demonstrates both "top gallant" and "under deck" in its levels of meaning, so does the next in the collection, and it is the only one that is unequivocally addressed to "J.P." In "An Invitation, To J.P. Written Extempore,"[54] PP asks James Pickering to join her for tea with "Lovely Miss L. and N.," "Mr. J. W. and likewise S.P." "Miss L." is most likely Maria Lloyd, and "Miss N." is probably "Miss Rebecca Nowell" from the subscription list. She is possibly the daughter of James Newell, Peruke Maker, Prince's St. Chester, or William or Robert Newell, Skinners and Corn Dealers, Lower Bridge St. Chester, or William Newill Victualler, Foregate St. Chester. "S.P." is probably Steven Palin, the Postmaster, from Northgate Street, Chester and "J.W." either John Watson, Excise Officer, Queen's Street, Chester, or John Wright, Tanner, Foregate Street, Chester, all from the subscription list and Bailey's Directory.

It is probable that all three men of the group were unmarried and over thirty: they are successful and listed in Bailey's Directory as professionals or as the proprietors of businesses. PP was unmarried and twenty-nine or thirty, and so, probably, were the other two women in the party. James Pickering is asked to bring his "*German* flute" as PP "has promis'd to sing," and the party looks very sedate and aboveboard. However, once again, the poem gives away more about PP's feelings for James Pickering than the scene suggests.

First, we must note that this is the only invitation of the five to have been published in the volume, which would suggest it was special to PP. Second, the invitation ends with the lines:

> Adieu, I'm in haste to dress for these Smarts,
> If I please but their eyes, I'll unseen steal their hearts:
> Perhaps you will say I've no right but to one,
> But you've nothing to fear, as your own, Sir, is gone.[55]

This suggests that James Pickering's heart is engaged and possibly by PP, but they are not unequivocal. His heart is "gone" but not "mine," and the poet has flirtatiously suggested that if she dresses well she can, though blind, "steal" the hearts of the other two men at the party. Perhaps James Pickering has told her that he loves someone else, or this is further reference to his relationship with his mother: both are possible reasons for this curious use of the word "gone." But we can take the reading no further, other than to suggest that the animosity between James Pickering's mother and PP was the impediment and the reason why they waited until 1780 to marry.

Whatever the future might hold, the next poem in the collection marks a change of heart in PP and brings a note of resignation in her attitude toward its addressee. "A Valentine, Extempore; On drawing a young Gentleman three times successively,"[56] dramatizes the Valentine's Day tradition of drawing names from a lottery of handwritten names to find the one who will become your sweetheart for a year. It is most probably addressed to James Pickering as it recalls the poem in PP's second collection mentioned above, where she draws "J.P.'s" name on four consecutive years.[57] However, in this poem PP draws a name three times in one day:

> Believe me, Sir, Dame Fortune does decree,
> That none but you my Valentine must be;

> Amidst a score your name I careless threw,
> And from that number thrice your name I drew.[58]

Giving the choice of her sweetheart to "Dame Fortune" is somewhat ironic since Fortuna, like PP, is blind. But the choice of the blind goddess as guide for the blind woman both gives and takes away from the fact that James Pickering's name has been drawn three times. That "Dame Fortune" has chosen the name suggests both a vain hope that it might confirm that the person drawn is really in love with her as well as the resignation that drawing valentines is only a game and the blind goddess can see nothing of the future. The two thoughts read together through the rest of the poem suggest desperation, so much so that, rather than developing new thoughts about love, the poem is separated between reiterating PP's themes of the benefits of friendship over love:

> 'Tis friendship, Sir, glows in my virgin breast,
> No affectation e'er my soul possess'd.

and the preference of a woman for the single life, where:

> No blustring husband then can cry Obey,
> Or over me rule with tyrannic sway.

With this new resolution, PP now turns her poems to addressing advice to a niece on entering her teens and retires to the country.[59] It may well be to the woman with whom she stayed on her country retreat that the lines about her "wonderful defect" were composed. Thus, her description of her mood swings from "under decks" to "top gallant" may be a reference to her hope and disappointment in her relationship with James Pickering.

It may or may not be valid to read the poems as a diary in the order in which they appear in the collection, but I believe we can because of the logic of the poems as verse epistles concerning specific people in specific situations and because a logic of narrative and context has begun to appear in those poems addressed to James Pickering that on wider consideration appears to be consistent throughout, if consistent in the inconsistency of their love.

Thus, the narrative of the collection suggests it is safe to argue that it was only after her retreat to the country that PP addressed him once more. This very fact suggests that she had been extremely upset by what had happened between them and that the valentine had been bravado. The final poem she wrote to him, "The following Advice to a gay Bachelor, upon the Marriage State,"[60] suggests he find someone else to marry while holding a hint of regret.

> But while you emulate the Bee,
> Real happiness you ne'er will see;
> Wed, Strephon, then, ere 'tis too late,
> And you shall own, in single state,
> A joy that's true you never found,
> 'Till you in HYMEN's bands were bound;
> There mutual friendship ever dwell
> Beyond what I have skill to tell:[61]

After leaving Chester, PP stayed for a few months in Staffordshire at a house called Biana,[62] returned home to Lichfield, from which she wrote of being in a convent because she was separated from James Pickering by distance as well as by inclination:

> So long a Convent now hath been my lot,
> Folly and men by me are quite forgot;
> For Nuns devotion must prefer to all,
> Nay scorn those cheats the world does pleasure call;
> At this methinks I hear you warmly cry,
> Prissy a Nun! no, rather first she'll die;[63]

But we must pause at these lines. PP is adamant that she "Hates it [pleasure] and Men, as Misers do their gold," but the simile is an odd one: misers love their gold but hate to spend it. The suggestion appears to be that PP is still enamored of James Pickering despite being distanced from him because of the intervention of both their mothers.

If this reasoning gestures toward the truth, it would follow that her purchase of a house in Saughall, which is mentioned in the poem "A Journal from Lichfield to Chester,"[64] was made not just so PP could live near her Chester relatives (the poem is addressed to her niece) and her friend

Maria Lloyd, but so that she can be near, although not too near, James Pickering. Thus, it is probable that PP's Mamma died first, releasing her from her Lichfield convent, and she bought the house near Chester to be far enough away from James Pickering's mother. Evidence suggests that the house was bought before PP was married: in "A Journal" she calls it "My house at Saughall then my care," and it was from this house that the wedding party set off in "Letter to a Sister Giving an Account of the Author's Wedding-Day,"[65] whence the same poem tells of their return to "our house." This latter house must be in Chester rather than Saughall as it would be inconvenient for a tradesman like James Pickering to live five miles away from his work.

These poems both come from the 1794 collection, which does not offer up its riches so readily to a biographical narrative. A brief study of its genesis accounts for the arrangement, form, and content of the poems being so different from the 1770 collection. The 1770 collection was printed in Birmingham "for the Author" by T. Warren, whose other publications date between 1733 and 1770. The 1794 collection was edited by Joseph Weston, printed in Birmingham by E. Piercy, "And Sold by J. Johnson, St Paul's Churchyard, London." Why PP chose to publish the second collection in Birmingham when she lived in Chester, some one hundred miles away, is mysterious. There was a logic to publishing the first in the geographical center of her subscription tour, but there was no such tour for the second collection. Joseph Weston, the editor, explains in his preface that PP had approached him before the death of her husband with a letter of recommendation from John Morfitt asking him to "forward her subscription, to the utmost of my power." Apparently, Weston did nothing about it until PP visited him again after James Pickering died, this time to ask Weston to "prepare [her] works for the Press." But the publication was "retarded by obstacles almost insurmountable."[66] Rather than going on tour and reciting her work, this time PP is recorded as having relied on passing copies of her poems around to potential subscribers: a much less efficacious business model. There is no subscription list printed in the second collection, although Weston writes that the book had to be published, and in the form it appeared to satisfy subscribers. In the event, passing around the copies of her poems meant "that the fatal THUMB had made more havoc with *words* than its redoubted NAMESAKE with *Giants*. Numbers were mutilated, and numbers destroyed."[67] Furthermore, Weston complains of having the gout, which prevented him from doing the transcriptions, additions, and emendations. For this reason, PP's choice of Birmingham for printing is the more curious. There were printers in Chester capable of the job, and where manuscripts were illegible she could have recited her poems again to an amanuensis with both near at hand to the printer.

Who Joseph Weston was is also uncertain. I cannot locate his name anywhere else in eighteenth-century publishing, and he was unknown to PP before her introduction by John Morfitt. Weston records that PP approached him, saying, "I have not a Friend in the world, who can undertake the office, unless you will prove that Friend."[68] It is likely therefore that Weston had been known to John Morfitt as an editor. The poems Weston added to the collection, some of which were reconstructions of copies of PP's poems that were so damaged as to be unreadable, demonstrate that he was not untalented in his own right. It is very probable that his other publications were from Birmingham and will be rediscovered in due course.

John Morfitt was an attorney, the author of a number of king-and-country pamphlets under the pseudonym of "Job Nott, button burnisher," who regularly attacked Joseph Priestley in the press as he does in one of the poems in this collection.[69] What is difficult to determine is his relationship with PP. He may have been the Pointon family lawyer, he may have drawn up some sort of legal document for the first subscription list, he may have been trustee of the money collected, but this must remain a surmise for the present. Weston tells us that Morfitt originally offered nineteen poems to fill up the collection but was prevailed upon to add a further twenty-four. Weston himself mended four of PP's verses and added a further seven of his own. In all, the book is made up of sixty-eight pages of poems by PP, seventy-nine by John Morfitt, and thirty-six by Joseph Weston, each separately paginated.

Further differentiating the 1794 collection from the earlier is the lack of the authorial voice in the long titles which in effect turned nearly all the 1770 poems into verse epistles by providing the contexts of utterance, the situation of the addressee, and the author's state of mind when she replied. In the later collection, we do not have, for example, the vehement avowal that she was the author of a poem she recited that someone had claimed was not her own, which was followed by a poem full of hurt pride, from which the authorship of the disputed poem could not be ascertained.[70] Nevertheless, when in the preface to the second collection Weston draws our attention to the question over her authorship of the two poems addressed to her niece, we get a nugget of biographical fact. His excuse for publishing the second of the disputed poems, which is certainly not PP's,[71] is that James Pickering was "unwilling that one couplet of his beloved Wife's should be lost to the world."[72] The statement tells us more about the marriage than it does about the authorship of the verses, giving us James Pickering's unfaltering pride in his wife's work, albeit she only smoothed out some of the original poem's bumpy meter.

The level of James Pickering's pride in his wife's work adds a new aspect to our reading of their faltering steps to marriage. Why would he, who was so blind to criticism of PP, not marry her the instant they met? Their wedding day is described in detail in "Letter to a Sister Giving an Account of the Author's Wedding Day,"[73] which tells of a full day's celebrations beginning at Saughall, the short journey to St. Michael, Shotwick, for the ceremony, and the longer journey to Parkgate for the wedding breakfast before going home to Chester via the village of Two Mills. But in the lines addressing her sister, there are clues as to why the two may not have married earlier, and they tell of a new set of obstacles from those apparent in the earlier collection. PP begins the poem admonishing her sister for not attending the wedding or even writing to congratulate her:

> Your silence, Dear Sister, I justly will chide,
> Since ten months ago I became I.P's bride;
> Nor need I to doubt but the same you must know;
> Each Paper through Britain announc'd it was so
> Which made me expect you wou'd congratulate,
> In Sister-like manner, my new change of state.[74]

PP is distressed by her sister's failure to attend, but we are told the reason why in the final lines of the same poem—snobbery:

> Methinks, I by this, hear you cry with a sneer,
> "Lord bless me! what wonders one may live to hear!
> "That thus my gay Sister should sudden'y change!"
> Get married, Maria,—you'll not think it strange;
> The old maxim you'll find to hold good, I am sure,
> That "Home still is Home, be it ever so poor;"
> But, if it's a good one, what can we wish more?[75]

In Maria Pointon's snobbish mind, to marry a tradesman was beneath her sister. To be sure, James Pickering's parlous financial status is raised in a poem addressed to "my friend" which appears later in the collection. "The Author's Choice of a Husband," describes a man of education and moderation but ends with the lines:

> I hear you, at this, methinks, sneeringly say,
> Can merit supply all our wants every day—
> That frequently thread-bare is known to appear?
> Have Patience; I'd wish him five hundred a year.[76]

PP continued to try to convince her sister that she should be friends with James Pickering. "Extempore Epistle Occasioned by my Sister neither Writing nor Coming agreeably as promised" begins: "You said, Maria, that you would be here, / Before the summer had expir'd my dear!"[77] The couplet would suggest that Maria Pointon answered the marriage verse epistle saying she would come but failed once again to be as good as her word. What galls PP the more in this verse epistle is that Maria's silence manifested itself as rudeness to her husband:

> And since my consort kindly wrote to you,
> And said he should rejoice to see you too,
> To him at least you might have sent a line;
> If I've offended all the fault was mine:[78]

The exchange of letters between the sisters sets up the question: Would a family which (putatively) boasted a captain, a ship's surgeon, and the wife of a landowning gentleman among its members regard the marriage of a blind sibling to a tradesman as socially awkward?[79] In the poem about her wedding, none of her own family is mentioned as being in attendance. Nevertheless, the wedding poem notes one significant change which suggests that my earlier idea that PP and James Pickering were not married as he was advised against it by his mother may indeed be correct: "And my Husband's Step-Mother attended the Bride."[80]

It may have been that PP and James Pickering waited for his father to remarry before they tied the knot. Courses of events seldom happen for a single reason, and a combination of the two—the pride of the wife's family and the prejudice of the husband's mother—might easily account for lovers being kept apart for ten years. Once again, I would argue that this is not a version of the cultural model of disability but an account of what did happen to PP.

And marry they did, though they appear to have lived in penury. PP's line about wishing her husband "five hundred a year" impresses the suggestion that the couple were probably in financial difficulties when the second collection was commissioned. If James Pickering Senior married again, he might have had a young family to look after, and with four other "sadlers" trading in Chester, there might not have been enough business. The subscription for the first collection had brought in nearly £400, from which she had been able to buy a house, but the remainder cannot have been enough to keep the couple even if it had been well invested. Furthermore, PP's poem "On the Deadness of Trade in Birmingham"[81] suggests that a similar economic downturn might have happened in Chester: a recession which would have affected both her husband's business and her own investments, if she had any. Whatever caused her financial difficulties, Joseph Weston describes her in a "desolate situation" after "her irremediable calamity,"[82] James Pickering's death.

It would appear, then, that we can construct a narrative about the publication of the second collection of poems. PP approached John Morfitt at the suggestion of her husband, who was "unwilling that one couplet of his beloved Wife's should be lost to the world." Morfitt introduced her to Joseph Weston, whom she visited before and again after her husband's death, whence the collection and its potential revenues were more necessitous. Weston took up his pen only when gout allowed him to hold it, more than a year after PP's visit. He had been given a number of damaged copies of poems from which he made fair copies of thirty-six, which was not enough to publish as a collection. He mended four more that were added to his own six as "Additional Poems," which along with the forty-two "Poetical Sketches" by John Morfitt made up the volume. This meant that the book, although sold as *Poems by Mrs. Pickering,* was, in fact, weighted more to Weston and Morfitt, for the sole reason that PP continued to live in Chester and out of easy reach of Weston, to whom she might have dictated more.

The process was exacerbated by the state of the copies that were given to him; however, where Weston suggests that PP's poems were illegible because they had been passed around to potential subscribers, it is quite as likely that some were early versions or alternate versions of poems published as early as the first collection. For example, the two poetic invitations to James Pickering, one in each collection and each placed at page 33, appear to be versions of one another.

I have noted above the ironic tone of the one in the 1770 collection, with its reminder to James Pickering that his heart is "gone." That in the 1794 collection shares the same rhythmic and rhyme pattern of four beats a line in couplets, and the first part of each, if not identical, uses the same ideas and groups of words: "Crown'd with glee," "your German flute," PP's singing, music's charms, "wit," and dressing up. The endings are not similar: the first tells how PP will flirt with the other men and take their hearts; the second evokes Urania, the muse of astronomy and philosophy, over Venus, the goddess of love, in order that she can remain chaste like Diana. Both ask James Pickering to reply, the first with its ironic edge, and the second telling "Strephon" he must come "Lest you sigh, when too late, for neglecting the fair." Neither poem can therefore be called unalloyed in its conviction of how the summons will be received and acted upon by its recipient, and what differentiates them is that in the first, PP determines to play the flirt, whereas in the second, she will maintain chastity, which will grant her poetic skill. It is in these respects, I would argue, that the poems might be read as variations of each other and, further, might be argued to give us an understanding of the way in which PP composed her poems.

Whereas sighted writers tend to compose with paper and pen, crossing out wrong directions, PP's composition was "Extempore," that is, unscripted, but not, I would argue, unplanned. The two invitations use not only the same rhythmic pattern and couplets but also the same ideas at the beginning and end equivocally, and to that formula PP adds particulars from a stock of ideas she was wont to use. In the 1770 invitation, we have recourse to initials of names, "Miss L.," "Miss N.," "J.W.," and "S.P."; in the one from 1794, we have the use of the idea that if she remains chaste she will not lose her poetic gift. It is as though PP made up her poems from a common stock, threading the ideas like ready-made beads to make a whole with rhythm that varied only in the number of beats in a line and in rhyming couplets. What we have of her poetry, then, is a series of records of moments in the lives of each poem as they changed and metamorphosed, that have by chance been copied down by an amanuensis. Their lack of originality, it might be argued, suggested that PP lacked poetic vision, and this is in reality exactly so: she does not write sighted verse that she can review word for word, but as she goes through her life with its repeated birthdays and parties that call forth a verse, she reminds us that these occasions are all versions of one another.

An Invitation to Mr. J.P. Written Extempore. 1770
As it's holiday-time, if you'll come we'll be gay,
Lovely Miss L. and N. I expect them at tea.
Mr. J.W. and likewise S.P.
You will meet them both here, my friend, crown'd with glee.
If agreeable, Sir, your *German* flute bring,
And a music-book too, since I've promis'd to sing;
For music's soft charms can enliven the soul,
Whilst the fair sprightly' Wit makes old TIME rapid roll:
In this joyous summons you dare to attend,
In verse, or in prose, a line quickly send.
Adieu, I'm in haste to dress for these Smarts,
If I please but their eyes, I'll unseen steal their hearts:
Perhaps you will say I've no right to but one,
But you've nothing to fear, as your own, Sir, is gone.

Invitation to the Author's Birth-day. 1794.
If you to my Birth-day politely will come,
Crown'd with glee and good humour, you'll find me at home.
Your German Flute with you I wish you would bring,
As it's sweet soothing strains may invite me to sing.
But, if with my voice I can't charm you, my friend,
I'll invoke all the graces their magic to lend;
Whilst with wit and good humour my converse I'll change,
Through all nature and art I'll endeavour to range.
Minerva, frown not, if I dare to aspire
To what virtue must love and what wisdom admire;
But deign with thy garlands my temples to bind,
And with graces internal embellish my mind!
And, would bright Urania but make me her care,
Proud Venus's gifts I will ne'er sigh to share;
Tho' beauty her lilies and roses may boast:
But charms that ne'er fade sure merit the toast.
To Diana's chaste altar my tribute I'll bring,
And deep will I drink of fair virtue's pure spring.
O Hasten then, Strephon, to friendship's fair court,
Where Mirth and where innocence, smiling resort;
Nor, sordidly, cry—you've no leisure to spare:
take counsel, be wise, and make merit your care—
Lest you sigh, when too late, for neglecting the fair.

Likewise, the two valentines to James Pickering already discussed, one in the 1770 and one in the 1794 collection, the first of which recalled drawing his name three times from the valentine lottery in one year, and the second drawing him in four consecutive years. Once again, each poem works with the same stock of ideas, the request to pardon the presumption of a woman courting a man, favoring intellect over beauty, the offer of friendship, the problem of marriage (Hymen and the Gordian knot), and a warning against how a couple might change for the worse when married. Once again, each poem is filled in with other ideas from PP's stock of images, for example the measuring of James Pickering's wealth being of the mind and not of the mining town (Potosi), in the 1794 valentine.

If this description of PP's method of writing is accurate, it may also be the reason why she felt she had to go to an editor with the copy for the second collection and gave Joseph Weston permission to "alter, expunge, and add whatsoever I thought proper."[83] For PP, as a blind poet, her verse was never fixed to an endpoint that was learned and recited; it was a set of ideas in her head that came out in rhythm and rhyme to fit with one of a series of similar but different situations, and in effect was always a verse epistle with addressor, addressee, and date. Where Jess Domanico argues that Pointon's "Consolatory Ode" on her blindness, of which we have three versions, "relies heavily on revising language to craft the poetic narrative of her experience as a blind poet,"[84] I would go further and suggest that for PP, the blind poet, language is not so much in "revision" (which suggests a visual metaphor) but is always malleable: it is always capable of being hammered into the shape of a verse with the addition of rhythm and rhyme to fit a new circumstance. For this reason, I would argue that we should reclassify all PP's poetry as verse epistles as they are all situational: all hammered into shape for an occasion.

Thus, we can find PP's place of safety in the form of her house in Saughall, five miles outside the bustle of Chester:

> Sigh not, my soul, though from gay life retired,
> Leave that for those by whom gay life's admired;
> While others boast the pleasures of the town,
> In rural life contented I'll sit down;
> Beneath the spreading oak there take my seat,
> With sportive lambs enjoy the calm retreat;
> Whilst tuneful songsters swell their willing throats,
> As if they meant to charm me with their notes;
> I'm pleas'd to smell the odours shed around,
> Whilst others view the gay enamell'd ground;
> For cou'd I see the butterfly appear,
> I then might think some shining Belle was near:
> Yet soon we find the flutterer disappear;

> In Contemplation let my minutes pass,
> And then I'll envy not the City Lass;
> Of all those joys, she with such rapture tells;
> In rural life, to me, more pleasures dwells.[85]

Similar to Maxwell and Gills, PP's place of safety was away from urban bustle of a big town; like Maxwell's, it lay in the sounds of the birds and the smells of the flowers, and like the places of safety of each of the other two, it lay in her own choosing.

In Lieu of a Cultural Model for Disability

If it were to be argued that each of the lives of the three blind people presented here was an example of the cultural model of disability since it is society's response to impaired people that makes them disabled, I would argue that this makes all people disabled. Society does not offer anyone smooth pathways to financial success, love, and happiness. Each of us must work toward what we want in whatever way we can, using the unique gifts we have. And we have read of Thomas Gills, John Maxwell, and Priscilla Pointon using their gifts of blindness to work toward their own personal goals and achieving them.

Nor can we discern any other pattern of social attitudes that shaped these three blind people's lives. Gills and Maxwell were religious and benefited from the help of their religious communities. Pointon was not religious, or rather appears to have found religion restricting, and got on with her life despite it. Maxwell was financially independent. Gills and Pointon found some financial success but were always struggling to make ends meet, though none of the three expected to be the beneficiaries of charitable giving. There is little evidence from any of these three cases that there was a general trend that suggested their blindness "got in the way" or made other people "feel discomfort or awkwardness," nor even that they "needed to be cared for" or were "not as productive as" sighted people. While there is not a sense that they were "the same as everyone else,"[86] their uniqueness and their own attitudes to their uniqueness were always the way they defined themselves, and the way other people defined them. But this was never carried on in terms of ocularcentrism or ocularnormativity. None of these three blind people were expected to be able-bodied, or expected their blindness could be cured. No theory can account for these lives or produce a history of the blind from them. There are only individual lives.

NOTES

1. Philosophy, Sight, and Blindness

1. Michel Foucault, *The Birth of the Clinic*, trans. A. M. Sheridan (London: Tavistock, 1973), 65 (translation significantly modified from the original French).
2. Oliver Goldsmith, *The citizen of the world; or letters from a Chinese philosopher, residing in London, to his friends in the east* (London: John Newbery, 1762).
3. Karl Philipp Moritz, *Travels, chiefly on foot, through several parts of England, in 1782. Described in letters to a friend, by Charles P. Moritz, a literary gentleman of Berlin* (London: G. G. and J. Robinson, 1795).
4. See the account of couching given on pages <oo>.
5. Variability understood this way is not a theory. But nor is it a principle or an idea (which imports too much of the Lockean). If it were a principle, it would need to inform or guide critique—but that is not the claim I am making. Instead, I am claiming that—like, for example, deconstruction—the expectation of Variability is unconditional and will be the case whether you do anything about it or not. This is not the same as being a principle, as critiques guided by principles blind themselves to the condition of Variability. Variability's unconditionality allows for an unravelling of "principled" critique. Furthermore, as an expectation, Variability can always be proved wrong and its conclusions temporary, as the corrections to my former work in the chapter on Thomas Gills suggest.
6. Dwight Christopher Gabbard, "Disability Studies and the British Long Eighteenth Century," *Literature Compass* 8, no. 2 (2011): 80–94.
7. Gabbard, "Disability Studies and the British Long Eighteenth Century," 80.
8. *OED Online*, s.v. "empiric, n. and adj.," accessed 19 December 2016.
9. Francis Bacon, *Sir Francis Bacon his apologie, in certaine imputations concerning the late Earle of Essex VVritten to the right Honorable his very good Lord, the Earle of Deuonshire, Lord Lieutenant of Ireland* (London: Felix Norton, 1604), 57–58.
10. P. L., *A letter from an apothecary in London, to his friend in the country; concerning the present practice of physick, in regard to empiricks, empirical methods of cure, and nostrums [. . .]* (London: M. Cooper, 1752).

11. Robert Rutson James, *Studies in the History of Ophthalmology in England Prior to the Year 1800* (1933; repr., Cambridge: Cambridge University Press, 2013).
12. *Annals of the Royal College of Surgeons* 25, no. 4 (November 1959): 264, http://www.ncbi.nlm.nih.gov/pmc/articles/PMC2413917/pdf/annrcse00354-0058a.pdf.
13. Rutson James, *Studies in the History of Ophthalmology*, preface unpaginated.
14. Peter Kennedy, *Ophthalmographia; or, a treatise of the eye* [. . .] (London: Bernard Lintott, 1713).
15. Peter Kennedy, *A supplement to Kennedy's Ophthalmographia; or, treatise of the eye* [. . .] (London: T. Cooper, 1739).
16. Rutson James, *Studies in the History of Ophthalmology*, 89.
17. Kennedy, *Supplement*, 89–92.
18. Rutson James, *Studies in the History of Ophthalmology*, 90.
19. Chapter 2 of this volume gives a more detailed account of this operation.
20. The chapters on John "Chevalier" Taylor and John Taylor, oculist of Hatton Garden, are by George Coats, a Scottish ophthalmologist (1876–1915). Coats gave his name to a rare vascular retinal condition.
21. Rutson James, *Studies in the History of Ophthalmology*, 222.
22. Rutson James, *Studies in the History of Ophthalmology*, 223.
23. Roy Porter, *Health for Sale: Quackery in England, 1660–1850* (Manchester: Manchester University Press, 1989), 61.
24. Rutson James, *Studies in the History of Ophthalmology*, 89.
25. Rutson James, *Studies in the History of Ophthalmology*, 89.
26. I have explored this problem with regard to Priscilla Pointon in an essay, "Blind Woman on the Rampage: Priscilla Pointon's Grand Tour of the Midlands and the Question of the Legitimacy of Sources for Biography," in *Voice and Context in Eighteenth-Century Verse: Order in Variety*, ed. Joanna Fowler and Allan Ingram, 230–47 (Basingstoke: Palgrave, 2015).
27. Optical Character Recognition (OCR) is the name for the way text is prepared for electronic searching. The digital image is scanned to recognize letters and numbers, but the process often results in garbled text when used with hand-carved fonts. For example, a completely random search for "William Read" brought forth this: ". . . J^earn imt ap. prehend that they cannot fpare time futticient from theit necefl'ary Bufinefs, he gives notice, that he yjlf Read, as is pra&lfed in London* only, . . ."

2. Blindness Is Not a "Disability"

1. Peter Singer, *Practical Ethics* (Cambridge: Cambridge University Press, 1980). All quotes are taken from the iBooks edition (which is the third edition dating from 2011), so no page numbers are cited. Quotes may be located using the search function, so thoughtfully added to this computer program, but at the expense of page numbers.
2. Peter Singer uses the word "reasonable" eighteen times in the book, each time in a way that suggests that the ethical response is always reasonable. I used the iBooks search function to find out this fact.
3. Singer, *Practical Ethics*.
4. Singer, *Practical Ethics*.

5. Singer, *Practical Ethics*.
6. Alison Kafer, *Feminist, Queer, Crip* (Bloomington: Indiana University Press, 2013), 2.
7. Singer, *Practical Ethics*.
8. Singer, *Practical Ethics*.
9. Rosemarie Garland-Thomson, "A Habitable World: Harriet McBryde Johnson's 'Case for My Life,'" *Hypatia: A Journal of Feminist Philosophy* 30, no. 1 (Winter 2015): 302.
10. I remember, when I was an undergraduate in 1982, David Wood organizing a series of seminars in which all the heads of the other departments at Warwick University came to "confess" to the Philosophy Department that their subjects were no more than stories.
11. Michel Foucault, *The Archaeology of Knowledge*, trans. A. M. Sheridan Smith (London: Routledge, 2002), 142. Originally published in French in 1969.
12. Foucault, *Archaeology*, 143.
13. For example, in *Histoire de la folie à l'âge classique—Folie et déraison* (Paris: Plon, 1961), translated as *Madness and Civilization: A History of Insanity in the Age of Reason* by R. Howard (London: Tavistock, 1965), Foucault describes such a gesture as "the realm in which the man of madness and the man of reason, moving apart, are not yet disjunct; and in an incipient and very crude language, antedating that of science, begin the dialogue of their breach, testifying in a fugitive way that they still speak to each other."
14. For those of you who are sighted, Alex, for example, pauses slightly before a word in scare quotes so a hearing-only reader can tell the difference between these two forms of a word.
15. *OED Online*, s.v. "disabled, adj. and n.," accessed 3 October 2106.
16. I choose the Burney Collection as newspapers give a snapshot of the popular, rather than the technical, uses of words.
17. *Daily Gazetteer* (London ed.), no. 122, Tuesday, 18 November 1735.
18. *London Evening Post*, no. 1438, 1 February 1737–3 February 1737.
19. *General Advertiser* (1744) (London), no. 4072, Saturday, 14 November 1747.
20. *Public Advertiser* (London), no. 5842, Thursday, 19 July 1753.
21. See, for example, Patrick Wallis, "Introduction: The Growth of the Early Modern Medical Economy," in "Changes in Medical Care," special issue, *Journal of Social History* 49, no. 3 (2016): 477–83.
22. Les Invalides, like the Chelsea Hospital, was built as an army veterans' respite home.
23. John Griffin, *Proposals for the relief and support of maimed, aged, and disabled seamen, in the merchants service of Great Britain. Humbly offer'd to all Lovers of their Country, and to all true Friends to Trade and Navigation By John Griffin, Mariner* (London, 1745), 4.
24. *OED Online*, s.v. "able, adj., adv., and n.," accessed 10 October 2016, S2.
25. Thanks to Teresa Michals, and her work on amputee admirals in particular, for alerting me to this aspect of life in the navy.
26. John Atkins, *The navy surgeon; or, practical system of surgery. With a dissertation on cold and hot mineral springs; and physical observations on the coast of Guiney* (London: J. Hodges, 1742).
27. A portrait of Galfridus Walpole without his arm was made by Charles Gervas (see http://www.bridgemanimages.com/fr/asset/86920/jervas-charles-1675-1739/portrait-of-galfridus-walpole-c-1683-1726-oil-on-canvas).

28. Atkins, *The navy surgeon*, 133–37.
29. Atkins, *The navy surgeon*, 142–43.
30. *London Evening Post*, no. 6158, 16 April 1767–18 April 1767.
31. Jane Austen, *Mansfield Park*, iBooks ed., https://itun.es/gb/rp2Kx.l.
32. Other crew ratings, such as Landsmen, Ordinary Seamen, and Ship's Boy, might be understood to have hoped to be promoted to the rating of Able-Seamen.
33. Brian Lavery, *Royal Tars: The Lower Deck of the Royal Navy, 875–1850* (Annapolis, MD: Naval Institute Press, 2010), 267–68. My thanks to Teresa Michals for drawing my attention to this information.
34. Lennard J. Davis, ed., *The Disability Studies Reader*, 5th ed. (New York: Routledge, 2017). References are taken from the Kindle edition and so have no page numbers. While Kindle does have a search function, continuous electronic reading out loud is not so easy and might be improved.
35. Davis, *Disability Studies Reader*, 5th ed.
36. Davis, *Disability Studies Reader*, 5th ed.
37. Davis, *Disability Studies Reader*, 5th ed.
38. Davis, *Disability Studies Reader*, 5th ed.
39. Davis, *Disability Studies Reader*, 5th ed.
40. Davis, *Disability Studies Reader*, 5th ed.
41. Davis, *Disability Studies Reader*, 5th ed.
42. Lennard J. Davis, *Disability Studies Reader*, 1st ed. (New York: Routledge, 1997), 10.
43. The image can be found at http://www.bridgemanimages.com/fr/search?filter_text=François-Andre+Vincent%2C+Zeuxis+&filter_group=all&filter_region=GBR.
44. Davis's own "Constructing Normalcy: The Bell Curve, the Novel, and the Invention of the Disabled Body in the Nineteenth Century"; "Deaf and Dumb in Ancient Greece," by M. Lynn Rose; and "A Silent Exile on this Earth: The Metaphoric Construction of Deafness in the Nineteenth Century," by Douglas Baynton.
45. "Spoken Daggers, Deaf Ears, and Silent Mouths: Fantasies of Deafness in Early-Modern England," by Jennifer L. Nelson and Bradley S. Berens; "Disability and Society before the Eighteenth Century: Dread and Despair," by Margaret A. Winzer; and Davis's own "Universalizing Marginality: How Europe Became Deaf in the Eighteenth Century."
46. Davis, *Disability Studies Reader*, 1st ed., 111.
47. Davis, *Disability Studies Reader*, 4th ed. (New York: Routledge, 2013), 2.
48. Raymond Williams, *Marxism and Literature* (Oxford: Oxford University Press, 1977).
49. Davis, *Disability Studies Reader*, 1st ed., 118.
50. Davis, *Disability Studies Reader*, 1st ed., 114, my emphasis.
51. Davis, *Disability Studies Reader*, 1st ed., 115.
52. Jaap Maat, 'Teaching Language to a Boy Born Deaf in the Seventeenth Century: The Holder-Wallis Debate," *History and Philosophy of the Language Sciences*, https://hiphilangsci.net/2013/11/06/teaching-language-to-a-boy-born-deaf-in-the-seventeenth-century-the-holder-wallis-debate.
53. Leila Frances Monaghan, *Many Ways to Be Deaf: International Variation in Deaf Communities* (Washington, DC: Gallaudet University Press, 2013), 40.
54. Monaghan, *Many Ways to Be Deaf*, 40.

55. "Part of a Letter from Richard Waller, Esq; S.R.S. to Dr. Hans Sloane, R.S. Secr. concerning Two Deaf Persons, Who can Speak and Understand What is Said to Them by the Motion of the Lips," *Philosophical Transactions of the Royal Society* 25 (1706): 2468–69.
56. *Post Boy* (1695) (London), no. 4697, 1 September 1719–3 September 1719, contains the first advertisement for *Life and Surprizing Adventures* and explains that the book will be published soon and that he resides "in the Spring Gardens, at the backside of the Ship Tavern." *Weekly Journal or Saturday's Post* (London), no. 51, Saturday, 21 November 1719, describes the book which is to be published by subscription, "imprinted with a new Letter, and on Imperial Paper," and offers subscriptions at half a guinea. When it was published, it was sold only by the notorious bookseller Edmund Curll. *Evening Post* (1709) (London), no. 2096, 1 January 1723–3 January 1723, contains the first advertisement of the second edition of *Life and Surprizing Adventures* for sale at 5s.
57. (London: printed for J. Peele at Mr. Locke's-Head in Pater-Noster-Row, 1724). First advertised in *British Journal* (1722) (London), no. 13, Saturday, 15 December 1722. The first edition was advertised in the *Daily Journal* (London), no. 989, Monday, 23 March 1724. It was unattributed and sold at Burton's Coffee-House. A second edition was advertised in the *Daily Post* (London), issue 1530, Friday, 21 August 1724. This was "revised by Mrs Eliza Haywood" and published by Thomas Corbett. Two further printings are extant; the third version is dated 1724, "revised by Mrs Eliza Haywood," and was sold by "J. Peele." I can find no advertisements for this version. The fourth version is dated 1725, was advertised in the *Daily Post* (London), no. 1668, Friday, 29 January 1725. It is also "revised by Mrs. Eliza Haywood" and was sold by Ellis, Brotherton, Batley, Woodward and Fox. All four versions were printed with the same plates, as the ornaments are identical, and there is a consistent error in the page numbers in the contents page, where "89" is printed instead of "98." The book, which, at about 260 pages, is slightly shorter than Campbell's Biography, was always sold at 3s 6d.
58. London: W. Ellis, J. Roberts, Mrs Bilingsly, A. Dod and J. Fox, 1725.
59. *Evening Post* (1709) (London), no. 1636, 23 January 1720–26 January 1720, explains that Campbell can now be found at "his House in Exeter-Court."
60. *Daily Post* (London), no. 184, Wednesday, 4 May 1720.
61. Eliza Haywood, *The Dumb Projector: Or, a Trip to Holland made by Mr. Duncan Campbell* (London: W. Ellis, J. Roberts, Mrs Bilingsly, A. Dod and J. Fox, 1725), 36.
62. Haywood, *The Dumb Projector*, 37
63. David T. Mitchell and Sharon L. Snyder, *Narrative Prosthesis: Disability and the Dependencies of Discourse* (Ann Arbor: University of Michigan Press, 2001).
64. See, for example, http://www.nineteenthcenturydisability.org/bibliography.
65. Vin Nardizzi, "Disability Figures in Shakespeare," in *The Oxford Handbook of Shakespeare and Embodiment: Gender, Sexuality and Race,* ed. Valerie Traub (Oxford: Oxford University Press, 2016), 459.
66. Pierre Desloges, *Observations d'un sourd et muèt, sur un cours élémentaire d'éducation des sourds et muèts* (Amsterdam and Paris: B. Morin, 1779).
67. The service can be found at gallica.bnf.fr.
68. Harlan Lane, ed., *The Deaf Experience: Classics in Language and Education,* trans. Franklin Philip (Cambridge: Harvard University Press, 1984).

69. Davis, *The Disability Studies Reader*, 1st ed., 120.
70. Davis, *The Disability Studies Reader*, 1st ed., 120.
71. Desloges, *Observations d'un sourd et muèt,* avertissement, 4–5. The editor's notes are paginated separately from the rest of the text.
72. Daniel Defoe, *The Fortunes and Misfortunes of the Famous Moll Flanders* (London: Chetwood and Edling, 1721[2]), iv.
73. Defoe, *The Fortunes and Misfortunes of the Famous Moll Flanders*, A2.
74. Desloges, *Observations d'un sourd et muèt,* avertissement, 5.
75. Desloges, *Observations d'un sourd et muèt,* 6.
76. Desloges, *Observations d'un sourd et muèt,* 3.
77. Davis, *The Disability Studies Reader*, 1st ed., 120.
78. Desloges, *Observations d'un sourd et muèt,* 3–4.
79. Anne Therese Quartararo, *Deaf Identity and Social Images in Nineteenth-Century France* (Washington, DC: Gallaudet University Press, 2008), see chap. 5.
80. Quartararo, *Deaf Identity and Social Images in Nineteenth-Century France,* http://gupress.gallaudet.edu/excerpts/DISIfive3.html
81. Davis, *The Disability Studies Reader*, 1st ed., 112.
82. Davis, *The Disability Studies Reader*, 1st ed., 111.
83. See *Mr Campbell's Packet for the Entertainment of Gentlemen and Ladies* (London: T. Bickerton, 1720).
84. Foucault, *Birth of the Clinic,* 65.
85. Davis, *The Disability Studies Reader*, 1st ed., 124.
86. Davis, *The Disability Studies Reader*, 1st ed., 124.

3. Text as Theory

1. See http://plato.stanford.edu/entries/condillac/.
2. The *Stanford Encyclopaedia* is using Condillac's spelling of Cheselden's name.
3. George Berkeley, *An Essay Towards a New Theory of Vision* (Dublin: printed by Aaron Rhames for Jeremy Pepyat, 1709 and 1710).
4. *Public Advertiser* (London), no. 6068, Tuesday, 9 April 1754.
5. *Public Advertiser* (London), no. 6850, Saturday, 2 October 1756.
6. *Public Advertiser* (London), no. 6902, Saturday, 20 November 1756.
7. *Public Advertiser* (London), no. 7198, Saturday, 19 November 1757.
8. *Public Advertiser* (London), no. 7225, Saturday, 24 December 1757.
9. *Public Advertiser* (London), no. 7484, Saturday, 4 November 1758.
10. *Public Advertiser* (London), no. 7918, Saturday, 22 March 1760.
11. *Public Advertiser* (London), no. 7970, Saturday, 24 May 1760.
12. *Gazetteer and London Daily Advertiser* (London), no. 10686, Monday, 13 June 1763.
13. *Public Advertiser* (London), no. 9155, Wednesday, 7 March 1764.
14. *Gazetteer and New Daily Advertiser* (London), no. 13413, Tuesday, 25 February 1772; issue repeated in *Public Advertiser* (London), no. 11649, Friday, 28 February 1772, where the name is given as Tinnamore.
15. *Daily Advertiser* (London), no. 13700, Thursday, 17 November 1774.

16. *Morning Chronicle and London Advertiser* (London), no. 2340, Tuesday, 19 November 1776.
17. *Daily Advertiser* (London), no. 14410, Saturday, 22 February 1777.
18. *Daily Advertiser* (London), no. 14742, Saturday, 28 March 1778, repeated in *Public Advertiser* (London), no. 13566, Thursday, 2 April 1778.
19. *Daily Advertiser* (London), no. 14880, Saturday, 5 September 1778.
20. *St. James's Chronicle or the British Evening Post* (London), no. 2976, 6 April 1780–8 April 1780.
21. *Public Advertiser* (London), no. 7066, Saturday, 18 June 1757.
22. *Daily Advertiser* (London), no. 13047, Friday, 16 October 1772.
23. Marjolein Degenaar, *Molyneux's Problem: Three Centuries of Discussion on the Perception of Forms* (Dordrecht: Kluwer Academic, 1996), 52.
24. John Locke, *Essay concerning Humane Understanding*, 2nd ed. (London: Thomas Dring and Samuel Manship, 1694), bk. 2, chap. 9, § 8, 67.
25. Laura Berchielli, "Colour, Space and Figure in Locke: An Interpretation of the Molyneux Problem," *Journal of the History of Philosophy* 40, no. 1 (2002): 48.
26. Berchielli, "Colour, Space and Figure," 49.
27. Charles William Wells, *An Essay on Single Vision with Two Eyes* (London: T. Cadell, 1792); John Crisp, *Observations on the Nature and Theory of Vision* (London: J. Sewell, 1796).
28. Desiree Park, "Locke and Berkeley on the Molyneux Problem," *Journal of the History of Ideas*, 30, no. 2 (April-June 1969): 254, 258.
29. Park, "Locke and Berkeley," 253.
30. Kate E. Tunstall, *Blindness and Enlightenment* (London: Continuum, 2011).
31. George Berkeley, *An Essay Towards a New Theory of Vision*, 2nd ed. (Dublin: printed by Aaron Rhames for Jeremy Pepyat, 1709), 197–98.
32. William Cheselden, "An Account of some Observations made by a young Gentleman, who was born blind, or lost his Sight so early, that he had no Rembrance of ever having seen, and was couch'd between 13 and 14 Years of Age. By Mr. Will. Chesselden, F.R.S. Surgeon to Her Majesty and to St. Thomas' Hospital," *Philosophical Transactions: Giving some accompt of the present undertakings, studies and labours of the ingenious in many considerable parts of the world* 35 (London: Royal Society, 1735): 447–50.
33. Cheselden, "An Account," 448.
34. Tunstall, *Blindness and Enlightenment*, 196.
35. Tunstall, *Blindness and Enlightenment*, 196–97.
36. Tunstall, *Blindness and Enlightenment*, 14.
37. London and Bath: S. Richardson, 1749.
38. It may well be that Locke did not answer Molyneux's problem directly because he had not yet met his "blind man made to see" and consequently thought that Molyneux was wrong.
39. Locke, *Essay* (1690), chap. 4, §19, 34.
40. Locke, *Essay* (1694), bk. 1, chap. 4, §20, 35.
41. Locke, Essay, bk. 2, chap. 5, 1st ed. 51; 2nd ed., 55.
42. Locke, *Essay*, bk. 2, chap. 1 §2, 40.

43. Tunstall's book begins with several accounts of the unveiling of a person whose eyes have been couched and argues that this became a typical Romantic device.
44. Cheselden, "An Account," 448.
45. L. Girard, "Dislocation of Cataractous Lens by Enzymatic Zonulolysis: A Suggested Solution to the Problem of the 18 Million Individuals Blind from Cataracts in Third-World Countries," *Ophthalmic Surgery* 26, no. 4 (1995): 343–45.
46. William Oldys, *Observations on the Cure of William Taylor, the Blind Boy of Ightham, in Kent* (London: E. Owen, 1753), 12.
47. David Hosack, "Observations on vision, Communicated by George Pearson M.D. F.R.S." *Philosophical Transactions* [London], [1794].
48. Hosack, "Observations on vision," 3.
49. Hosack, "Observations on vision," 4.
50. Degenaar, *Molyneux's Problem*, 59.
51. Degenaar, *Molyneux's Problem*, 59.
52. *Howle Howleglas deseyued a wynedrawer in Lubeke* (n.p., 1519), 2.
53. *Post Boy* (1695) (London), no. 219, 29 September 1696–1 October 1696.
54. Philosophical Society of Edinburgh, *Medical essays and observations, published by a society in Edinburgh* [. . .], vol. 4. The third edition, revised and enlarged by the authors (Edinburgh, 1747), 149.
55. Charles de Saint-Yves, one of the French pioneers of eye surgery, first mentions "couching spectacles" by name in his *New treatise of the diseases of the eye*, which appeared in English in 1741. The French first edition dates from 1722.
56. *Weekly Journal or British Gazetteer* (London), Saturday, 23 May 1724.
57. Michael Bruno and Eric Mandelbaum, "Locke's Answer to Molyneux's Thought Experiment," *History of Philosophy Quarterly* 27, no. 2 (April 2010): 167.
58. Park, "Locke and Berkeley," 253.
59. *Annotations upon the Holy Bible. Wherein the sacred text is inserted, and various readings annex'd; together with the parallel scriptures. The more difficult terms in each verse are explained. Seeming contradictions reconciled. Questions and doubts resolved. And the whole text opened. By the late Reverend and learned Divine. Mr. Matthew Poole. The fourth edition, with large contents before each chapter; truely corrected and amended: together with the harmony of the evangelists, by Mr. Sam. Clark, never done with Pool's annotations before. And what further shall be thought convenient, will be insert in the title page of the second volume*, vol. 1 (Edinburgh, 1700).

4. Unofficial Eye Care

1. "From the Italian montambanco, montimbanco (late 17th cent.), contracted form of monta in banco (1598 in Florio), lit. 'mount on bench.'"mountebank, n.," *OED Online*, accessed 16 April 2018.
2. List of sources reproduced from the *ODNB: Le Neve's Pedigrees of the knights*, ed. G. W. Marshall, Harleian Society, 8 (1873): 490–91; R. R. James, ed., *Studies in the history of ophthalmology in England prior to the year 1800* (1933), 122–9; L. S. King, *The medical world of the eighteenth century* (1958), 47–50; 'Some famous quacks: V., Sir William Read', *The Practitioner* 78 (1907): 416–21; TNA: PRO, A Prob 6/91, fol. 71 (146)r.; *Dr.*

Sacheverel turn'd oculist (1710) [copy at BL]; 'Post nubila Phoebus, nihil absque Deo' [handbill; copy at BL]; W. Read, 'Read's true and faithful experiments' (c. 1705); 'The Oculist: a poem address't to Sir W. Read' (1705) [copy at BL]; G. Everitt, *Doctors and doctors: some curious chapters in medical history and quackery* (1888), 254–5; W. Musgrave, Obituary prior to 1800, ed. G. J. Armytage, 5, *Harleian Society* 48 (1901), 121.

3. I can find no source for the idea that Read began as a tailor, and it may well be that since the couching operation was carried out with a needle, a folk legend grew up around him that he had been a tailor.
4. This information is transcribed in full from *Early English Books Online*, in which copy Jacques Guillemeau's name is not included on the title page, which suggests Banister did not openly acknowledge his source either.
5. Rutson James, *Studies in the History of Ophthalmology*, 124.
6. The date of the first edition, which I have not located, and which Savage-Smith calls *A Treatise of the Eye* (1705), is suggested by the comment in the third section of the second edition (which is probably Read's own work): "I had towards the latter end of the last Year 1705, several other Patients troubled with such violent Deflexions upon the Eyes, as quite to impart the Sight" (29). *A short but exact account of all the diseases incident to the eyes*, called in two versions "Second edition corrected," was advertised once in *Post Man and the Historical Account* (London), no. 1840, 5 January 1710–7 January 1710. It would appear that Read's *A Treatise of the Eye* may be a result of Arnold Sorsby calling his paper, reprinted from the *British Journal of Ophthalmology* in 1932, "Sir William Read's Treatise of the Eyes."
7. *Post Boy* (1695) (London), no. 2502, 24 May 1711–26 May 1711. The issue contains two separate affidavits for Read's cures: Mary Reynolds of Wade Mills in Hertfordshire, and Edward South of Harhaidge, near Bonningfield, also in Hertfordshire.
8. *Observator* (1702) (London), no. 30, 11 April 1711–14 April 1711. "Abel" is Abel Roper, the editor of the *Post Boy*, and "*Dr. Sacheverel*," Henry Sacheverell, the fashionable Anglican priest and author of many attacks on the Whigs for putting the church in danger.
9. Rutson James, *Studies in the History of Ophthalmology*, 124.
10. W. Pettis, *Some memoirs of the life of John Radcliffe* (London, 1715), 37.
11. *Weekly Journal or Saturday's Post* (London), no. 103, Saturday, 29 November 1718.
12. A. Sakula, "Dr John Radcliffe, Court Physician, and the Death of Queen Anne," *Journal of the Royal College of Physicians of London* 19 (1985): 255–60, 256.
13. For example: "Mr Bonnell's Life was written by Wm Harrington, who has publish'd a New Book of Mr Bonnells containing *Devotions* &c. wch is recommended to the world by Mr Jo. Strip. Mr. Sam. Palmer, &c all Whigs. Mr Bonnell himself who is so commended by these Pharisaical People, was of the Whiggish side" (Thomas Hearne, *Remarks and Collections*, 11 vols., ed. C. E. Doble [Oxford: Clarendon, 1885], 1:42–43).
14. *London Gazette*, no. 4144, 26 July 1705–30 July 1705.
15. *London Gazette*, no. 4145, 30 July 1705–2 August 1705.
16. Nevertheless, I find little reason for Curthoys to make the point about Hearne's acidity, as his entry for 1 August 1705, reads: "On July 27th last, ye Queen Knighted Dr Wm. Read, ye Oculist—On the 29th of the same Month She also Knighted Dr. Edw. Hannes the Physitian" (Hearne, *Remarks and Collections*, 1:21).

17. There is almost no evidence to be found about Agutter's life, except for an advertisement in *London Gazette,* no. 3116, 19 September 1695–23 September 1695, that Corelli's violin sonatas can be bought from him, and, of course, his exquisitely carved violins.
18. Originally the London residence of the archbishop of York.
19. A number of other addresses are mentioned, for example "at the Raven over against Exeter Exchange" and "at Shandios St. Covent Garden" (which I cannot locate) from where Read advertised briefly before the permanent move to Durham Yard. However, it is not possible to argue that Read was itinerant after 1704.
20. *Post Man and the Historical Account* (London), no. 216, 24 September 1696–26 September 1696.
21. *Collection for Improvement of Husbandry and Trade* (London), no. 87, Friday, 30 March 1694.
22. *Post Boy and Historical Account* (London), no. 23, 29 June 1695–2 July 1695, no.23.
23. *London Gazette,* no. 2449, 29 April 1689–2 May 1689.
24. Originally the London residence of the archbishop of Durham.
25. See *Survey of London, vol. 18, St Martin-in-The-Fields II: The Strand,* ed. G. H. Gater and E. P. Wheeler (London, 1937), British History Online, http://www.british-history.ac.uk/survey-london/vol18/pt2/pp84-98. The Adam brothers demolished the area to make way for the Adelphi Buildings, the first neoclassical structure in London, in 1768.
26. *London Gazette,* no. 2447, 22 April 1689–25 April 1689.
27. *Post Boy* (1695) (London), no. 464, 23 April 1698–26 April 1698.
28. *Post Man and the Historical Account* (London), no. 676, 11 November 1699–14 November 1699.
29. Advertised to be sold in *Post Man and the Historical Account* (London), no. 1439, 18 August 1705–21 August 1705.
30. *Post Man and the Historical Account* (London), no. 216, 24 September 1696–26 September 1696.
31. Rutson James, *Studies in the History of Ophthalmology,* 130.
32. Read, *A short but exact account of all the diseases incident to the eyes,* second pagination, 30.
33. Rutson James, *Studies in the History of Ophthalmology,* 126.
34. Read, *A short but exact account of all the diseases incident to the eyes,* second pagination, 4–5.
35. Read, *A short but exact account of all the diseases incident to the eyes,* second pagination, 5.
36. Read, *A short but exact account of all the diseases incident to the eyes,* second pagination, 6.
37. Read, *A short but exact account of all the diseases incident to the eyes,* second pagination, 6.
38. Read, *A short but exact account of all the diseases incident to the eyes,* second pagination 7.
39. Read, *A short but exact account of all the diseases incident to the eyes,* second pagination, 7.
40. Rutson James, *Studies in the History of Ophthalmology,* 97. Sharp's contribution to eye surgery was to have invented "a rather beak shaped knife" to improve success rates in Daviel's operation for cataracts.
41. Samuel Sharp, *A treatise on the operations of surgery, with a description and representation of the instruments used in performing them* (London: J. Brotherton &c, 1739), 157.

42. Read, *A short but exact account of all the diseases incident to the eyes,* second pagination, 3.
43. *Post Man and the Historical Account* (London), no. 216, 24 September 1696–26 September 1696.
44. History of Parliament online.
45. *Post Boy* (1695) (London), no. 1150, 24 September 1702–26 September 1702.
46. *ODNB,* s.v. Charles Bernard.
47. *London Gazette,* no. 3837, 17 August 1702–20 August 1702.
48. Sir Ambrose Heal, *The London Goldsmiths, 1200–1800: A Record of the Names and Addresses of the Craftsmen, Their Shop-Signs and Trade-Cards* (Cambridge: Cambridge University Press, 1935), 218. It is not out of the question that the Company of Goldsmiths' register found the address for Payne in Read's advertisement.
49. *London Gazette,* no. 3872, 17 December 1702–21 December 1702.
50. *London Gazette,* no. 4101, 26 February 1705–1 March 1705.
51. *Post Man and the Historical Account* (London), no. 216, 24 September 1696–26 September 1696.
52. *Flying Post or The Post Master* (London), no. 475, 26 May 1698–28 May 1698.
53. *Flying Post or The Post Master* (London), no. 477, 31 May 1698–2 June 1698; *Flying Post or The Post Master* (London), 16 June 1698–18 June 1698.
54. *Flying Post or The Post Master* (London), no. 512, 20 August 1698–23 August 1698.
55. *London Gazette,* no. 3728, 31 July 1701–4 August 1701.
56. *Daily Courant* (London), no. 182, Monday, 16 November 1702.
57. *London Gazette,* no. 3931, 12 July 1703–15 July 1703.
58. His last continuous use of the title "sworn Servant to His late Majesty" was in *London Gazette,* no. 3837, 17 August 1702–20 August 1702.
59. Rutson James, *Studies in the History of Ophthalmology,* 123–24.
60. *London Gazette,* no. 4039, 24 July 1704–27 July 1704.
61. *Daily Courant* (London), no. 547, Monday, 17 January 1704; *Daily Courant* (London), no. 566, Monday, 7 February 1704.
62. *Post Man and the Historical Account* (London), no. 1239, 10 February 1704–12 February 1704.
63. *London Gazette,* no. 4002, 16 March 1704–20 March 1704.
64. *Post Man and the Historical Account* (London), no. 1260, 4 April 1704–6 April 1704; *Daily Courant* (London), no. 617, Friday, 7 April 1704.
65. For example, *Daily Courant* (London), no. 605, Friday, 24 March 1704 (claims to have cured 100 poor since last Christmas); *Daily Courant* (London), no. 636, Saturday, 29 April 1704 (claims "hundreds resort to his house"); *London Gazette,* no. 4014, 27 April 1704–1 May 1704.
66. *London Gazette,* no. 4039, 24 July1704–27 July 1704; *London Gazette,* no. 4040, 27 July 1704–31 July 1704.
67. *Daily Courant* (London), no. 797, Friday, 3 November 1704.
68. *Post Man and the Historical Account* (London), no. 1239, 10 February 1704–12 February 1704.
69. *Daily Courant* (London), no. 636, Saturday, 29 April 1704.
70. *Post Man and the Historical Account* (London), no. 1239, 10 February 1704–12 February 1704.

71. The church was demolished in 1841 to make way for the Royal Exchange building (Aram Bakshian, "The French Church in Threadneedle St.," *History Today* 43, no. 5 [May 1993]).
72. *ODNB*.
73. John Aikin and William Johnson, *General Biography* (London: John Stockdale &c, 1814).
74. *Daily Courant* (London), no. 605, Friday, 24 March 1704.
75. *Daily Courant* (London), no. 941, Saturday, 21 April 1705; *London Gazette*, no. 4118, 26 April 1705–30 April 1705.
76. *Daily Courant* (London), no. 973, Tuesday, 29 May 1705; *London Gazette*, no. 4128, 31 May 1705–4 June 1705.
77. *Post Man and the Historical Account* (London), no. 1441, 25 August 1705–28 August 1705. The advertisement names "Jo. Haler, Governor" and "D. Crauford, Lieut. Governor" of the Chelsea Hospital.
78. *London Gazette*, no. 4145, 30 July 1705–2 August 1705.
79. *Post Man and the Historical Account* (London), no. 1699, 4 January 1709–6 January 1709.
80. *Post Man and the Historical Account* (London), no. 1239, 10 February 1704–12 February 1704.
81. Removal of bladder stones, or lithotomy. The figure of 200 guineas is given in the *ODNB*.
82. Porter, *Health for Sale*, 61.
83. *London Gazette*, no. 4228, 16 May 1706–20 May 1706.
84. *Post Man and the Historical Account* (London), no. 1629, 22 June 1706–25 June 1706.
85. *Post Man and the Historical Account* (London), no. 1680, 1 October 1706–3 October 1706.
86. *Post Man and the Historical Account* (London), no. 1752, 25 March 1707–27 March 1707; *Post Man and the Historical Account* (London), no 1780, 13 May 1707–15 May 1707.
87. *Post Boy* (1695) (London), no. 1894, 3 July 1707–5 July 1707.
88. I cannot locate this advertisement.
89. *London Gazette*, no. 4385, 17 November 1707–20 November 1707.
90. *Daily Courant* (London), no. 2071, Friday, 8 October 1708.
91. *Post Man and the Historical Account* (London), no. 1961, 7 October 1708–9 October 1708.
92. *London Gazette*, no. 4002, 16 March 1704–20 March 1704.
93. *Daily Courant* (London), no. 605, Friday, 24 March 1704.
94. *Post Man and the Historical Account* (London), no. 1637, 11 July 1706–13 July 1706.
95. *London Gazette*, no. 4228, 16 May 1706–20 May 1706.
96. *Daily Courant* (London), no. 4180, Friday, 18 March 1715.
97. *London Gazette*, no. 4548, 9 June 1709–13 June 1709.
98. For example, the first advertisement in the *Tatler* (1709) (London), no. 107, 13 December 1709–15 December 1709.
99. *Norwich Gazette or The Loyal Packet*, Saturday, 26 January 1712.
100. *Post Boy* (1695) (London), no. 2642, 15 April 1712–17 April 1712.
101. *Evening Post* (1709) (London), no. 959, 27 September 1715–29 September 1715.

102. *Flying Post or The Post Master* (London), no. 688, 5 October 1699–7 October 1699.
103. *Tatler* (1709) (London), no. 109, 17 December 1709–20 December 1709.
104. (London: Thomas Marshe, 1575), 98.
105. (London: Thomas Childe, 1703), 140.
106. See the preface to Robert Eaton, *An Account of Dr. Eaton's Styptick Balsam* (London, 1723), v.
107. "Some Observations upon Dr. Eaton's Styptick by Dr. Sprengell, R.S.S. Coll. Med. Lond. Lic," *Philosophical Transactions* 33 (1724): 381–91, 108–14.
108. The operation was also reported in "Post nubila Phoebus, nihil absque Deo" and was performed before the Duke of Northumberland, who was an active soldier, presumably to demonstrate Read's skill in field amputations and the effectiveness of his Styptick-Water.
109. *Daily Courant* (London), no. 905, Saturday, 10 March 1705.
110. Peter Paxton, *An essay concerning the body of man, wherein its changes or diseases are consider'd, and the operations of medicines observ'd* (London: Richard Wilkin, 1701), 256.
111. Congenitally split lip and twisted head position.
112. *Weekly Packet* (London), no. 132, 8 January 1715–15 January 1715.
113. *British Weekly Mercury* (London), no. 517, 21 May 1715–28 May 1715.
114. *Weekly Journal with Fresh Advices Foreign and Domestick* (London), Saturday, 21 May 1715.
115. *Weekly Journal with Fresh Advices Foreign and Domestick* (London), Saturday, 28 May 1715.
116. John Banister *A needefull, new, and necessarie treatise of chyrurgerie briefly comprehending the generall and particular curation of vlcers, drawen foorth of sundrie worthy wryters, but especially of Antonius Calmeteus Vergesatus, and Ioannes Tagaltius, by Iohn Banister . . . Hereunto is anexed certaine experiments of mine ovvne inuention, truely tried, and daily of me practised* (London: Thomas Marshe, 1575), 101.
117. Konrad Gesner, *The newe iewell of health wherein is contayned the most excellent secretes of phisicke and philosophie, deuided into fower books [. . .]* (London: Henrie Denham, 1576), 100.
118. John Aikin. *A manual of materia medica, containing a brief account of all the simples directed in the London and Edinburgh dispensatories, with their several preparations and the principal compositions into which they enter* (Yarmouth, Downes and March, 1785), 188.
119. See Henry Yule, *The Book of Ser Marco Polo* (London: John Murray, 1871), 118.
120. Benedict Duddell, *A treatise of the diseases of the horny-coat of the eye, and the various kinds of cataracts. To which is prefix'd, a method, entirely new, of scarifying the eyes for several disorders. With remarks on the practice of some oculists both at home and abroad.* (London: John Clark, 1729), 33, 59.
121. George Chandler, *A treatise of a cataract, its nature, species, causes and symptoms [. . .]* (London: Cadell, 1775), 42.
122. The *ODNB* article suggests that neither replied to the summons of the college.
123. Samuel Garth, *The dispensary a poem, in six canto's* (London: John Nutt, 1699).
124. *Weekly Journal or Saturday's Post* (London), no. 83, Saturday, 12 July 1718.
125. *Mist's Weekly Journal* (London), no. 56, Saturday, 21 May 1726.

126. *Weekly Journal or British Gazetteer* (London), Saturday, 13 December 1718.
127. *Weekly Journal with Fresh Advices Foreign and Domestick* (London), Saturday, 4 June 1715.
128. *Weekly Journal with Fresh Advices Foreign and Domestick* (London), Saturday, 11 June 1715.
129. *Weekly Journal with Fresh Advices Foreign and Domestick* (London), Saturday, 9 July 1715.
130. *Weekly Journal or Saturday's Post* (London), no. 126, Saturday, 29 April 1721.
131. *Weekly Journal or Saturday's Post* (London), no. 157, Saturday, 2 December 1721.
132. *Weekly Journal or Saturday's Post* (London), no. 164, Saturday, 20 January 1722.
133. *Weekly Journal or Saturday's Post* (London), no. 215, Saturday, 8 December 1722.
134. *Weekly Journal or Saturday's Post* (London), no. 222, Saturday, 26 January 1723.
135. *Weekly Journal or Saturday's Post* (London), no. 97, Saturday, 18 October 1718.
136. *Mist's Weekly Journal* (London), no. 132, Saturday, 28 October 1727.
137. *Weekly Journal or Saturday's Post* (London), no. 71, Saturday, 9 April 1720.
138. *Weekly Journal or Saturday's* Post (London), Saturday, 6 June 1719 (no issue number available).
139. For example, *Weekly Journal or Saturday's Post* (London), no. 104, Saturday, 26 November 1720.
140. *Weekly Journal or Saturday's Post* (London), no. 304, Saturday, 22 August 1724.
141. *Weekly Journal or Saturday's Post* (London), no. 309, Saturday, 26 September 1724. The alteration was made after two weeks in no. 306, but the available image is not of good quality.
142. For example, *Country Journal or The Craftsman* (London), no. 149, Saturday, 10 May 1729.
143. *Country Journal or The Craftsman* (London), no. 167, Saturday, 13 September 1729.
144. *Country Journal or The Craftsman* (London), no. 189, Saturday, 14 February 1730.
145. *Country Journal or The Craftsman* (London), no. 787, Saturday, 1 August 1741.
146. *Mist's Weekly Journal* (London), no. 151, Saturday, 9 March 1728.
147. *Mist's Weekly Journal* (London), no. 162, Saturday, 25 May 1728.
148. *Mist's Weekly Journal* (London, no. 114, Saturday, 24 June 1727.
149. *London Evening Post* (London), no. 116, 3 September 1728–5 September 1728.
150. *Weekly Journal or Saturday's Post* (London), no. 103, Saturday, 29 November 1718.
151. *Weekly Journal or Saturday's Post* (London), no. 49, Saturday, 7 November 1719.
152. Thomas Sydenham, *The compleat method of curing almost all diseases to which is added an exact description of their several symptoms/written in Latin by Dr. Thomas Sydenham; and now faithfully Englished* (London: printed and are to be sold by Randal Taylor [. . .], 1694), 13, 14, 16.
153. See *ODNB*.

5. Official Eye Care

1. Alexander Pope, *First epistle of the first book of Horace imitated* (London: R. Dodsley, 1738), 7.
2. Cheselden, "An Account," 447–50.

3. The *ODNB* reports: "In the sixth edition of [*The anatomy of the humane body*] 1741 he recorded that of 213 public lithotomies twenty had died, several from smallpox and whooping cough; no fewer than 105 were under ten years of age, mainly male, of whom three died. The death rate increased in older age groups but was astonishingly low by previous standards, given that neither anaesthesia nor asepsis was available. Alexander Pope wrote to Dr Swift in 1736: 'he is the most noted and deserving man in the whole of the profession of Chirurgery: and has saved the lives of thousands by his manner of cutting for the stone.'"
4. None of Cheselden's other reports to the Royal Society concerned sight: "Some Anatomical Observations," *Philosophical Transactions* 28, no. 337 (1712): 281–82; "A Remarkable Case of a Person Cut for Stone in the New Way, Commonly Called Lateral," *Philosophical Transactions* 44, no. 478 (1746): 33–35; "A Relation of a Scirrhous Tumour," *Philosophical Transactions* 28, no. 337 (1712): 276–78; "Dimensions of Some Human Bones, *Philosophical Transactions* 27, no. 333 (1710): 436; "Effects of Lixivium Saponis," *Philosophical Transactions* 44, no. 478 (1746): 325–36; "Observations on the Eclipse of the Moon," *Philosophical Transactions* 34, no. 392 (1726): 37–38; "A Remarkable Cure . . . of a . . . Large Fracture and Depression of the Skull," *Philosophical Transactions* 41, no. 452 (1739): 495–500.
5. See William Cheselden, *Syllabus, sive index humani corporis partium anatomicus, in XXXV prolectiones distinctus. In usum theatri anatomici Wilhelmi Cheselden, chirurgi* (London, 1711), which is Cheselden's syllabus for his lecture course.
6. William Cheselden, *The anatomy of the humane body* (London: N. Cliff, D. Jackson and W. Innys, 1713).
7. *Post Boy* (1695) (London), no. 2843, 28 July 1713–30 July 1713; *Evening Post* (1709) (London), no. 621, 30 July 1713–1 August 1713; *Post Boy* (1695) (London), no. 2848, 8 August 1713–11 August 1713; *Post Boy* (1695) (London), no. 2888, 10 November 1713–12 November 1713; *Post Boy* (1695) (London), no. 2890, 14 November 1713–17 November 1713; *Post Boy* (1695) (London), no. 2930, 16 February 1714–18 February 1714; *Post Boy* (1695) (London), no. 2932, 20 February 1714–23 February 1714; *Daily Courant* (London), no. 3918, Saturday, 15 May 1714; *Daily Courant* (London), no. 3924, Saturday, 22 May 1714.
8. It must be borne in mind that the numbers I am working with describe the advertisements recoverable by electronic searches in each case, so they record far fewer advertisments than were actually placed.
9. *Daily Courant* (London), no. 3846, Saturday, 20 February 1714; (London: D.Browne, W. Taylor and J. Browne, 1714).
10. *London Evening Post*, no. 1954, 17 August 1734–20 August 1734.
11. London: W. Bowyer, 1730.
12. William Cheselden, *Appendix to the fourth edition of The anatomy of the humane Body* (London: William Bowyer, 1730), 8.
13. Cheselden, *Appendix*, 8.
14. Cheselden, *Appendix*, 17.
15. Cheselden, *Appendix*, 18.
16. Cheselden, *Appendix*, 19.
17. Cheselden, "An Account," 447–50.

18. London: William Bowyer, 1733.
19. Allister Neher, "The Truth about Our Bones: William Cheselden's *Osteographia*," *Medical History* 54, no. 4 (October 2010): 517.
20. *London Evening Post*, no. 1566, 26 November 1737–29 November 1737.
21. Anon., "Eloge de M. Georges Mareschal," in *Mémoires de l'Académie Royale de Chirurgie*, vol. 2 (Paris: Delaguette, 1753), 31–42.
22. Anon, *Mémoire pour le sieur François La Peyronie premier chirurgien du roy, . . . et les prevosts & collége des maîtres en chirurgie de Paris; contre les doyen & docteurs-régens de la Faculté de médecine de Paris, et contre l'Université de Paris* (Paris: Imp. de Charles Osmont, 1746).
23. A slightly different account of the split between the Barbers and Surgeons, which is based on parliamentary reports rather than Cheselden's experience with the French, is given in Margaret Pelling's "Corporationalism or Individualism: Parliament, the Navy, and the Splitting of the London Barber Surgeons' Company in 1745," in *Guilds and Associations in Europe, 900–1900*, ed. Ian A. Gadd and Patrick Wallace (London: Centre for Metropolitan History, 2006), 57–82, 64.
24. John Ranby, *The Method of Treating Gun-Shot Wounds* (London: John and Paul Knapton, 1744), dedication.
25. There is some irony here since at the Battle of Dettingen the Hanoverian and British allies fought the French.
26. Confusingly, the Company of Barbers still occupies a building called the Barber-Surgeons' Hall and has a membership of 39 percent surgeons.
27. An irony here is that the Royal College of Physicians in London gained its Royal Charter twelve years after the Royal College of Surgeons of Edinburgh, which incorporated barbers and surgeons.
28. To this day, surgeons in Britain still use the title "Mr.," "Mrs.," "Miss," or "Ms." rather than "Dr."
29. London: John and Paul Knapton, 1745.
30. Literally this means "Lye that dissolves stones."
31. This is mentioned in Ranby, *Narrative of the last illness of the Earl of Orford, from May 1744 to the day of his decease, 18 March following* (London: John and Paul Knapton, 1745), 3, 22, 23, 27, 28, 36.
32. Ranby, *Narrative*, 39.
33. Ranby, *Narrative*, 33.
34. Ranby, *Narrative*, 12.
35. Ranby, *Narrative*, 39.
36. Ranby, *Narrative*, first page of preface, unpaginated.
37. James Jurin, *An epistle to John Ranby, Esq; Principal Serjeant Surgeon to His Majesty, And F.R.S. on the subject of his Narrative of the last illness of the late Earl of Orford, as far as it relates to Sir Edward Hulse, Dr Jurin, and Dr Crowe* (London: Jacob Robinson, 1745), 6.
38. Duddell, *Treatise*.
39. Duddell, *Treatise*, vii.
40. Duddell, *Treatise*, vii–viii.
41. Benedict Duddell, *An appendix to the treatise of the horney-coat of the eye, and the cata-*

ract. With an answer to Mr. Cheselden's appendix, relating to his new operation upon the iris of the eye (London: E. Howlatt, 1733).
42. Kennedy, Supplement.
43. Daily Courant (London), no. 4180, Friday, 18 March 1715.
44. Kennedy, Ophthalmographia; or, a treatise of the eye.
45. See advertisement in Reconciler (London), no. 2, Friday, 1 May 1713.
46. William Cheselden, The anatomy of the humane body. With XXXIV copper-plates. By W. Cheselden, Surgeon to St. Thomas's-Hospital, And Fellow of the Royal Society, 3rd ed. (London: William Bowyer, 1726); William Cheselden, The anatomy of the human body. By William Cheselden, Surgeon to Her Majesty, F.R.S. And Surgeon to St. Thomas's-Hospital, 4th ed. With the addition of an appendix, which also is printed separately for the use of those who have the former editions (London: William Bowyer, 1730).
47. Kennedy, Supplement, 71–72.
48. (London: R. Dodsley, 1738), 7.
49. Peter Kennedy, An essay on external remedies. Wherein it is considered, whether all the curable distempers incident to human bodies, may not be cured by outward means. [. . .] (London Andrew Bell, 1715). See preface, unpaginated
50. Kennedy, An essay on external remedies, preface, unpaginated.
51. Kennedy, Ophthalmographia, or, a treatise of the eye, preface, unpaginated.
52. Kennedy, Ophthalmographia, or, a treatise of the eye, preface, unpaginated.
53. Antoine Maitre-Jean, Traité des maladies de l'oeil (Paris: Jacques Lefebvre, 1707).
54. Pierre Brisseau, Traité de la cataracte et du glaucoma (Paris: Laurent d'Houry, 1709).
55. Kennedy, Ophthalmographia, or, a treatise of the eye, preface, unpaginated.
56. Kennedy, Ophthalmographia, or, a treatise of the eye, 42. Alumen ustum (burned alum) and vitriolum album (white vitriol = zinc sulphate) are both astringents. Aerugo (verdigris = copper carbonate) is known to irritate the eye unless irrigated, so is an odd element of the powder.
57. Kennedy, Supplement, 74.
58. Kennedy, Supplement, 74–75.
59. Kennedy, Supplement, 76.
60. Amsterdam, 1685.
61. The anatomy of humane bodies . . . Illustrated with large explications, containing many new anatomical discoveries and chirurgical observations: to which is added an introduction explaining the animal economy (Oxford: Samuel Smith and Benjamin Walford, 1698).
62. Kennedy, Supplement, 73–74.
63. Kennedy, Supplement, 84–85.
64. Kennedy, Supplement, 86.
65. Kennedy, Supplement, 86, 89.
66. Kennedy, Supplement, 89–90.
67. Kennedy, Supplement, 91.
68. Kennedy, Supplement, 92.
69. Kennedy, Supplement, 87–88.
70. Kennedy, Supplement, 93n.
71. Kennedy, Supplement, 94–95.
72. Kennedy, Supplement, 94.

73. Cheselden, *Anatomy*, 6th ed., 299–100.
74. Cheselden, *Anatomy*, 4th ed., 255.
75. Cheselden, *Anatomy*, 6th ed., 317.
76. Cheselden, *Anatomy*, 6th ed., 317.
77. Cheselden, *Anatomy*, 6th ed., 300.
78. Kennedy, *Supplement*, 71.
79. Kennedy, *Supplement*, 95–96.
80. Kennedy, *Supplement*, 96.
81. Kennedy, *Supplement*, 99.
82. Kennedy, *Supplement*, 72.
83. Kennedy, *Supplement*, 73.
84. Kennedy, *Supplement*, 73.
85. Kennedy, *Supplement*, 93.
86. These are high numbers of advertisements for any book, and particularly high numbers for a medical work.
87. *General Advertiser* (1744) (London), no. 4513, Monday, 17 April 1749.
88. London: J. Hooke and J. Graves, 1721; and a *Supplement* (London: T. Bickerton, 1721).
89. *London Journal* (1720), no. 225, Saturday, 16 November 1723.
90. Kennedy, *Supplement*, 73.
91. Kennedy, *External Remedies,* preface, unpaginated.

6. A Profession of Couching

1. Porter, *Health for Sale;* Daniel M. Albert and Sarah L. Atzen, *Chevalier John Taylor, England's Early Oculist: Pretender or Pioneer?* (Madison, WI: Parallel, 2012).
2. Lorenz Christoph Mizler, *Musikalische Bibliothek*, vol. 4 (1754); and, most recently, Nikolaus Forkel, *Johann Sebastian Bach: His Life, Work and Art,* trans. Charles Sandford Terry (New York: Harcourt Brace, 1920), 27.
3. Bert Lenth, "Bach and the English Oculist," *Music & Letters* 19, no. 2 (April 1938): 182–98.
4. *London Chronicle*, no. 542, 14 June 1760–17 June 1760. Handel had been couched on 3 November 1752 by William Bromfield (*General Advertiser* [1744] [London], no. 5622, Saturday, 4 November 1752), who was "not a particularly gifted surgeon" (*ODNB*) and who had no track record of couching operations.
5. *Public Advertiser* (London), no. 7426, Thursday, 24 August 1758.
6. Charles de Saint-Yves, *A new treatise of the diseases of the eyes. Containing proper remedies, and describing the chirurgical operations requisite for their cures* [. . .] (London: Crokatt, Osborne and Smith, 1741).
7. Cheselden died in 1752, so any patent on his operation would have died with him. This is the only record I have found of the Chevalier operating in this way.
8. According to the *Public Advertiser* (London), no. 13310, Tuesday, 10 June 1777, "Baron de Wenzel, Oculist to his Britannick Majesty, is arrived at his House in Pall-Mall, where he continues to perform the Operation of extracting the Cataract on the Poor Gratis." Below this advertisement is another: "A few days ago Hannah Steele, recommended by Mr Phillips and Mr Sutton, Churchwardens of St Martin's in the Fields

was restored to Sight by Mr Taylor, Oculist of Hatton Garden." The advertisements would suggest that the *ODNB* entry may be in error. John Taylor the fourth states in his own unreliable *Records of My Life* ([New York: J.&J. Harper, 1833], 15) that the post was to go to his father, but the Duke of Bedford, having had a cataract couched by the baron, persuaded the king to take him on in favor of John Taylor, oculist of Hatton Garden.

9. Peter Billings, *Folly Predominant* (London: H. Carpenter, 1755).
10. I have located about six hundred advertisements for each of the Chevalier and John Taylor, oculist of Hatton Garden, which span their careers.
11. John Taylor, *An account of the mechanism of the eye. Wherein its power of refracting the rays of light, and causing them to converge at the retina, is consider'd* [. . .] (Norwich: Henry Cross-Grove, 1727), 23, 24, 26.
12. There is a Green Plaque confirming "the printer" Henry Cross-Grove's dates as 1696–1744 on the Three-Tuns Public House in Earlham Road, Norwich.
13. As Roy Porter suggests, "it made better sense for the irregular doctor to be itinerant (mobility . . . gave the unscrupulous the advantage of being able to make himself scarce before his failures became obvious to all)" (*Health for Sale*, 61).
14. *Norwich Gazette*, no. 1848, 27 February 1742–6 March 1742.
15. *Norwich Gazette*, no. 1849, 6 March 1742–13 March 1742.
16. *Norwich Gazette*, no. 1850, 13 March 1742–20 March 1742.
17. *Norwich Gazette or The Loyal Packet*, Saturday, 26 January 1712.
18. *Philosphical Transactions* 35, no. 402 (1727–28).
19. Taylor, *An account of the mechanism of the eye*, 23–24.
20. Taylor, *An account of the mechanism of the eye*, 24.
21. Taylor, *An account of the mechanism of the eye*, 25–26.
22. John Taylor, *The History of the Travels and Adventures of the Chevalier John Taylor, Opthalmiater* (London: J. Williams, 1762), 1:9–10.
23. *London Evening Post*, no. 1174, 27 May 1735–29 May 1735.
24. *Daily Journal* (London), no. 5424, Tuesday, 15 July 1735.
25. BL catalogue lists: John Taylor, *Traite sur les maladies de l'organe immediat de la vue* (Paris, 1735). Benedict Duddell, *Supplement to the Treatise of the Horny Coat of the Eye*, 16, mentions he has seen this book and does not approve of it. He also mentions several translations.
26. John Taylor, *An impartial inquiry into the seat of the immediate organ of sight: viz. whether the retina or choroïdes. Being the subject of a lecture, in a course lately given on the nature and cure of the diseases of the eye* (London: M. Cooper, 1742), Wellcome Library.
27. *Daily Journal* (London), no. 5429, Monday, 21 July 1735.
28. London: T. Cooper, 1742.
29. *Daily Journal* (London), no. 5429, Monday, 21 July 1735.
30. Benedict Duddell was one of those who were present at the demonstration and who believed that the Chevalier was a quack, as I shall explore below.
31. *London Daily Post and General Advertiser*, no. 283, Monday, 29 September 1735.
32. *Daily Gazetteer* (London ed.), no. 118, Wednesday, 12 November 1735.
33. *Grub-Street Journal* (London), no. 307, Thursday, 13 November 1735.
34. *Grub-Street Journal* (London), no. 307, Thursday, 13 November 1735.

35. *Grub-Street Journal* (London), no. 307, Thursday, 13 November 1735.
36. The header of the first number, where the quote is taken from Pope's *Dunciad. Grub-Street Journal* (London), no. 1, Thursday, 8 January 1730.
37. Bertrand A. Goldgar, "Pope and the *Grub-Street Journal*," *Modern Philology* 74, no. 4 (May 1977): 366–80.
38. Goldgar, "Pope and the *Grub-Street Journal*," 375.
39. The *Treatise* was advertised in the *General Evening Post* (London), no. 348, 20 December 1735–23 December 1735, and in two subsequent numbers of the same newspaper. Also in the *London Evening Post*, no. 1265, 25 December 1735–27 December 1735.
40. *London Daily Post and General Advertiser*, no. 357, Wednesday, 24 December 1735.
41. John Taylor, *Treatise on the diseases of the Chrystalline Humour of a Human Eye* (London: James Roberts, 1736), ii.
42. Taylor, *Treatise*, ii.
43. Taylor, *Treatise*, ii.
44. Taylor, *Treatise*, iv.
45. Taylor, *Treatise*, 47.
46. Taylor, *Treatise*, 49.
47. Taylor, *Treatise*, 51.
48. Taylor, *Treatise*, 60.
49. *Grub-Street Journal* (London), no. 316, Thursday, 15 January 1736.
50. Taylor, *Treatise*, 8.
51. *Grub-Street Journal* (London), no. 317, Thursday, 22 January 1736.
52. Kennedy, *Supplement*, 71–72.
53. Kennedy, *Supplement*, 96.
54. Kennedy, *Supplement*, 97.
55. The sector was a hinged metal instrument which closed the two edges of the incision together.
56. Kennedy, *Supplement*, 98.
57. For example, in *Stamford Mercury* (Lincolnshire, England), Thursday, 22 January 1736; *Newcastle Courant* (Tyne and Wear, England), Saturday, 14 February 1736.
58. For example, *Caledonian Mercury* (Midlothian, Scotland), Tuesday, 1 June 1736, and *Derby Mercury*, (Derby, England), Thursday, 3 June 1736, note: "To-morrow Morning Dr Taylor begins his Progress to Bath, Bristol and Gloucester that the Country People may reap the Benefit of his expertise." Also, *Daily Gazetteer* (London ed.), no. 392, Tuesday, 28 September 1736, notes that the Chevalier is in Oxford.
59. George Coats, "The Chevalier Taylor," *Royal London Ophthalmic Hospital Reports* 20 (May 1913), reprinted in Robert Rutson James, *Studies in the History of Ophthalmology Prior to the Year 1800* (1933; repr., Cambridge: Cambridge University Press, 2013), 132–219.
60. For example, Anon., *The English Impostor Detected* (Dublin, 1732). Coats calls this "a work without Merit" (Rutson James, *Studies in the History of Ophthalmology*, 162). The piece, in English prose, Latin and English verse, is an attempt to copy Swift's style and reads the Chevalier as an English invader of Ireland, putting these words into his mouth: "O *Ireland*, thou land of Fools, doom'd to be the Prey of every Knave; how prosperously does Imposture thrive in thy fruitful Soil!" (10).

61. Fiona Haslam, *From Hogarth to Rowlandson: Medicine in Art in Eighteenth-Century Britain* (Liverpool: Liverpool University Press, 1996), 54.
62. *London Daily Post and General Advertiser*, no. 450, Saturday, 10 April 1736.
63. *Daily Gazetteer* (London ed.), no. 528, Saturday, 5 March 1737.
64. *Caledonian Mercury* (Midlothian, Scotland), no. 2555, Tuesday, 17 August 1736, and no. 2559, Thursday, 26 August 1736; *Stamford Mercury* (Lincolnshire, England), no. 220, Thursday, 26 August 1736; *Newcastle Courant* (Tyne and Wear, England), no. 592, Saturday, 28 August 1736. I cannot locate the poem in any of the London newspapers, but this is probably because the issues are missing or the OCR is unreadable.
65. *Grub-Street Journal* (London), no. 257, Thursday, 28 November 1734, lists twelve cases, where Ward's drop had caused such heavy purging that several patients had died.
66. Joshua Ward might be labeled a quack for having little or no official British medical training, but since he was exiled to France for sixteen years, and no one has researched what studies he might have carried out there, we might as easily give him the benefit of the doubt.
67. *Grub-Street Journal* (London), Thursday, no. 257, 28 November 1734.
68. *London Daily Post and General Advertiser*, no. 549, Wednesday, 4 August 1736.
69. It is not, but the *Ipswich Journal* of Saturday, 7 August 1736, describes the operation thus: "Mrs. Mapp perform[ed] an Operation on the Daughter of the Widow Armstead, a Shoemaker in Gracechurch Street, a young Woman about 14 Years of Age, whose Shoulder, Elbow and Wrist were out, . . . so much to his Lordship's [Lord Baltimore] Satisfaction, that he gave her five Guineas."
70. Haslam, *Hogarth to Rowlandson*, 54.
71. *London Daily Post and General Advertiser*, no. 603, Wednesday, 6 October 1736; *London Daily Post and General Advertiser*, no. 604, Thursday, 7 October 1736.
72. *London Daily Post and General Advertiser*, no. 605, Friday, 8 October 1736; *London Daily Post and General Advertiser*, no. 606, Saturday, 9 October 1736.
73. *Daily Journal* (London), no. 5819, Monday, 18 October 1736.
74. *Ipswich Gazette* (Suffolk, England), no. 845, Friday, 15 October 1736–Friday, 22 October 1736.
75. *Newcastle Courant* (Tyne and Wear, England), no. 501, Saturday, 30 October 1736.
76. *Daily Gazetteer* (London ed.), no. 409, Monday, 18 October 1736.
77. Anon., *The Operator* (London: T. Payne, 1740).
78. *London Evening Post*, no. 1923, 8 March 1740–11 March 1740. The advertisement for publication states: "This Play, contrary to the usual Custom of acting before it be known whether the Piece will bear it, is submittal to the candid Censure of the Publick, and then design'd to be exhibited on the Stage."
79. For example, on Thursday, 20 September 1736, the Chevalier's operations in Oxford were observed by Drs. Frewen and Frampton.
80. *Daily Advertiser* (London), no. 3745, Wednesday, 19 January 1743.
81. London: M. Cooper, 1761.
82. Anon., *The Life and Extraordinary History of the Chevalier John Taylor* (London: M. Cooper, 1761), 1:114–15.
83. Anon., *The Life and Extraordinary History*, passim.
84. Anon., *The Life and Extraordinary History*, 1:9.

85. Anon., *The Life and Extraordinary History*, 1:46–47.
86. He is baptized a Jew (Anon., *The Life and Extraordinary History*, 1:61).
87. His library, listed in Anon., *The Life and Extraordinary History*, 1:192–93, includes "Gavan's Master-Key to Popery; Hobb's Leviathan; . . . The Solemn League and Covenant [and] . . ."
88. John Philips, *The Splendid Shilling* (London: Thomas Bennet, 1705), 2.
89. Anon., *The Life and Extraordinary History*, 1:81–82.
90. *Tatler*, no. 249, 1710.
91. Joseph Addison, *An Essay on the Georgics*, in John Dryden, *The works of Virgil containing his Pastorals, Georgics and Aeneis: Adorn'd with a hundred sculptures, translated into English verse by Mr. Dryden* (London: Jacob Tonson, 1693), unpaginated.
92. *Oxford Dictionary of National Biography* (2004), s.v. "Taylor, John (1703–1772)," by Roy Porter.
93. Taylor, *Travels and Adventures*, 1:ii.
94. Taylor, *Travels and Adventures*, 1:iii.
95. Taylor, *Travels and Adventures*, 1:iv–vi.
96. Taylor, *Travels and Adventures*, 1:vi–xi.
97. Anon., *The Life and Extraordinary History*, unpaginated.
98. *Public Advertiser* (London), no. 7391, Wednesday, 5 July 1758.
99. *Public Advertiser* (London), Thursday, no. 8466, 24 December 1761.
100. *Lloyd's Evening Post and British Chronicle* (London), no. 727, 10 March 1762–12 March 1762.
101. *Lloyd's Evening Post and British Chronicle* (London), no. 784, 21 July 1762–23 July 1762; *London Chronicle*, no. 879, 10 August 1762–12 August 1762. *Lloyd's Evening Post and British Chronicle* (London), no. 794, 13 August 1762–16 August 1762.
102. *Lloyd's Evening Post and British Chronicle* (London), no. 784, 21 July 1762–23 July 1762; *London Chronicle*, no. 879, 10 August 1762–12 August 1762; *Lloyd's Evening Post and British Chronicle* (London), no. 794, 13 August 1762–16 August 1762.
103. Signed "T.S." and dated "Cheapside, June 24 1762." *St. James's Chronicle or the British Evening Post* (London), no. 207, 6 July 1762–8 July 1762.
104. *Lloyd's Evening Post* (London), no. 991, 16 November 1763–18 November 1763.
105. *Bath Chronicle and Weekly Gazette*, vol. 1, no. 35, Thursday, 11 June 1761.

7. Free and Accessible Eye Care for All

1. Both are described as "Itinerant Oculist" in the *ODNB*.
2. Rutson James, *Studies in Ophthalmology*, 122–219. Porter, *Health for Sale*, 61–79.
3. Oldys, *Observations on the Cure of William Taylor*, 5.
4. *Public Advertiser* (London), no. 8201, Monday, 16 February 1761.
5. *Public Advertiser* (London), no. 8476, Monday, 4 January 1762.
6. John Taylor, *An Account of some of the many Remarkable Cures of Various Diseases of the Eyes, performed by John Taylor, Oculist of Hatton Garden, who practiced for upwards of thirty years in London only* (repr., London, 1777).
7. *ODNB*.
8. *Lloyd's Evening Post* (London), no. 991, 16 November 1763–18 November 1763.

9. Oldys, *Observations of the Cure of William Taylor*, iv.
10. *General Advertiser* (1744) (London), no. 5202, Saturday, 22 June 1751.
11. The incident of the pawned diamond cross in Edinburgh is noted above. The Chevalier was also mentioned as a "Fugitive surrendered to the Warden of His Majesty's Prison of the FLEET" during the scandal about the spurious *Life* (*London Gazette*, no. 10155, 7 November 1761–10 November 1761.
12. There is no contemporary short form to indicate "John Taylor, oculist of Hatton garden," and I don't want to call him "John Taylor" because his grandfather, father, and son were also "John Taylor." I'm using the diminutive "Junior" because in many ways he was a cadet version of his father, the Chevalier, and unlike his own son, he remained in the family business.
13. *Daily Advertiser* (London), no. 4015, Wednesday, 30 November 1743, repeated verbatim in *Daily Advertiser* (London), no. 4027, Wednesday, 14 December 1743.
14. *ODNB*. Once again this information is derived from John Taylor, *Records of My Life*, which is simply the recounting of family stories and gossip, and claims for itself no accuracy to date and detail.
15. *General Advertiser* (1744) (London), no. 4488, Saturday, 18 March 1749.
16. *London Evening Post*, no. 3594, 1 November 1750–3 November 1750.
17. There is no record of the Chevalier being accepted into the Company of Surgeons, who licensed apprenticeships.
18. *Daily Advertiser* (London), no. 4066, Saturday, 28 January 1744, repeated in *Daily Advertiser* (London), no. 4078, Saturday, 11 February 1744.
19. *Daily Advertiser* (London), no. 4120, Saturday, 31 March 1744.
20. *Daily Advertiser* (London), no. 4150, Saturday, 5 May 1744; *London Evening Post*, no. 2582, 24 May 1744–26 May 1744; *London Evening Post*, no. 2587, 5 June 1744–7 June 1744.
21. *London Evening Post*, no. 2591, 14 June 1744–16 June 1744.
22. *London Evening Post*, no. 2446, 12 July 1743–14 July 1743; advertisement for *An Impartial Enquiry into the Seat of the Immediate Organ of Sight*.
23. *Daily Advertiser* (London), no. 4198, Saturday, 30 June 1744.
24. *Daily Advertiser* (London), no. 4378, Saturday, 3 November 1744.
25. *Daily Advertiser* (London), no. 4402, Saturday, 1 December 1744.
26. *Daily Advertiser* (London), no. 4432, Saturday, 5 January 1745; *Daily Advertiser* (London), no. 4450, Saturday, 26 January 1745; *Daily Advertiser* (London), no. 4414, Saturday, 9 March 1745; *London Evening Post*, no. 2711, 21 March 1745–23 March 1745; *Daily Advertiser* (London), no. 4432, Saturday, 30 March 1745; *Daily Advertiser* (London), no. 4450, Saturday, 20 April 1745; *Daily Advertiser* (London), no. 4462, Saturday, 4 May 1745.
27. *George Faulkner the Dublin Journal* (Ireland), no. 1896, 7 May 1745–11 May 1745.
28. *George Faulkner the Dublin Journal* (Ireland), no. 1904, 4 June 1745–8 June 1745.
29. *George Faulkner the Dublin Journal* (Ireland), no. 1905, 8 June 1745–11 June 1745.
30. *Daily Advertiser* (London), no. 4548, 20 July 1745.
31. *General Advertiser* (1744) (London), no. 3730, Saturday, 11 October 1746.
32. *George Faulkner the Dublin Journal* (Ireland), no. 2100, 28 April 1747–2 May 1747, notes the Chevalier is still in Dublin and has perfected an operation to correct squinting.

General Evening Post (London), no. 2219, 26 December 1747–29 December 1747, reports that the Chevalier returning to London via Liverpool "and is expected at Queen's Street from Bristol in a few Days."

33. *London Evening Post*, no. 3153, 16 January 1748–19 January 1748; *London Evening Post*, no. 3236, 28 July 1748–30 July 1748; *London Evening Post*, no. 3251, 1 September 1748–3 September 1748; *London Evening Post*, no. 3269, 13 October 1748–15 October 1748; *London Evening Post*, no. 3270, 15 October 1748–18 October 1748; *General Advertiser* (1744) (London), no. 4366, Saturday, 22 October 1748.

34. *General Advertiser* (1744) (London), no. 4371, Friday, 28 October 1748, First Lecture; *General Advertiser* (1744) (London), no. 4374, Monday, 31 October 1748; Second Lecture; *London Evening Post*, no. 3276, 29 October 1748–1 November 1748, Third Lecture; *General Advertiser* (1744) (London), no. 4375, Wednesday, 2 November 1748; *General Advertiser* (1744) (London), no. 4376, Thursday, 3 November 1748, Subscription Book for the whole series of 30 lectures; *General Advertiser* (1744) (London), no. 4383, Friday, no. 4383, 11 November 1748, First Lecture, this day; *General Advertiser* (1744) (London), no. 4384, Saturday, 12 November 1748; *General Advertiser* (1744) (London), no. 4388, Thursday, 17 November 1748; *General Advertiser* (1744) (London), no. 4389, Friday, 18 November 1748; *General Advertiser* (1744) (London), no. 4390, Saturday, 19 November 1748, Lecture, and a new lecture at Mercers' Hall next Monday; *General Advertiser* (1744) (London), no. 4391, Monday, 21 November 1748; *General Advertiser* (1744) (London), no. 4392, Tuesday, 22 November 1748; *General Advertiser* (1744) (London), no. 4394, Thursday, 24 November 1748; *General Advertiser* (1744) (London), no. 4396, Friday, 25 November 1748, Fourth Lecture; *General Advertiser* (1744) (London), no. 4396, Saturday, 26 November 1748, Theological lecture on Sunday; *General Advertiser* (1744) (London), no. 4397, Monday, 28 November 1748, Mercers' Hall Lecture tonight; *General Advertiser* (1744) (London), no. 4398, Tuesday, 29 November 1748, mentions 100 cures; *General Advertiser* (1744) (London), no. 4400, Thursday, 1 December 1748; *General Advertiser* (1744) (London), no. 4401, Friday, 2 December 1748; *General Advertiser* (1744) (London), no. 4402, Saturday, 3 December 1748; *London Evening Post*, no. 3290, 1 December 1748–3 December 1748, two cures from the tour and two lectures;*General Advertiser* (1744) (London), no. 4417, Friday, 23 December 1748, possibly spurious lecture advertisement mentioning the imitator: Foote.

35. *General Advertiser* (1744) (London), no. 14401, Friday, 2 December 1748, Auction 40, "And an Oration in Praise of Sight, as at Edinburgh, Oxford, Cambridge, Dublin and Foreign Universities"; *General Advertiser* (1744) (London), no. 4404, Tuesday, 6 December 1748, Auction 41, "And an Oration in Praise of Sight, as at Edinburgh, Oxford, Cambridge, Dublin and Foreign Universities"; *General Advertiser* (1744) (London), no. 4407, Friday, 9 December 1748, Auction 42, "And an Oration in Praise of Sight, as at Edinburgh, Oxford, Cambridge, Dublin and Foreign Universities. With a DANCE in CHARACTER"; *General Advertiser* (1744) (London), no. 4412, Thursday, 15 December 1748, Auction 44, "And an Oration in Praise of Sight, as at Edinburgh, Oxford, Cambridge, Dublin and Foreign Universities. With a DANCE in CHARACTER"; *General Advertiser* (1744) (London), no. 4412, Saturday, 17 December 1748, Auction 45, "By DESIRE. . . . And an Oration in Praise of Sight, as at Edinburgh, Oxford, Cambridge, Dublin and Foreign Universities. With a DANCE in CHARACTER"; *General Advertiser*

(1744) (London), no 4415, Wednesday, 21 December 1748, Auction 46, "By DESIRE.... And an Oration in Praise of Sight, as at Edinburgh, Oxford, Cambridge, Dublin and Foreign Universities. With a DANCE in CHARACTER.... Mr FOOTE, having read Yesterday Dr TAYLOR'S Paragraph, is determined to pay his Compliments to him on Friday next, and will emend his Conduct in Regard to that Imitation"; *General Advertiser* (1744) (London), no. 4417, Friday, 23 December 1748, Auction 47, "By DESIRE.... And an Oration in Praise of Sight, as at Edinburgh, Oxford, Cambridge, Dublin and Foreign Universities. With a DANCE in CHARACTER"; *General Advertiser* (1744) (London), no. 4420, Tuesday, 27 December 1748, Auction 48, "By DESIRE.... And an Oration in Praise of Sight, as at Edinburgh, Oxford, Cambridge, Dublin and Foreign Universities. With a DANCE in CHARACTER.... (Being positively the last Time of performing this Season)"; *General Advertiser* (1744) (London), no. 4422, Thursday, 29 December 1748, Auction 49 "By DESIRE.... And an Oration in Praise of Sight, as at Edinburgh, Oxford, Cambridge, Dublin and Foreign Universities. With a DANCE in CHARACTER"; *General Advertiser* (1744) (London), no. 4429, Wednesday, 4 January 1749, Auction 50, "By DESIRE.... And an Oration in Praise of Sight, as at Edinburgh, Oxford, Cambridge, Dublin and Foreign Universities. With a DANCE in CHARACTER"; *General Advertiser* (1744) (London), no. 4433, Monday, 9 January 1749, Auction 51, "An ORATION in Praise of SIGHT &c"; *General Advertiser* (1744) (London), no. 4436, Thursday, 12 January 1749, Auction 52, "An ORATION in Praise of SIGHT &c."; *General Advertiser* (1744) (London), no. 4439, Monday, January 23, 1749, Auction "by Desire ... An ORATION in Praise of SIGHT &c."; *General Advertiser* (1744) (London), no. 4442, Friday, 27 January 1749, Auction 54, no further references to Taylor.

36. *General Advertiser* (1744) (London), no. 3730, Saturday, 11 October 1746.
37. *General Advertiser* (1744) (London), no. 4366, Saturday, 22 October 1748.
38. *Bath Chronicle*, no. 1413, Thursday, 27 December 1787, Dr Hodson, purveyor of Persian Drops; *Gazetteer and London Daily Advertiser*, no. 9894, Wednesday, 31 December 1760, Dr. Lowther Anti-Scorbutic medicine, treatments for nervous disorders &c. No 14 Hatton Garden; *Gazetteer and New Daily Advertiser* (London), no. 12059, Wednesday, 28 October 1767, Mrs. Gibson's Medicine for Conception; *London Daily Advertiser and Literary Gazette*, no. 228, Saturday, 23 November 1751, Dr Horseman, elector of the College of Physicians; *London Evening Post*, no. 4570, 19 February 1757–22 February 1757, Dr Butler, "Eminent Physician"; *Morning Herald* (London), Monday, no. 1756, 12 June 1786, advertises a hospital called the Universal Medical Asylum; *Morning Herald* (London), 2268, Tuesday, 29 January 1788, Dr. Fothergill's [Fothergels] Medicine for nervous Complaints; *Public Advertiser* (London), no. 9733, Friday, 10 January 1766, Mr. Gibson's hair removal creams; *Public Advertiser* (London), no. 8804, Thursday, 20 January 1763, Dr. Blackwood's tincture for sale at Mr Hodge's Little Kirby St., Hatton Garden; *Public Advertiser* (London), no. 10593, Tuesday, 11 October 1768, Hamilton's Toothache tincture; *Public Advertiser* (London), no. 6961, Wednesday, 16 February 1757, Dr. Chapman practitioner in Venereal Disease; *Whitehall Evening Post or London Intelligencer*, 16 January 1755–18 January 1755, Peter Billings, Professor of Lunacy; *Whitehall Evening Post or London Intelligencer*, no. 663, 10 May 1750–12 May 1750, Dr Henry, practitioner in Nervous Disorders; *Whitehall Evening Post or London Intelligencer*, no. 2101, 4 September 1759–6 September 1759. Dr Rayment, practitioner in

nervous disorders; *Whitehall Evening Post or London Intelligencer*, no. 1304, 21 September 1754–24 September 1754. Mr. Hewitt, Surgeon; *Weekly Journal with Fresh Advices Foreign and Domestick* (London), Saturday, 28 May 1715, David Povey, Dentist; *Whitehall Evening Post or London Intelligencer*, no. 1534, 23 December 1755–25 December 1755, Benjamin Bosanquet, Physician.

39. *General Advertiser* (1744) (London), no. 5273, Saturday, 14 September 1751.
40. *London Evening Post*, no. 2820, 30 November 1745–3 December 1745.
41. *General Advertiser* (1744) (London), no. 4787, Sunday, 26 February 1749.
42. *General Advertiser* (1744) (London), no. 4488, Saturday, 18 March 1749.
43. *London Evening Post*, no. 3594, 1 November 1750–3 November 1750.
44. *General Advertiser* (1744) (London), no. 5135, Friday, 5 April 1751.
45. *General Advertiser* (1744) (London), no. 5143, Monday, 15 April 1751.
46. *General Advertiser* (1744) (London), no. 5144, Tuesday, 16 April 1751, repeated in *London Evening Post*, no. 3666, 18 April 1751–20 April 1751.
47. *General Advertiser* (1744) (London), no. 5202, Saturday, 22 June 1751.
48. *London Daily Advertiser and Literary Gazette*, no. 216, Saturday, 9 November 1751; *London Daily Advertiser and Literary Gazette*, no. 218, Tuesday, 12 November 1751; *London Evening Post*, no. 3759, 21 November 1751–23 November 1751; *London Evening Post*, no. 3762, 28 November 1751–30 November 1751.
49. *Daily Advertiser* (London), no. 6595, Wednesday, 26 February 1752; *General Advertiser* (1744) (London), no. 4554, Saturday, 11 April 1752.
50. John Taylor, *Records of My Life*, 17. This is the autobiography of the fourth John Taylor, 1757–1832, son of John Taylor of Hatton Garden. It was published in New York by J&J Harper in 1833.
51. Rutson James in *Studies* writes that "Oldys' account of the blind boy of Ightham cured by Taylor is greatly inferior to Cheselden's" (232). But this is probably because he does not recognise that the mistakes the boy makes were consonant with Berkeley's expectation that distance was learned from experience. Nor, strangely, does Rutson James make much of the idea of founding the first English hospital for the blind.
52. John Taylor, *Records of My Life*, suggests that Monsey was "one of my father's [Junior's] earliest and warmest friends" (19) and that Monsey had called him in when Godolphin needed to be bled (54).
53. As was William Cheselden.
54. London: E. Newbery, 1791. There were at least eight editions.
55. John Taylor, *Records of My Life*, 27.
56. Oldys, *Observations of the Cure of William Taylor*, v.
57. Oldys, *Observations, of the Cure of William Taylor*, v.
58. Oldys, *Observations, of the Cure of William Taylor*, vi.
59. *London Daily Advertiser*, no. 552, Saturday, 16 December 1752.
60. *London Evening Post*, no. 3930, 4 January 1753–6 January 1753.
61. *Public Advertiser* (London), no. 5699, Friday, 2 February 1753.
62. *London Daily Advertiser*, no. 623, Friday, 9 March 1753; *Public Advertiser* (London), no. 5736, Saturday, 17 March 1753.
63. Which would account for Rutson James's disparaging comment about it.
64. Oldys, *Observations of the Cure of William Taylor*, 9–10.

65. Oldys, *Observations of the Cure of William Taylor*, 5.
66. *London Evening Post*, no. 3594, 1 November 1750–3 November 1750.
67. Oldys, *Observations of the Cure of William Taylor*, 7.
68. Oldys, *Observations of the Cure of William Taylor* 7.
69. *Norwich Gazette*, no. 1848, 27 February 1742–6 March 1742.
70. Oldys, *Observations of the Cure of William Taylor*, 11.
71. See pages <oo> in chapter 1 of this volume.
72. Oldys, *Observations of the Cure of William Taylor*, 20.
73. *ODNB*.
74. The *ODNB* tells us that Boyce set many songs for the stage, as well as internal music.
75. Oldys, *Observations of the Cure of William Taylor*, 25–26.
76. *London Daily Advertiser*, no. 662, Tuesday, 24 April 1753. Cure Thomas Arne. Arne wrote music for Frederick Prince of Wales, including "Rule Britannia!" while Boyce wrote for the king, and probably most notably "Heart of Oak"!
77. *London Daily Advertiser and Literary Gazette*, no. 216, Saturday, 9 November 1751.
78. John Taylor, *Records of My Life*, 30. It is not out of the bounds of possibility that Junior trained Jonathan Wathen, who developed eye surgery in the late eighteenth century along with his apprentice James Ware. Wathen was apprenticed to his brother Samuel Wathen, but he had no other formal medical training. Together the brothers worked on venereal diseases, but why Jonathan Wathen turned to eye surgery after 1777 and who taught him is not known. However, it must be remembered that Junior's profession was winding down in 1777, and there is no record of him operating after 1780.
79. John Taylor, *Records of My Life*, 14.
80. *Public Advertiser* (London), no. 5781, Wednesday, 9 May 1753.
81. Samuel Sharp, "A Description of a New Method of Opening the Cornea, in Order to Extract the Crystalline Humour; By Mr. Samuel Sharp, Surgeon to Guy's Hospital, and F.R.S," *Philosophical Transactions* 48 (1753): 161–63.
82. Samuel Sharp, "A Second Account of the New Method of Opening the Cornea, for Taking away the Cataract; By Samuel Sharp, Surgeon to Guy's Hospital, and F.R.S." *Philosophical Transactions* 48 (1753): 322–31.
83. *Public Advertiser* (London), no. 5964, Saturday, 8 December 1753.
84. *Public Advertiser* (London), no. 6068, Tuesday, 9 April 1754; "Master Smith . . . after being deemed incurable"; *Public Advertiser* (London), no. 6142, Saturday, 6 July 1754, "Mr James Johnson, a Prisoner in the Fleet, received a Blow on his Right Eye, which not only deprived him of his sight, but brought on an Eversion of the lower Eye-lip, attended with a Tumour the size of a large Wallnut"; *Public Advertiser* (London), no. 6226, Saturday, 12 October 1754, "Joseph Ingram in the Work-House upon Saffron Hill . . . who had been blind twenty five Years"; *Public Advertiser* (London), no. 6850, Saturday, 2 October 1756, "Daughter of Mr Hargraft . . . was restored to Sight"; *Public Advertiser* (London), no. 6902, Saturday, 20 November 1756, "Daughter of Captain Cuite . . . who had labored under a violent Inflammation, and loss of Sight for several Weeks, . . . quite recovered."
85. *Public Advertiser* (London), no. 7460, Saturday, 23 September 1758.
86. *Public Advertiser* (London), no. 7478, Saturday, 28 October 1758.

87. I cannot locate a contemporary copy of the *Proposal*, but the substance of it appears to be that reprinted in a slightly altered form in *An Account of some of the many Remarkable Cures... Performed by John Taylor, Oculist of Hatton Garden* (London: "Reprinted," 1777). I do not know what "Reprinted" means exactly, but many advertisements use the phrase "Pamphlet of cures gratis," which I believe to be a version of this final pamphlet. The 1777 book itself reprints a number of the advertisement formulae that had been used in newspapers.
88. John Taylor, *An Account of some of the many Remarkable Cures* [...], 3–4.
89. John Taylor, *An Account of some of the many Remarkable Cures* [...], 4–5.
90. *Public Advertiser* (London), no. 10084, Thursday, 26 February 1767.
91. *Gazetteer and New Daily Advertiser* (London), no. 12641, Wednesday, 6 September 1769; *Public Advertiser* (London), no. 10874, Friday, 8 September 1769.
92. *Public Advertiser* (London), no. 0278, Saturday, 17 March 1759.
93. *Public Advertiser* (London), no. 8233, Wednesday, 25 March 1761.
94. *Public Advertiser* (London), no. 8404, Monday, 12 October 1761.
95. *Gazetteer and London Daily Advertiser*, no. 10384, Wednesday, 4 August 1762.
96. *Public Advertiser* (London), no. 8931, Friday, 17 June 1763.
97. *Gazetteer and New Daily Advertiser* (London), no. 12941, Wednesday, 22 August 1770; *Gazetteer and New Daily Advertiser* (London), no. 12943, Friday, 24 August 1770; *Gazetteer and New Daily Advertiser* (London), no. 12949, Friday, 31 August 1770.
98. *Gazetteer and New Daily Advertiser* (London), no. 12259, Friday, 17 June 1768; *Public Advertiser* (London), no. 10503, Saturday, 25 June 1768.
99. *Public Advertiser* (London), no. 10503, Tuesday, 28 June 1768.
100. The earliest date for this addition to parish recommendation is in an advertisement in the *Public Advertiser* (London), no. 7953, Saturday, 3 May 1760. The advertisement claims that the subscription "will soon be filled... [and] the List may be seen at his House."
101. *Public Advertiser* (London), no. 8938, Saturday, 25 June 1763.
102. Although there is no evidence, it is quite likely that he and his father divided their practice in 1748, with the Chevalier taking the country, and Junior, the city.
103. John Taylor, *Records of My Life*, 14.
104. *London Evening Post*, no. 6682, 13 September 1770–15 September 1770; *Bingley's Weekly Journal Or the Universal Gazette* (London), Saturday, no. 16, 22 September 1770.
105. *Public Advertiser* (London), no. 8169, Friday, 9 January 1761. The "large room" does not appear on Rocque's 1746 Map of London, though the Dog and Duck does, on Lambeth Road, roughly where the Imperial War Museum now stands. The Asylum, according to John Entick, "is a Modern Charity... or house of refuge for orphans and other deserted girls of the poor, under 12 years of age, to preserve them from the miseries and dangers to which they would be exposed, and from the guilt of prostitution: proposed by Sir John Fielding, Knt., and supported by private charities" (Entick, *A new and accurate history and survey of London, Westminster, Southwark, and places adjacent; containing whatever is most worthy of notice in...* [London: Edward and Charles Dilly, 1766], 386–87).
106. Its drink license was taken away after a long legal wrangle between 1781 and 1799. It is no surprise that Rev. John Entick does not mention it in his comprehensive survey

107. *London Evening Post*, no. 5014, 22 December 1759–25 December 1759, New Cure for Birth Blindness.
108. *Daily Advertiser* (London), no. 13047, Friday, 16 October 1772.
109. *Gazetteer and New Daily Advertiser* (London), no. 11791, Saturday, 20 December 1766.
110. *Lloyd's Evening Post and British Chronicle* (London), no. 647, 4 September 1761–7 September 1761.
111. *Lloyd's Evening Post* (London), no. 975, 10 October 1763–12 October 1763; *Public Advertiser* (London), no. 9087, Saturday, 17 December 1763.
112. *Gazetteer and New Daily Advertiser* (London), no. 11561, Tuesday, 1 April 1766; *Gazetteer and New Daily Advertiser* (London), no. 11575, Thursday, 17 April 1766.
113. *World and Fashionable Advertiser* (London), no. 213, Wednesday, 19 September 1787.
114. It is interesting that James Jurin's treatment of Robert Walpole's bladder stones using soap continued to his death because of Walpole's fear of William Cheselden's "Lateral" operation, so might be classed as complementary medicine.

8. Thomas Gills of St. Edmunds-Bury and the Itinerant Giver

1. There is some confusion about his name, since only three of his pamphlets bear the name "Gills" while seven call him "Gill," and two do not use his name. However, one "Thomas Gills, A blind Man" was buried at St. Mary's Church, St. Edmunds-Bury on 15 January 1715 (Bury St. Edmunds Record Office, 545/4/3), and it is from this record that I chose to give his name the final "s."
2. Chris Mounsey, "'God grant us Grace, that we may take due Pains, / To practice what this Exercise contains; / To which, if we apply our best Endeavour, / We shall be happy here, and bless'd for ever.' Thomas Gills: An Eighteenth-Century Blind Poet and the Language of Charity," in *The Idea of Disability in the Eighteenth Century*, ed. Mounsey (Lewisburg, PA: Bucknell University Press, 2014), 225.
3. Olwen Hufton, *The Poor of Eighteenth Century France 1750–1789* (Oxford: Clarendon, 1974); Steven King and Alana Tomkins, eds., *The Poor in England 1700–1850* (Manchester: Manchester University Press, 2003).
4. In this argument I followed Thomas Sokoll, *Essex Pauper Letters 1731–1837* (Oxford: Clarendon, 2001) and explored the two poems by Gills along with the catechism available on ECCO, "Upon the Recovery of his Sight and the Second loss thereof," which was printed with a more general lamentation "On the Misery of Blindness" and dated 1710 with no evidence.
5. For the discovery of these works, I am indebted to Bridget Keegan and John Goodridge and the Nottingham Trent University Laboring Class Poets Online project (https://lcpoets.wordpress.com/introtobibliography/).
6. J.O., Thomas Gill, the Blind Man of St. Edmundsbury, in *Notes and Queries*, vol. s1-V, no. 139 (June 1852): 608.
7. National Library of Scotland, Call number: CWN 301 (1–8).
8. Both printed in London and dated 1709.

9. There is no date or place of publication.
10. Copies of *New-year's gift* and *The Blind man's case* are both recorded in the Yale Beinecke Library, but I have not examined these.
11. Mounsey, "God Grant us Grace," 227.
12. Gills, *Blind man's case*, 3.
13. Gills, *Blind man's case*, 6.
14. Gills, *Blind man's case*, 8.
15. Bury St. Edmunds Record Office, 545/4/3.
16. See http://www.clockswatches.co.uk/index.php.
17. Worldcat gives the spelling of this word as "Circumsision" for both the Beinecke and the National Library of Scotland (NLS) editions of this poem, but that at the NLS is spelled correctly.
18. Whether or not these Janeways were related to the Richard Janeways father and son is not certain, but the name is not common, and the publication list of Janeway Senior suggests that they were.
19. For example, Richard Baxter, *Which is the True Church?* (London: printed, and are to be sold by Richard Janeway, in Butcher-Hall Lane, 1679); Samuel Bold, *A Plea for moderation towards Dissenters* (London: R. Janeway in Queen's Head Alley, in Pater-Noster Row, 1683); Increase Mather, *A narrative of the miseries of New England, by reason of the arbitrary government erected there* (London: printed for Richard Janeway in Queen's Head-Court in Pater Noster Row . . . , 1688).
20. Anon., *A true narrative of the Duke of Monmouth's late journey into the west* (London: printed and to be sold by Richard Janeway in Queen's-Head Alley in Pater-Noster Row, 1680). That year Janeway published twelve additional, more-or-less sensational four-page pamphlets; cf. Francis Nicholson, *The confession of Francis Nicholson (who committed the most barbarous murther upon the body of John Dimbleby, servant to Mr. Marriot) at the place of execution which was upon the green over against Hampton Court, and near the place where he did the murther on Wednesday last, it being the 27th of October 1680* (London: printed and to be sold by Richard Janeway, 1680).
21. *The acceptable sacrifice, or, The excellency of a broken heart shewing the nature, signs, and proper effects of a contrite spirit / being the last works of that eminent preacher and faithful minister of Jesus Christ, Mr. John Bunyan of Bedford* (London: printed by Rich. Janeway, Jun. for John Gwillim . . . , 1698); *The barren fig-tree: or The doom and downfal of the fruitless professor. Shewing that the day of grace may be past with him long before his life is ended. The signs also by which such miserable mortals may be known. / By John Bunyan . . . ; To which is added, his Exhortation to peace and unity among all that fear God. Exhortation to peace and unity among all that fear God. Exhortation to peace and unity among all that fear God* (London: printed by R. Janeway, jun. for Jonathan Robinson, at the Golden Lion in St. Paul's Church-Yard, 1698).
22. For example, Francis Bugg, *Some reasons humbly offered to the honourable House of Commons, why the Quakers principles and practices should be examined, and censured or suppressed,* (London: printed for the author, by Rich. Janeway, Jun. on Addle-Hill, near Doctors-Commons, and sold by J. Robinson, at the Golden-lion, in St. Paul's Church-yard; where also may be had his other books, 1699).
23. A. J., *A compleat account of the Portugueze language. Being a copious dictionary of English*

with *Portugueze, and Portugueze with English* [. . .] (London: printed by R. Janeway, for the Author, 1701).
24. *The Celestial Envoy: or, a scene not yet Acted. Containing some short notations on the 10th chapter of the Book of Apocalypse. Humbly inscrib'd to the E—of OX—D* (London: printed by R. Janeway, in Dogwel-Court in White Friars, for the Author, 1713).
25. Gills, *Upon the circumcision*, 4.
26. Gills, *Upon the circumcision*, 5.
27. Gills, *Upon the circumcision*, 5–6.
28. Gills, *Upon the Circumcision*, 7.
29. Gills, *Upon the circumcision*, 6.
30. Gills, *Upon the Nativity*, 1.
31. Robert Nelson, *A companion for the festivals and fasts of the Church of England: With collects and prayers for each solemnity* (London: printed by W.B. for A. and J. Churchill, at the Black Swan in Pater Noster Row, 1704).
32. Nelson, *Companion*, x.
33. Nelson, *Companion*, xix.
34. Nelson, *Companion*, xxii.
35. Gills, *Upon the Nativity*, 3.
36. Gills, *Upon the Nativity*, 7.
37. Gills, *Upon the Nativity*, 8.
38. *Examiner or Remarks upon Papers and Occurrences* (London), no. 4, 13 November 1712–20 November 1712.
39. On 8 March 1711, a French refugee, the former abbé La Bourlie (better known by the name of the Marquis de Guiscard) was being examined before the Privy Council on a charge of treason, when he stabbed Harley in the breast with a penknife.
40. *Oxford Dictionary of National Biography*, s.v. "Hamilton, James, fourth duke of Hamilton and first duke of Brandon (1658–1712)," by Rosalind K. Marshall, accessed 1 July 2015.
41. Gills, *Lamentation*, 1.
42. Gills, *Lamentation*, 3.
43. Gills, *Lamentation*, 3.
44. Gills, *Lamentation*, 3.
45. Gills, *Lamentation*, 4.
46. *Tatler* (1709) (London), no. 238, 14 October 1710–17 October 1710.
47. Brendan O'Hehir, "Meaning of Swift's 'Description of a City Shower,'" *English Literary History* 27, no. 3 (September 1960): 202.
48. Thomas Gills, *The Blind man's case at London: or, a character of that city. Sent in a letter to his friend in the country* (London, 1711), shelved at National Library of Scotland, Cwn.301 (8).
49. Both are available on ECCO.
50. The only known copy is in the National Library of Scotland, shelved at NLS Cwn 301 (2).
51. Both are available on ECCO.
52. Worldcat likewise suggests there are two editions of *Upon the Recovery of his Sight, and the Second Loss thereof* in 1705 and 1710 (the ECCO version has no date), and two edi-

tions of *The Blind man's case* in 1711 and 1712 (the latter being the date of the Beinecke catalogue).
53. The only known copy is in the National Library of Scotland, shelved at NLS Cwn 301 (3).

9. John Maxwell

1. John Maxwell, *The reflection* (York: Thomas Gent, 1743), 3.
2. Alexander Pope, *Windsor Forest* (London: Bernard Lintott, 1713)
3. Alexander Pope, *An Essay on Criticism* (London: W. Lewis, W. Taylor, T. Osborn, J. Graves, 1711), 10.
4. John Dryden, *Alexander's Feast; or the Power of Musique. An Ode for St Cecilia's Day* (London: Tonson, 1697).
5. Pope, *Essay on Criticism*, 21.
6. Pope, *Essay on Criticism*, 23.
7. Cambridge: J. Bentham, 1743.
8. N.p: n.p., 1751.
9. Earl R. Wasserman, "Pope's Ode for Musick," *English Literary History* 28, no. 2 (June 1961): 163. Wasserman is trying to change critics' minds about the poem in this paper, but it makes a useful starting point for my argument.
10. Alexander Pope, *Ode for Musick* (London: Bernard Lintott, 1713), 8.
11. Elkanah Settle, *Thalia Triumphans* (London, 1715, 1716, 1722).
12. John Dryden, *Eleonora* (London: Jacob Tonson, 1692), 20.
13. Garth, *The dispensary*, canto IV, 45. A "Jakes" is a toilet.
14. Milton, *Paradise Lost*, bk. VIII (London: Peter Parker and Robert Boulter, 1667), unpaginated.
15. Stephen Duck, *Poems on Several Occasions* (London: J. Roberts, 1730).
16. Maxwell, *The reflection*, 4.
17. Maxwell, *The reflection*, 4–5. The only way the last line in this quote scans is if the word "contemplates" is read with a strong Yorkshire accent as two iambs "con-tem" and "pul-ates."
18. Maxwell, *The reflection*, 5.
19. Maxwell, *The reflection*, 5.
20. Maxwell, *The reflection*, 6.
21. Maxwell, *The reflection*, 21.
22. Maxwell, *The reflection*, 21.
23. Maxwell, *The reflection*, 13.
24. The Royal Martyr may be King Charles I, who was beheaded at the Banqueting House in 1648, or James II, whose removal from office was widely regarded in the eighteenth century as "Dry Martyrdom" since his head was not cut off.
25. Maxwell, *The reflection*, 28.
26. Maxwell, *The reflection*, 16.
27. For example in *The miscellaneous works in prose and verse of Mrs. Elizabeth Rowe*, 2 vols. (London: R. Hett & R. Dodsley, 1739), 1:21.
28. Maxwell, *The reflection*, 13.

29. London: Henry Herringman, 1668.
30. London: Jacob Tonson, 1685.
31. London: Henry Herringman, 1676.
32. (London: T.H. &c, 1710), 185.
33. London: Henry Herringman, 1671.
34. English translation: London: H. Rhodes, 1683.
35. London: John Harding and Richard Wilkin, 1696.
36. London: Jacob Tonson, 1693.
37. *Five New Plays* (London: Henry Herringman, Jacob Tonson &c., 1692).
38. London: Humphrey Moseley and Thomas Dring, 1653.
39. London: H. Rhodes, 1683.
40. London: Jacob Tonson, 1703.
41. London: A. Millar & R. Dodsley, 1755.
42. London: James Magnes, 1678.
43. 3 vols. (London: R. Bentley, 1695) or 6 vols. (London: Jacob Tonson, 1717–18, 1725).
44. Maxwell, *The reflection*, 11.
45. The same register gives the name of a son as "Umfra," which may be "Humphrey."
46. Francis Drake, *Eboracum: or the History and Antiquities of the City of York* (London: William Bowyer, 1739), 304.
47. (Leeds: Leeds Mercury Office, 1823), 54.
48. North Yorkshire County Archive, Northallerton, zym ii 2/1 mic 3069 /0001.
49. The Minute Book notes *ex gratia* payments of 10 shillings to two people who were "half-blind."
50. Drake, *Eboracum*, 304.
51. See *Register of the Freemen of the City of York, vol. 2, 1559–1759*, ed. Francis Collins (Durham, 1900), British History Online, http://www.british-history.ac.uk/york-freemen/vol2/pp262-289.
52. All other recipients of money were in benefit until they died.
53. S. L. Ollard and P. C. Walker, eds., *Archbishop Herring's visitation returns, 1743* (Leeds: Yorkshire Archeological Society, 1928), 5 vols., 4:204. Winifrede Maxwell is also mentioned on this page.
54. London, 1740.
55. ODNB.
56. Challoner, *Garden of the Soul*, 19.
57. Thomas Seaton, *The devotional Life render'd familiar, easy, and pleasant, in several hymns upon the most common occasions of human life* (London: J. Roberts, 1734).
58. London: J. Downing, 1716.
59. Maxwell, *The faithful pair*, 4.
60. Maxwell, *The faithful pair*, 11.
61. Latin verse was usually written in hexameters.
62. Maxwell, *The faithful pair*, 13.
63. Maxwell, *The faithful pair*, 13–14.
64. Maxwell, *The faithful pair*, 25–26.
65. Maxwell, *The faithful pair*, 26.
66. Maxwell, *The faithful pair*, 27.

67. Ovid, *Ovid's Metamorphoses, in fifteen books. Translated by Mr. Dryden. Mr. Addison.* [. . .], 2 vols. 2nd ed. (London, 1720), 2:156.
68. The play became famous, and would have been known to Maxwell, because it was plagiarized by George Powell's *The Imposture Defeated, or, A Trick to Cheat the Devil* (London, 1697).
69. Ovid, *Metamorphoses*, trans. Dryden, 159.
70. John Vanbrugh, *The Relapse, or virtue in Danger* (London: John Briscoe, 1697), 48.
71. Mary Pix, *The Deceiver Deceiv'd* (London: R. Basset, 1698), 14.
72. Maxwell, *The faithful pair*, 38.

10. Priscilla Pointon Gets Married

1. The poem was first republished by Roger Lonsdale in his *Eighteenth-Century Women Poets: An Oxford Anthology* (Oxford: Oxford University Press, 1989), and now Pointon is a standard addition to lists of eighteenth-century poets.
2. Priscilla Pointon, *Poems on Several Occasions* (Birmingham: T. Warren, 1770), 31.
3. As Jess Domanico points out, the "Consolatary Ode" exists in three forms: as an excerpt in the *Birmingham Gazette* for 12 September 1768; in a short form purportedly "the first Poetical Composition of the Author's," aged thirteen, in *Poems on Several Occasions*, 11; and as "Consolatory Reflections, that have Occasionally occurred on that most lamentable Incident, My Loss of Sight: with Some few Alterations and Additions, to what I had at first composed upon this melancholy Subject," in *Poems on Several Occasions*, 99 (Jess Domanico, "Reading the Blind Poetess of Lichfield: The Consolatory Odes of Priscilla Poynton," in *The Idea of Disability in the Eighteenth Century*, ed. Chris Mounsey, 203–22 [Lewisburg, PA: Bucknell University Press, 2014]).
4. Mounsey, "Blind Woman on the Rampage."
5. Simon Dickie, *Cruelty and Laughter: Forgotten Comic Literature and the Unsentimental Eighteenth Century* (Chicago: University of Chicago Press, 2011), 86.
6. PP, *Poems on Several Occasions*, 1770, 100.
7. PP, *Poems on Several Occasions*, 1770, 100.
8. PP, *Poems on Several Occasions*, 1770, 101.
9. PP, *Poems on Several Occasions*, 1770, 42–43.
10. PP, *Poems on Several Occasions*, 1770, 48, Extempore Advice, by the Author to her Brother, when newly appointed Surgeon to a Man of War.
11. These are discussed in more detail below.
12. PP, *Poems on Several Occasions*, 1770, 15.
13. PP, *Poems on Several Occasions*, 1770, 13.
14. PP, *Poems on Several Occasions*, 1770, 36. "The following lines by the Author, To her cousin Miss M.B. of Chester, On entering her Teens. Written Extempore."
15. PP, *Poems on Several Occasions*, 1770, 48.
16. PP, *Poems on Several Occasions*, 1770, 47.
17. Jess Domanico, "Reading the Blind Poetess of Lichfield," 205.
18. Bill Overton, "Journeying in the Eighteenth Century: British Verse Epistle," *Studies in Travel Writing* 13, no. 1 (2009): 3–25.
19. PP, *Poems on Several Occasions*, 1770, 13, 27, 81, 86, 100.

20. PP, *Poems, on Several Occasions* 1770, 8, 15, 40, 50, 68, 83, 91, 95.
21. PP, *Poems on Several Occasions*, 1770, 26, 82, 83, 84.
22. PP, *Poems on Several Occasions*, 1770, 14.
23. PP, *Poems on Several Occasions*, 1770, 23. He is attacked once again on page 92, for not returning the copy of her Consolatory Ode she had sent him.
24. PP, *Poems on Several Occasions*, 1770, 26.
25. PP. *Poems on Several Occasions*, 1770, 32.
26. PP, *Poems on Several Occasions*, 1770, 39.
27. PP, *Poems on Several Occasions*, 1770, 87.
28. PP, *Poems on Several Occasions*, 1770, 88.
29. PP, *Poems on Several Occasions*, 1770, 45.
30. PP, *Poems on Several Occasions*, 1770, 58.
31. PP, *Poems on Several Occasions*, 1770, 60.
32. *Adams's Weekly Courant* (Chester, England), no. 1743, Tuesday, 10 April 1770; *Adams's Weekly Courant* (Chester, England), no. 2479, Tuesday, 15 August 1780.
33. Cheshire016_RS00013140_4018452_4018452_00716-PICKERING_JAMES.
34. PP, *Poems on Several Occasions*, 1770, 33.
35. PP, *Poems by Mrs. Pickering* (Birmingham: E. Piercy, 1794), 26.
36. PP, *Poems by Mrs. Pickering*, 1794, 27.
37. PP, *Poems on Several Occasions*, 1770, 20, 45.
38. PP, *Poems on Several Occasions*, 1770, 25.
39. PP, *Poems on Several Occasions*, 1770, 25.
40. PP, *Poems on Several Occasions*, 1770, 25.
41. PP, *Poems on Several Occasions*, 1770, 25.
42. PP, *Poems on Several Occasions*, 1770, 31–32.
43. There are some MS notes in the 1794 collection of poems by Dr. Parr, one of which suggests that PP was never clean. In sum the notes amount to no more than a nasty commentary defacing the book of poems, which makes me wonder why ECCO chose that copy to use when there is another, clean copy in the British Library.
44. Eliza Haywood, *The Adventures of Miss Betsy Thoughtless*, 4 vols. (London: Thomas Gardiner, 1751), 1:280–81.
45. Haywood, *Betsy Thoughtless*, 1:281.
46. PP, *Poems on Several Occasions*, 1770, 32.
47. Haywood, *Betsy Thoughtless*, 4:252.
48. Haywood, *Betsy Thoughtless*, 4:312.
49. Jemmy is a shortened form of James, Jeremy, or Jeremiah.
50. PP, *Poems on Several Occasions*, 1770, 33.
51. Eliza Haywood, *The History of Jemmy and Jenny Jessamy*, 3 vols. (London, 1753), 2:98.
52. PP, *Poems on Several Occasions*, 1770, 33.
53. Haywood, *Jemmy and Jenny Jessamy*, 2:46.
54. PP, *Poems on Several Occasions*, 1770, 33.
55. PP, *Poems on Several Occasions*, 1770, 34.
56. PP, *Poems on Several Occasions*, 1770, 34.
57. PP, *Poems by Mrs. Pickering*, 1794, 64, "To Mr J.P. On Drawing him Four Years Successively for a Valentine."

58. PP, *Poems on Several Occasions*, 1770, 33–34.
59. PP, *Poems on Several Occasions*, 1770, 36, 37, "The following lines by the Author, To her cousin Miss M.B. of Chester, On entering her Teens. Written Extempore," and "The following Lines on Retirement, which occurred to the Author during a short Visit in the Country."
60. PP, *Poems on Several Occasions*, 1770, 45.
61. PP, *Poems on Several Occasions*, 1770, 46.
62. PP, *Poems on Several Occasions*, 1770, 56. "The following Lines made extempore on Leaving Biana in Staffordshire, where the Author spent several agreeable months."
63. PP, *Poems on Several Occasions*, 1770, 82.
64. PP, *Poems by Mrs. Pickering*, 1794, 35.
65. PP, *Poems by Mrs. Pickering*, 1794, 20.
66. PP, *Poems by Mrs. Pickering*, 1794, iii.
67. PP, *Poems by Mrs. Pickering*, 1794, iii.
68. PP, *Poems by Mrs. Pickering*, 1794, iii.
69. The poem has been explored by A. V Simcock in "'Reason's Dim Telescope': A Poetic Tirade against Joseph Priestley, F.R.S.," *Notes and Records of the Royal Society of London* 49, no. 1 (January 1995): 79–84.
70. PP, *Poems on Several Occasions*, 1770, 26.
71. I have located the poem, "Verses addrest to my Niece, Miss S.N of Chester, Upon her Marriage," PP, *Poems by Mrs. Pickering*, 1794, 48, in several other places. The first suggests it was written too early to have been PP's own: Anon., *The Muse in a Moral Humour, By Several Hands*, 2 vols. (London, 1757), 2:249. Billed as "An Original Piece," it was sold separately as *Friendly Hints; which, being rightly observed, may prove very conducive to mutual happiness of both sexes in the married state* (Northampton, 1787). It is also passed off as the work of Esther Lewis, in *Poems moral and entertaining, written long since by Miss Lewis, then of Holt, now, for thirty years past wife of Mr Robert Clark of Tetbury* (Bath, 1789), 83. Although the poem also appears in Mr. Addison, *Interesting Anecdotes, memoirs, allegories, essays and poetic fragments, tending to amuse the fancy, and inculcate morality*, 12 vols. (London: 1794), 2:225, there is no reason to believe the poem is Addison's, and it does not appear under his name until this publication.
72. PP, *Poems by Mrs. Pickering*, 1794, iv.
73. PP, *Poems by Mrs. Pickering*, 1794, 20.
74. PP, *Poems by Mrs. Pickering*, 1794, 20.
75. PP, *Poems by Mrs. Pickering*, 1794, 23.
76. PP, *Poems by Mrs. Pickering*, 1794, 58.
77. PP, *Poems by Mrs. Pickering*, 1794, 24.
78. PP, *Poems by Mrs. Pickering*, 1794, 24.
79. PP's sister is memorialized in the third poem addressed to her "On the Death of the Author's Sister, Mrs Woolaston, of the Groves, near Enville." A Mr. Woolaston of Apley, Salop subscribed to the first collection, and Apley is one of the greatest houses in Shropshire, but it was the home of the Whitmore family. The National Archives mention one "Mr Henry Wollaston of the Groves p. Enfield," and even modern maps show a farm called "The Groves."
80. PP, *Poems by Mrs. Pickering*, 1794, 21.

81. PP, *Poems by Mrs. Pickering*, 1794, 45.
82. PP, *Poems by Mrs. Pickering*, 1794, iii.
83. PP, *Poems by Mrs. Pickering*, 1794, *Additional Poems*, 2.
84. Jess Domanico, "Reading 'The Blind Poetess of Lichfield': The Consolatory Odes of Priscilla Poynton," in *The Idea of Disability in the Eighteenth Century*, ed. Chris Mounsey (Lewisburg, PA: Bucknell University Press, 2013), 215.
85. PP, *Poems on Several Occasions*, 1770, 37–38.
86. These quotes are taken from the UK Government Report "Public Perceptions of Disabled People," https://www.gov.uk/government/uploads/system/uploads/attachment_data/file/325989/ppdp.pdf.

SELECTED BIBLIOGRAPHY

A. J., *A compleat account of the Portugueze language. Being a copious dictionary of English with Portugueze, and Portugueze with English. Together With an Easie and Unerring Method of its Pronunciation, by a distinguishing Accent, and a Compendium of all the necessary Rules of Construction and Orthography digested into a Grammatical Form. To which is Subjoined by way of appendix Their usual Manner of Correspondence by Writing, being all suitable, as well to the Diversion and Curiosity of the Inquisitive Traveller, as to the Indispensible Use and Advantage of the more Industrious Trader and Navigator to most of the known Parts of the World. By A. J.* London: printed by R. Janeway, for the Author, 1701.

Addison, Joseph. *An Essay on the Georgics.* In *The works of Virgil containing his Pastorals, Georgics and Aeneis: Adorn'd with a hundred sculptures, translated into English verse by Mr. Dryden,* by John Dryden. London: Jacob Tonson, 1693.

Aikin, John. *A manual of materia medica, containing a brief account of all the simples directed in the London and Edinburgh dispensatories, with their several preparations and the principal compositions into which they enter.* Yarmouth, Downes and March, 1785.

Aikin, John, and William Johnson. *General Biography.* London: John Stockdale &c, 1814.

Albert, Daniel M., and Sarah L. Atzen. *Chevalier John Taylor, England's Early Oculist: Pretender or Pioneer?* Madison, WI: Parallel, 2012.

Anon. *The Celestial Envoy: or, a scene not yet Acted. Containing some short notations on the 10th chapter of the Book of Apocalypse. Humbly inscrib'd to the E—of OX—D.* London: printed by R. Janeway, in Dogwel-Court in White Friars, for the Author, 1713.

Anon. "Eloge de M.Georges Mareschal." In *Mémoires de l'Académie Royale de Chirurgie,* vol. 2. Paris: Delaguette, 1753.

Anon. *The Life and Extraordinary History of the Chevalier John Taylor.* London: M. Cooper, 1761.

Anon. *Mémoire pour le sieur François La Peyronie premier chirurgien du roy . . . et les prevosts & collége des maîtres en chirurgie de Paris; contre les doyen & docteurs-régens de la Faculté de médecine de Paris, et contre l'Université de Paris.* Paris: Imp. de Charles Osmont, 1746.

Anon. *The Operator.* London: T. Payne, 1740.

Anon. "Part of a Letter from Richard Waller, Esq; S.R.S. to Dr. Hans Sloane, R.S. Secr. concerning Two Deaf Persons, Who can Speak and Understand What is Said to Them by the Motion of the Lips." *Philosophical Transactions of the Royal Society* 25 (1706): 2468–69.

Atkins, John. *The navy surgeon; or, practical system of surgery. With a dissertation on cold and hot mineral springs; and physical observations on the coast of Guiney.* London: J. Hodges, 1742.

Austen, Jane. *Mansfield Park.* iBooks ed. https://itun.es/gb/rp2Kx.l.

Bacon, Francis. *Sir Francis Bacon his apologie, in certaine imputations concerning the late Earle of Essex VVritten to the right Honorable his very good Lord, the Earle of Deuonshire, Lord Lieutenant of Ireland.* London: Felix Norton, 1604.

Banister, John. *A needefull, new, and necessarie treatise of chyrurgerie briefly comprehending the generall and particuler curation of vlcers, drawen foorth of sundrie worthy wryters, but especially of Antonius Calmeteus Vergesatus, and Ioannes Tagaltius, by Iohn Banister . . . Hereunto is anexed certaine experiments of mine ovvne inuention, truely tried, and daily of me practised.* London: Thomas Marshe, 1575.

Berchielli, Laura. "Colour, Space and Figure in Locke: An Interpretation of the Molyneux Problem." *Journal of the History of Philosophy* 40, no. 1 (2002): 47–65.

Berkeley, George. *An Essay Towards a New Theory of Vision.* Dublin: printed by Aaron Rhames for Jeremy Pepyat, 1709 and 1710.

Bidloo, Govard. *Anatomia humani corporis.* Amsterdam, 1685.

Billings, Peter. *Folly Predominant.* London: H. Carpenter, 1755.

Brisseau, Pierre. *Traité de la cataracte et du glaucoma.* Paris: Laurent d'Houry, 1709.

Bruno, Michael, and Eric Mandelbaum. "Locke's Answer to Molyneux's Thought Experiment." *History of Philosophy Quarterly* 27, no. 2 (April 2010): 165–80.

Burney Collection. Selected Newspapers

Challoner, Richard. *The garden of the soul: or, a manual of spiritual exercises and instructions for Christians who (living in the world) aspire to devotion.* 6th ed., corrected. London: T.Meighan, 1751.

Chandler, George. *A treatise of a cataract, its nature, species, causes and symptoms, With A Distinct Representation of the operations by couching and extraction: and Mr. Daviel's comparative view of their respective merits; together with Some Hints concerning Means for preventing its Formation, and superseding the Necessity of either Operation; Extracted from the best Authors.* London: Cadell, 1775.

Cheselden, William. *The anatomy of the humane body.* London: N. Cliff, D. Jackson, and W. Innys, 1713.

Cheselden, William. *The anatomy of the humane body. With XXXIV copper-plates. By W. Cheselden, Surgeon to St. Thomas's-Hospital, and Fellow of the Royal Society.* 3rd ed. London: William Bowyer, 1726.

Cheselden, William. *The anatomy of the humane body. By William Cheselden, Surgeon to Her Majesty, F.R.S. and Surgeon to St. Thomas's-Hospital.* 4th ed. With the addition of an appendix, which also is printed separately for the use of those who have the former editions. London: William Bowyer, 1730.

Cheselden, William. *The anatomy of the humane body. By W. Cheselden, Surgeon to his Majesty's Royal Hospital at Chelsea Fellow of the Royal Society and Member of the Royal Academy of Surgeons at Paris.* 5th ed. With forty copper plates engrav'd by Ger: Vandergucht. London, 1740.

Cheselden, William. *The anatomy of the humane body. By W. Cheselden, Surgeon to his Majesty's Royal Hospital at Chelsea Fellow of the Royal Society and Member of the Royal Academy of*

Surgeons at Paris. 6th ed. With forty copper plates engrav'd by Ger: Vandergucht. London, 1741.

Cheselden, William. *Appendix to the fourth edition of The anatomy of the humane body for the use of those who have the former editions*. London: William Bowyer, 1730.

Cheselden, William. *Syllabus, sive index humani corporis partium anatomicus, in XXXV prolectiones distinctus. In usum theatri anatomici Wilhelmi Cheselden, chirurgi*. London, 1711.

Coats, George "The Chevalier Taylor." *Royal London Ophthalmic Hospital Reports* 20 (May 1913). Reprinted in Robert Rutson James, *Studies in the History of Ophthalmology in England Prior to the Year 1800*. 1933. Cambridge: Cambridge University Press, 2013.

Crisp, John. *Observations on the Nature and Theory of Vision*. London: J. Sewell, 1796.

Davis, Lennard J., ed. *The Disability Studies Reader*. 1st ed. New York: Routledge, 1997.

Davis, Lennard J., ed. *The Disability Studies Reader*. 4th ed. New York: Routledge, 2013.

Davis, Lennard J., ed. *The Disability Studies Reader*. 5th ed. New York: Routledge, 2017.

Defoe, Daniel. *The Fortunes and Misfortunes of the Famous Moll Flanders*. London: Chetwood and Edling, 1721[2].

Degenaar, Marjolein. *Molyneux's Problem: Three Centuries of Discussion on the Perception of Forms*. Dordrecht: Kluwer Academic, 1996.

Desloges, Pierre. *Observations d'un sourd et muèt, sur un cours élémentaire d'éducation des sourds et muèts*. Amsterdam and Paris: B. Morin, 1779.

Dickie, Simon. *Cruelty and Laughter: Forgotten Comic Literature and the Unsentimental Eighteenth Century*. Chicago: University of Chicago Press, 2011.

Domanico, Jess. "Reading the Blind Poetess of Lichfield: The Consolatory Odes of Priscilla Poynton." In *The Idea of Disability in the Eighteenth Century*, edited by Chris Mounsey, 203–22. Lewisburg, PA: Bucknell University Press, 2014.

Drake, Francis. *Eboracum: or the History and Antiquities of the City of York*. London: William Bowyer, 1739.

Dryden, John. *Alexander's Feast; or the Power of Musique. An Ode for St Cecilia's Day*. London: Tonson, 1697.

Dryden, John. *Eleonora*. London: Jacob Tonson, 1692.

Duck, Stephen. *Poems on Several Occasions*. London: J. Roberts, 1730.

Duddell, Benedict. *An appendix to the treatise of the horney-coat of the eye, and the cataract. With an answer to Mr. Cheselden's appendix, relating to his new operation upon the iris of the eye*. London: E. Howlatt, 1733.

Duddell, Benedict. *A treatise of the diseases of the horny-coat of the eye, and the various kinds of cataracts. To which is prefix'd, a method, entirely new, of scarifying the eyes for several disorders. With remarks on the practice of some oculists both at home and abroad. By Benedict Duddell, Surgeon and Oculist*. London: printed for John Clark at the Royal Exchange, and sold by J. Roberts in Warwick-Lane, 1729.

Eaton, Robert. *An Account of Dr. Eaton's Styptick Balsam*. London, 1723.

Forkel, Nikolaus. *Johann Sebastian Bach: His Life, Work and Art*. Translated by Charles Sandford Terry. New York: Harcourt Brace, 1920.

Foucault, Michel. *The Archaeology of Knowledge*. Translated by A. M. Sheridan Smith. London: Routledge, 2002.

Foucault, Michel. *The Birth of the Clinic*. Translated by A. M. Sheridan. London: Tavistock, 1973.

Foucault, Michel. *Naissance de la clinique*. Paris: Presses Universitaires de France, 1963.
Gabbard, Dwight Christopher. "Disability Studies and the British Long Eighteenth Century." *Literature Compass* 8, no. 2 (2011): 80–94. 10.1111/j.1741-4113.2010.00771.x.
Garland-Thomson, Rosemarie. "A Habitable World: Harriet McBryde Johnson's 'Case for My Life.'" *Hypatia: A Journal of Feminist Philosophy* 30, no. 1 (Winter 2015): 300–306.
Garth, Samuel. *The dispensary a poem, in six canto's*. London: John Nutt, 1699.
Gesner, Konrad. *The newe iewell of health wherein is contayned the most excellent secretes of phisicke and philosophie, deuided into fower bookes. In the which are the best approued remedies for the diseases as well inwarde as outwarde, of all the partes of mans bodie: treating very amplye of all dystillations of waters, of oyles, balmes, quintessences, with the extraction of artificiall saltes, the vse and preparation of antimonie, and potable gold. Gathered out of the best and most approued authors, by that excellent doctor Gesnerus. Also the pictures, and maner to make the vessels, furnaces, and other instrumentes therevnto belonging. Faithfully corrected and published in Englishe, by George Baker, chirurgian*. London: Henrie Denham, 1576.
Gills, Thomas. *Advice to youth: or, instructions for young men and maids. By Thomas Gill, the blind man of St. Edmonds-Bury, Suffolk*. London, 1709.
Gills, Thomas. *The Blind man's case at London: or, a character of that city. Sent in a letter to his friend in the country*. London, 1711.
Gills, Thomas. *Instructions for children, in verse*. London, 1707.
Gills, Thomas. *Instructions for children, in verse. By Thomas Gills [. . .]*. London, 1709.
Gills, Thomas. *Lamentation on the death of His Grace Duke Hamilton. By Thomas Gill, the blindman of St. Edmund's-Bury, Suffolk*. London, 1712.
Gills, Thomas. *New-year's gift: or, a poem upon the circumsision [sic] of our Blessed Lord and Saviour Jesus Christ. By Thomas Gill [. . .]*. London, 1710.
Gills, Thomas. *Practical catechism: or, instructions for children, in verse. By Thomas Gill [. . .]*. London, 1710
Gills, Thomas. *Questions and answers. In verse, upon the creation of the world, the fall of man, the flood, and several other passages out of the Old Testament. By Thomas Gill, blindman, of St. Edmund's-Bury, Suffolk*. London, 1712.
Gills, Thomas. *Thomas Gills of St. Edmund's Bury in Suffolk, upon the recovery of his sight, and the second loss thereof*. London, 1710.
Gills, Thomas. *Useful and delightful instructions by way of dialogue between the master & his scholar, containing the duty of children. Composed in verse [. . .]*. London, 1712.
Gills, Thomas. *Useful and delightful instructions, by way of dialogue between the master & his scholar. Containing the duty of children. Composed in verse [. . .]*. London, 1716.
Girard, L. "Dislocation of Cataractous Lens by Enzymatic Zonulolysis: A Suggested Solution to the Problem of the 18 Million Individuals Blind from Cataracts in Third-World Countries." *Ophthalmic Surgery* 26, no. 4. (July-August 1995): 343–45.
Goldgar, Bertrand A. "Pope and the *Grub-Street Journal*." *Modern Philology* 74, no. 4 (May 1977): 366–80.
Goldsmith, Oliver. *The citizen of the world; or letters from a Chinese philosopher, residing in London, to his friends in the east*. London: John Newbery, 1762.
Griffin, John. *Proposals for the relief and support of maimed, aged, and disabled seamen, in the merchants service of Great Britain. Humbly offer'd to all Lovers of their Country, and to all true Friends to Trade and Navigation. By John Griffin, Mariner*. London, 1745.

Hartley, David. *Observations on Man, his Frame, his Duty, and his Expectations.* London and Bath: S. Richardson, 1749.
Haslam, Fiona. *From Hogarth to Rowlandson: Medicine in Art in Eighteenth-Century Britain.* Liverpool: Liverpool University Press, 1996.
Haywood, Eliza. *The Adventures of Miss Betsy Thoughtless.* 4 vols. London: Thomas Gardiner, 1751.
Haywood, Eliza. *The Dumb Projector: Or, a Trip to Holland made by Mr. Duncan Campbell.* London: W. Ellis, J. Roberts, Mrs Bilingsly, A. Dod and J. Fox, 1725.
Haywood, Eliza. *The History of Jemmy and Jenny Jessamy.* 3 vols. London: Thomas Gardiner, 1753.
Haywood, Eliza. *A Spy on the Conjurer.* London: printed for J. Peele at Mr. Locke's-Head in Pater-Noster-Row, 1724.
Hearne, Thomas. *Remarks and Collections.* 11 vols. Edited by C. E. Doble. Oxford: Clarendon, 1885.
Hosack, David. "Observations on vision, Communicated by George Pearson M.D. F.R.S." *Philosophical Transactions.* [London], [1794].
Hufton, Olwen. *The Poor of Eighteenth Century France 1750–1789.* Oxford: Clarendon, 1974.
J. O., "Thomas Gill, the Blind Man of St. Edmundsbury." *Notes and Queries* 1–5, no. 139 (June 1852): 608.
Jurin, James. *An epistle to John Ranby, Esq; Principal Serjeant Surgeon to His Majesty, And F.R.S. on the subject of his Narrative of the last illness of the late Earl of Orford, as far as it relates to Sir Edward Hulse, Dr Jurin, and Dr Crowe.* London: Jacob Robinson, 1745.
Kafer, Alison. *Feminist, Queer, Crip.* Bloomington: Indiana University Press, 2013.
Kennedy, Peter. *An essay on external remedies. Wherein it is considered, whether all the curable distempers incident to human bodies, may not be cured by outward means. Founded upon the certain Experience, Observation, and Practice, both of Antients and Moderns. Where it is also made plain by Simple Mechanical Reasonings, that it is not absolutely necessary for Medicines to be communicated by the Mouth, as Aliment, or common Nourishment. Together with the Methodical Prescriptions, or particular Manner, of Curing the said Distempers. To which is added, some thoughts on the manner of chirurgical remedies operating in wounds and ulcers, or other common Applications in Surgery; that from manifest Observations in Practice it seems highly probable, they operate after the same manner as when taken at the Mouth.* London: Andrew Bell, 1715.
Kennedy, Peter. *Ophthalmographia; or, a treatise of the eye, in two parts. Part I. Containing a New and Exact Description of the Eye; as also the Theory of the Vision considered, with its Diseases. Part II. Containing the Signs, Causes, and Cure of the Maladies incident to the Eye. To which is added an appendix of some of the diseases of the ear; wherein is observed the Communication between these Two Organs.* London: Bernard Lintott, 1713.
Kennedy, Peter. *A supplement to Kennedy's Ophthalmographia; or, treatise of the eye; in which is observ'd the plagiarism (from that treatise) contain'd in Dr. Bracken's Farriery. Remarks on Dr. Porterfield's Motions of the eye, in the Medical Essays, with the Difference in Opinions of Cataracts, explain'd and reconcil'd. Also on William Cheselden Esq; his Observations on the Eye, &c. in his Anatomy; and of the Improvements made in our Hospitals, &c. On Dr. P. Shaw, in his Practice of Physick; Dr. Jurin on Vision; and Mr. Sharp on the Operations of Surgery.* London: T. Cooper, 1739.

King, Steven, and Alana Tomkins, eds. *The Poor in England 1700–1850*. Manchester: Manchester University Press, 2003.

Lane, Harlan, ed. *The Deaf Experience: Classics in Language and Education*. Translated by Franklin Philip. Cambridge: Harvard University Press, 1984.

Lavery, Brian. *Royal Tars: The Lower Deck of the Royal Navy, 875–1850*. Annapolis, MD: Naval Institute Press, 2010.

Lenth, Bert. "Bach and the English Oculist." *Music & Letters* 19, no. 2 (April 1938): 182–98.

Locke, John. *Essay concerning Humane Understanding*. 1st ed. London: Thomas Dring and Samuel Manship, 1690.

Locke, John. *Essay concerning Humane Understanding*. 2nd ed. London: Thomas Dring and Samuel Manship, 1694.

Maat, Jaap. "Teaching Language to a Boy Born Deaf in the Seventeenth Century: The Holder-Wallis Debate." *History and Philosophy of the Language Sciences*. https://hiphilangsci.net/2013/11/06/teaching-language-to-a-boy-born-deaf-in-the-seventeenth-century-the-holder-wallis-debate.

Maitre-Jean, Antoine. *Traité des maladies de l'oeil*. Paris: Jacques Lefebvre, 1707.

Maxwell, John. *A continuation of a book, lately publish'd; call'd the polite assembly: or, the charms of solitude displayed*. York: Thomas Gent, 1759.

Maxwell, John. *The conversation: or, the lady's tale. A novel*. York: Thomas Gent, 1747.

Maxwell, John. *The faithful pair: or, virtue in Distress. A tragedy. By John Maxwell, being Blind*. York: Thomas Gent, 1740.

Maxwell, John. *A new tragedy, call'd, the loves of Prince Emilius and Lovisa*. York: Thomas Gent, 1755.

Maxwell, John. *A new tragedy: cali'd [sic], The distressed virgin*. York: Thomas Gent, 1761.

Maxwell, John. *The polite assembly: or, the Charms of Solitude Display'd*. York: Thomas Gent, 1757.

Maxwell, John. *The reflection. A poem*. York: Thomas Gent, 1743.

Maxwell, John. *The royal captive. A tragedy*. York: Thomas Gent, 1745.

Milton, John. *Paradise Lost*. London: Peter Parker and Robert Boulter, 1667.

Mitchell, David T., and Sharon L. Snyder. *Narrative Prosthesis: Disability and the Dependencies of Discourse*. Ann Arbor: University of Michigan Press, 2001.

Monaghan, Leila Frances. *Many Ways to Be Deaf: International Variation in Deaf Communities*. Washington, DC: Gallaudet University Press, 2013.

Moritz, Karl Philipp. *Travels, chiefly on foot, through several parts of England, in 1782. Described in letters to a friend, by Charles P. Moritz, a literary gentleman of Berlin*. London: G. G and J. Robinson, 1795.

Mounsey, Chris. "Blind Woman on the Rampage: Priscilla Pointon's Grand Tour of the Midlands and the Question of the Legitimacy of Sources for Biography." In *Voice and Context in Eighteenth-Century Verse: Order and Variety*, edited by Joanna Fowler and Allan Ingram, 230–47. Basingstoke: Palgrave, 2015.

Mounsey, Chris. "'God grant us Grace, that we may take due Pains, / To practice what this Exercise contains; / To which, if we apply our best Endeavour, / We shall be happy here, and bless'd for ever': Thomas Gills: An Eighteenth-Century Blind Poet and the Language of Charity." In *The Idea of Disability in the Eighteenth Century*, ed. Mounsey, 223–47. Lewisburg, PA: Bucknell University Press, 2014:

Nardizzi, Vin. "Disability Figures in Shakespeare." In *The Oxford Handbook of Shakespeare and Embodiment: Gender, Sexuality and Race*, edited by Valerie Traub. Oxford: Oxford University Press, 2016.

Neher, Allister. "The Truth about Our Bones: William Cheselden's *Osteographia*." *Medical History* 54, no. 4 (October 2010): 517–28.

Nelson, Robert. *A companion for the festivals and fasts of the Church of England: With collects and prayers for each solemnity*. London: printed by W.B. for A. and J. Churchill, at the Black Swan in Pater Noster Row, 1704.

Obituary of Robert Rutson James. *Annals of the Royal College of Surgeons* 25, no.4 (November 1959): 264. http://www.ncbi.nlm.nih.gov/pmc/articles/PMC2413917/pdf/annrcse00354-0058a.pdf.

O'Hehir, Brendan. "Meaning of Swift's 'Description of a City Shower.'" *English Literary History* 27, no. 3 (September 1960): 194–207.

Oldys, William. *Observations of the Cure of William Taylor, the Blind Boy of Ightham, in Kent*. London: E. Owen, 1753.

Overton, Bill. "Journeying in the Eighteenth Century: British Verse Epistle." *Studies in Travel Writing* 13, no. 1 (February 2009): 3–25.

Ovid. *Ovid's Metamorphoses, in fifteen books. Translated by Mr. Dryden. Mr. Addison. Dr. Garth. Mr. Mainwaring. Mr. Congreve. Mr. Rowe. Mr. Pope. Mr. Gay. Mr. Eusden. Mr. Croxall. And other eminent hands. Publish'd by Sir Samuel Garth, M.D. Adorn'd with sculptures*. 2 vols. 2nd ed. Vol. 2. London, 1720.

P. L., *A letter from an apothecary in London, to his friend in the country; concerning the present practice of physick, in regard to empiricks, empirical methods of cure, and nostrums. With remarks on Dr. Meads, Mr. Freke's, and Mr. Cheselden's method of cure for the itch, by externals only; setting forth the Dangerous Consequences of such a Method, if adhered to indiscriminately. Also some observations upon manna, shewing it to be a Composition though commonly supposed a Natural Production; with remarks on Dr. Mead's certain cure for the bite of a mad dog*. London: M. Cooper, 1752.

Park, Desiree. "Locke and Berkeley on the Molyneux Problem." *Journal of the History of Ideas* 30, no. 2. (April-June 1969): 253–60.

Paxton, Peter. *An essay concerning the body of man, wherein its changes or diseases are consider'd, and the operations of medicines observ'd*. London: Richard Wilkin, 1701.

Pelling, Margaret. "Corporationalism or Individualism: Parliament, the Navy, and the Splitting of the London Barber Surgeons' Company in 1745." In *Guilds and Associations in Europe, 900–1900*, edited by Ian A. Gadd and Patrick Wallace. London: Centre for Metropolitan History, 2006.

Pettis, W. *Some memoirs of the life of John Radcliffe*. London, 1715.

Philips, John. *The Splendid Shilling*. London: Thomas Bennet, 1705.

Pickering, Priscilla (nee Pointon). *Poems by Mrs. Pickering*. Birmingham: E. Piercy, 1794.

Pitt, Robert. *The Crafts and Frauds of Physic Expos'd*. London: Thomas Childe, 1703.

Pix, Mary. *The Deceiver Deceiv'd*. London: R. Basset, 1698.

Pointon, Priscilla. *Poems on Several Occasions*. Birmingham: T. Warren, 1770.

Pope, Alexander. *An Essay on Criticism*. London: W. Lewis, W. Taylor, T. Osborn, J. Graves, 1711.

Pope, Alexander. *First epistle of the first book of Horace imitated*. London: R. Dodsley, 1738.

Pope, Alexander. *Ode for Musick*. London: Bernard Lintott, 1713.
Pope, Alexander. *Windsor Forest*. London: Bernard Lintott, 1713.
Porter, Roy. *Health for Sale: Quackery in England, 1660–1850*. Manchester: Manchester University Press, 1989.
Quartararo, Anne Therese. *Deaf Identity and Social Images in Nineteenth-Century France*. Washington, DC: Gallaudet University Press, 2008.
Ranby, John. *The Method of Treating Gun-Shot Wounds*. London: John and Paul Knapton, 1744.
Ranby, John. *Narrative of the last illness of the Earl of Orford, from May 1744 to the day of his decease, 18 March following*. London: John and Paul Knapton, 1745.
Read, William. *A short but exact account of all the diseases incident to the eyes, with the causes, symptoms and cures. Also practical observations upon some extraordinary diseases of the eyes. By Sir William Read, Her Majesty's Oculist, and Operator in the Eyes in Ordinary*. London: printed, and sold by J. Baker, at the Black-Boy in Pater-Noster-Row, [1710?].
Rutson James, Robert. *Studies in the History of Ophthalmology in England Prior to the Year 1800*. 1933. Reprint, Cambridge: Cambridge University Press, 2013.
Saint-Yves, Charles, de. *A new treatise of the diseases of the eyes. Containing proper remedies, and describing the chirurgical operations requisite for their cures. With some new Discoveries in the Structure of the Eye, That demonstrate the immediate Organ of Vision. By M. de St. Yves, Surgeon Oculist of the Company of Paris. Together with the author's answer to M. Mouchard. Translated from the original French. By J. Stockton, M.D.* London: Crokatt, Osborne and Smith, 1741.
Sakula, A. "Dr John Radcliffe, Court Physician, and the Death of Queen Anne." *Journal of the Royal College of Physicians of London* 19, no. 4 (October 1985): 255–60.
Seaton, Thomas. *The devotional Life render'd familiar, easy, and pleasant, in several hymns upon the most common occasions of human life*. London: J. Roberts, 1734.
Settle, Elkanah. *Thalia Triumphans*. London, 1715, 1716, and 1722.
Sharp, Samuel. "A Description of a New Method of Opening the Cornea, in Order to Extract the Crystalline Humour; By Mr. Samuel Sharp, Surgeon to Guy's Hospital, and F.R.S." *Philosophical Transactions* 48 (1753): 161–63.
Sharp, Samuel. "A Second Account of the New Method of Opening the Cornea, for Taking Away the Cataract; By Samuel Sharp, Surgeon to Guy's Hospital, and F.R.S." *Philosphical Transactions* 48 (1753): 322–31.
Sharp, Samuel. *A treatise on the operations of surgery, with a description and representation of the instruments used in performing them*. London: J. Brotherton &c, 1739.
Simcock, A. V. "Reason's Dim Telescope": A Poetic Tirade against Joseph Priestley, F.R.S." *Notes and Records of the Royal Society of London* 49, no. 1 (January 1995): 79–84.
Singer, Peter. *Practical Ethics*. 1980. Reprint, Cambridge: Cambridge University Press, 2011.
Sokoll, Thomas. *Essex Pauper Letters 1731–1837*. Oxford: Clarendon, 2001.
Sprengell, "Dr." "Some Observations upon Dr. Eaton's Styptick By Dr. Sprengell, R.S.S. Coll. Med. Lond. Lic." *Philosophical Transactions* 33 (1724) 381–91, 108–14.
Sydenham, Thomas. *The compleat method of curing almost all diseases to which is added an exact description of their several symptoms / written in Latin by Dr. Thomas Sydenham; and now faithfully Englished*. London: printed and are to be sold by Randal Taylor, 1694.
Taylor, John. *An Account of some of the many Remarkable Cures of Various Diseases of the Eyes,*

performed by John Taylor, Oculist of Hatton Garden, who practiced for upwards of thirty years in London only. Reprint, London, 1777.

Taylor, John. *An account of the mechanism of the eye. Wherein its power of refracting the rays of light, and causing them to converge at the retina, is consider'd: With an Endeavour to ascertain the true Place of a Cataract, and to shew the good or ill Consequences of a Judicious or Injudicious Removal of it. By John Taylor, Surgeon in Norwich.* Norwich: Henry Cross-Grove, 1727.

Taylor, John. *The History of the Travels and Adventures of the Chevalier John Taylor, Opthalmiater.* London: J. Williams, 1762.

Taylor, John. *An impartial inquiry into the seat of the immediate organ of sight: viz. whether the retina or choroïdes. Being the subject of a lecture, in a course lately given on the nature and cure of the diseases of the eye.* London: M. Cooper, 1742.

Taylor, John. *Records of My Life.* New York: J&J Harper, 1833.

Taylor, John. *Treatise on the diseases of the Chrystalline Humour of a Human Eye.* London: James Roberts, 1736.

Tunstall, Kate E. *Blindness and Enlightenment.* London: Continuum, 2011.

Vanbrugh, John, *The Relapse, or virtue in Danger.* London: John Briscoe, 1697.

Wasserman, Earl R. "Pope's Ode for Musick." *English Literary History* 28, no. 2 (June 1961):163–86.

Wells, Charles William. *An Essay on Single Vision with Two Eyes.* London: T. Cadell, 1792.

Williams, Raymond. *Marxism and Literature.* Oxford: Oxford University Press, 1977.

Yule, Henry. *The Book of Ser Marco Polo.* London: John Murray, 1871.

INDEX

able seaman, 24, 25, 38
Académie Royale de Chirurgie, 111
Académie Royale des Sciences de Paris, 111
Addison, Joseph, 31, 68, 89, 157
amanuensis, 254, 256, 267, 272
American Civil War, 22, 33
Amyand, Serjeant Nicholas, 122, 146
Anne (queen of England), 6, 70, 78, 81
Arbuthnot, John, 118
Aristotle, 228
Arne, Thomas, 185
artificial pupil, 109, 130–31, 140
Austen, Jane, *Mansfield Park*, 24–25

Bach, J. S., 129
Bacon, Francis, 7–8, 77, 157
Banister, John, 93, 97
Banister, Richard, 66–67, 93
Baron Wenzel, 131, 194
Bartholomew Close, 73, 222
bee, 229, 265
Berkeley, George, 43, 48–53, 56–61, 105, 178
Blacklock, Thomas, 13, 239
blindness, 3–4, 7, 13–14, 20–21, 36–39, 40, 42, 47–53, 61–66, 74, 86, 99, 122–24, 183, 195, 199, 205, 209, 227–31, 241–42, 248–51, 256, 259–60, 274–76; born blind, 10, 43, 47–47, 52–55, 58, 68, 87, 91, 105, 109, 114, 113–33, 178, 183, 225
Boddington, Thomas, 192
Bosanquet, Samuel, 192
Boyce, William, 9, 183–86
Brisseau, Pierre, 7, 118, 143
Burney Collection of Seventeenth- and Eighteenth-Century Newspapers, 15, 22, 279
butterfly, 229, 274

Campbell, Duncan, 29–32, 35, 37–38, 41
care, free at the point of delivery, 12, 84, 94, 132, 189, 195
Cater, Mary, 6, 15, 89–104, 168, 176
Challoner, Richard, *Garden of the Soul*, 240–41
charity, 13, 23, 37, 39–40, 82, 84–86, 88, 180, 182, 190, 207, 210, 237–38, 249
Chelsea Hospital, 23, 46, 111, 180
Cheselden, William, 6, 9, 11–12, 42, 47, 51–59, 69, 86, 93, 105–35, 141–45, 150, 171–72, 178, 180–81; *The anatomy of the humane body*, 106, 110, 116–17, 119
Chester, 250, 252, 253, 255–56, 262, 265–68, 270–71, 274

Churchwarden, 45, 82, 84, 86, 188, 189, 237
color, 54, 57, 113, 225, 227–29, 233
colour, 54, 57, 122, 124, 158–59, 166–67, 227–28, 232
Company of Barbers and Surgeons, 11, 69, 78, 93, 95, 112–16, 172, 292
Company of Spectacle Makers, 59
Company of Surgeons, 69, 93, 112–13, 117
compulsory able-bodiedness, 4, 13–14, 16, 26, 33, 95, 199
Condillac, Etiènne, 6, 36, 42, 51
Condorcet, Marquis de, 36
consilio manuque, 10, 78, 99, 101
Coram, Thomas, 180, 184
couching, 3, 6, 9, 11–12, 42–43, 47, 53–60, 70, 75, 78–83, 86–87, 91, 93, 110–11, 123–28, 129–67, 171–72, 178, 185–88, 193
Crome, Mrs. (of Deptford), 9, 121–26
Cross-Grove, Henry, 132, 134, 183
cultural model of disability, 4–5, 12, 13–14, 18, 20, 23, 26–27, 32, 40–41, 62, 259, 270, 275
cure, 7–8, 10, 17–18, 23–24, 45–47, 53, 58, 61, 65–68, 70, 72, 74–92, 94–104, 109, 113, 116–20, 126–27, 130–34, 136, 138, 143, 150–55, 165, 169, 171, 173–83, 185, 188–95, 199, 229–30, 276

Daviel, Jacques, 186, 286
Davis, Lennard J., *Disability Studies Reader*, 26–38, 41
Daza de Valves, Benito, 59
de Lapeyronie, François Gigot, 112
de Saint Yves, Charles, 8, 130, 186
deafness, 4, 17, 25, 27–30, 32–38, 41–42
Defoe, Daniel, 29, 34–35, 42, 89
depression, 223, 246, 250, 251, 255, 256, 259, 262, 264
Desloges, Pierre, 33–36, 38, 42
Dickie, Simon, 250

Diderot, Denis, 36, 51
disability history, 22
disability studies, 5, 20, 22, 26–33, 38, 41, 62
disabled, 4, 13, 16–18, 22–26, 33, 42, 194, 200, 275
disease, 7, 9, 18, 44, 46, 66–67, 69, 74–76, 89, 91, 115–18, 123, 133, 137–40, 142, 155, 158, 171–73, 177–78, 182, 188–89, 193, 199
Dorothy Wilson Trust, 39, 237–38
Dryden, John, 225–26, 234–35, 246–47
Duck, Stephen, 227–28, 233
Duddell, Benedict, 97–98, 114–15, 122
Durham Yard, 10, 73, 79, 82, 88–91

empiricism, 48–49, 51–55, 178, 231
empirick, 7–8, 65, 135–36, 154
Enlightenment, 3, 37, 42, 47, 50
Eulenspiegel, Till (Howleglasse), 59

Foote, Samuel, 26, 174
Foucault, Michel, 3, 6, 20–22, 37, 42–43, 47, 52; historical a priori, 21–22, 26, 32, 37
Foundling Hospital, 10, 180–84
freeman, 13–14, 78, 237–39
Freke, John, 12, 86

Gabbard, Dwight Christopher, 5
Galen, 7, 97, 119
garden, 73, 224–25, 232–35, 239–45, 248–49
Garland-Thomson, Rosemarie, 5, 18–20, 22
Garrick, David, 184
Garth, Samuel, *The Dispensary*, 98, 227
Gent, Thomas, 233
George I, 6, 31, 69, 94, 112
George II, 69, 112
George III, 131
George IV, 131
Gills, Thomas, 13–14, 199–223, 275; *Advice to youth: or, instructions for young men and*

maids, 200, 222; *The Blind man's case at London or, a character of that city*, 214–21; *Instructions for children, in verse*, 200, 221, 223; *Lamentation on the death of His Grace Duke Hamilton*, 212–14; *New-year's gift: or, a poem on the circumcision of our Blessed Lord and Saviour Jesus Christ*, 205–9; *Practical catechism: or, instructions for children, in verse*, 200, 221–23; *Questions and answers. In verse, upon the creation of the world, the fall of man, the flood*, 200, 222–23; *Upon the Nativity of the Blessed Saviour*, 209–12
glaucoma, 7, 74–76, 78, 99, 118, 143
Goldgar, Bertrand, 140–41
Goldsmith, Oliver, 3
Gray, Thomas, 229
Great War, 22, 33
Griffin, John (mariner), 23,24
Grub Street Journal, 139–46, 149–50
gutta serena, 44, 74–75, 99, 153

Hamilton, 4th Duke of (James Hamilton), 201, 212–14
Handel, G. F., 25, 129–30, 183; *Messiah*, 10, 183
Hartley, David, 52
Haywood, Eliza, 31–32, 41, 260–62
hearing, 17, 29–31, 36–37, 53, 116, 217, 230, 254, 279
heaven, 52, 58, 157, 160, 167, 184, 211, 232–33, 242–43, 246, 252, 262
Herring, Thomas (archbishop of York), 236, 239, 241
Hogarth, William, *The Company of Undertakers*, 147–48, 150, 154
Holder, William (deaf educator), 30
Homer, 124, 254
Hosack, David, 58
Houlston, William, 192

idealism, 48–53, 58, 60, 232
impairment, 4, 17–26, 38, 41, 76, 233
iridotomy, 9
itinerancy, 10–12, 46, 66, 74, 76, 78, 86–87, 89, 129, 133–36, 142, 161–69, 194

Janeway, Richard (printer), 201, 203, 205–6, 212
Jones, Henry (bricklayer poet), 157–58
Jurin, James, 113–14, 150

Kennedy, Peter, 6, 8, 89, 115–27, 132, 141, 145–46, 154, 178; *Ophthalmographia*, 8, 116–19, 123, 126–27, 145; *Supplement to Kennedy's Ophthalmographia*, 8, 115–16, 126

Liberace, 6, 166
Lichfield, 253, 265–66
lithotomy, 105, 110–11, 113, 125–26, 150
Locke, John, 36–37, 47–61, 114, 277
love, 13, 141, 153, 206–7, 214–15, 224–26, 230, 233–34, 241–48, 256, 258–59, 262–65, 268, 270–73, 275
Lucas, Charles, 173

Maître-Jean, Antoine, 7, 118–19
Mapp, Sally (bonesetter), 147, 149–55
Mareschal, Georges, 111–12
marketing strategy, 71, 173–74, 178, 193, 221, 249
marriage, 221, 226, 237, 239, 252, 255–58, 261–62, 265, 268–69, 273
Martyn, John, 140–41
materialism, 48–51, 53, 57, 231
Maxwell, John, 13–14, 224–49, 275; *A continuation of a book, lately publish'd; call'd, the polite assembly; or, the charms of solitude display'd*, 235, 236, 239, 249; *The conversation, or, the lady's tale. A novel,*

Maxwell, John (*continued*)
234, 249; *The faithful pair: or, virtue in Distress. A tragedy*, 233–34, 241, 248; *A new tragedy cali'd* [sic] *The distressed virgin*, 235, 239; *A new tragedy call'd the loves of Prince Emilius and Lovisa*, 234–35; *The polite assembly, or, the Charms of Solitude Display'd*, 235–36, 249; *The reflection*, 225, 227, 229, 232, 234–35, 241, 249; *The royal captive*, 234

McBryde Johnson, Harriet, "Case for My Life," 18–20, 22

Mead, Richard, 105, 117, 127

medical model of disability, 4–5, 6, 12, 18, 20, 23, 25–27, 40, 194

memory, 54, 161, 242–25, 233, 242, 245

Messiah (Handel), 10, 183

Milton, John, 156, 227–28, 233, 254

Mohun, 4th Baron (Charles Mohun), 201, 212–14

Molyneux, William, 47–60

Monsey, Messenger, 46, 180–82

Moritz, Karl Philipp, 3

mountebank, 65–66, 69, 80, 131–32, 135, 154, 157, 161, 168

Nardizzi, Vin, 33, 38

Narrative Prosthesis: Disability and the Dependencies of Discourse, 32

National Library of Scotland, 200, 209, 240

Nelson, Horatio, Lord, 25

Nelson, Robert, 210–11

newspaper advertisements, 15, 23, 42, 45–47, 59, 66–70, 73–74, 76–91, 94–107, 116, 125–26, 132, 136–38, 146, 152, 155, 169–78, 181–82, 185, 188, 190–94, 201, 222, 256

Norwich Gazette, 132, 136

novel, 19, 28–29, 35, 42, 161, 234–35, 260, 262

optical character recognition, 15

Oldys, William, 179–86

overseers of the poor, 177, 188–89, 193–94

Overton, Bill, 254

Oxford Dictionary of National Biography (ODNB), 66, 71, 92, 109–10, 127, 131, 183, 212

patented operations, 9, 110, 141

patent remedies, 91–92, 95

patient, 6, 10, 12, 46, 57, 59–60, 65, 69, 74–75, 78, 82–89, 99, 101–2, 107, 109, 113–15, 120–21, 130–31, 139, 143, 145, 151–52, 161, 165–66, 168–69, 171, 178, 180–83, 186, 188–89, 194–95

Philosophical Transactions, 105, 110, 120, 123

Pickering, James (husband of Priscilla Pointon), 255–58, 260–66, 268–71, 273–74

Pix, Mary, 235, 247–48

plagiarism, 67, 116, 118, 119, 229

Plato, 242

Pointon, Priscilla, 13–14, 223, 239, 250–76, 278; "Address to a Bachelor, On a Delicate Occasion," 250, 254–55; "Consolatory Reflections," 251, 253, 274; *Poems by Mrs. Pickering* (1794), 239, 252, 257, 266–67, 271–75; *Poems on Several Occasions* (1770), 250

Pope, Alexander, 105–6, 117, 131, 140, 225–28; *An Essay on Criticism*, 225–26; *Windsor forest*, 225, 227

Popham, Alexander, 29–30

Porter, Roy, 10, 87, 169–70

Porterfield, William, 59

Pourfour du Petit, Francois, 7

Prince William, Duke of Cumberland, 69, 112

Pygmalion, 246–47

quack, 8–10, 65–66, 70, 74, 80, 83, 91–92, 94, 105, 118, 129, 135–36, 142, 146–54, 168, 171

Ranby, John, 12, 69, 93–94, 112–14
Read, William, 6, 10–12, 15, 43, 58, 65–94, 95, 97, 102–7, 126–27, 131, 134, 168, 176, 278
Reid, Thomas, 36–37
reputation, 70, 83, 111, 125, 132–45, 147, 154, 162, 180
Rousseau, Jean-Jacques, 36
Royal College of Physicians (Edinburgh), 59
Royal College of Physicians (London), 65, 71, 77, 83, 93, 113
Royal Society, 30, 42, 58, 93, 105, 109, 114, 140, 186, 188
Russel, Richard, 140–41
Rutson James, Robert, 8–12, 67, 70, 74–76, 81, 109

same only different, the, 4, 14, 19–22, 41
Sandford, Joseph, 112
Saunderson, Nicholas, 52
Scarlett, Edward (royal optician), 60
School for the Indigent Blind, 192
seamen, 23–25, 38, 68, 86, 89, 91
self-presentation, 70, 83, 95, 106, 168, 169, 170, 172, 200, 201
self-promotion, 128, 131–32, 135–36, 140–43, 153
Settle, Elkanah, 226
Sharp, Samuel, 76, 127, 165, 186, 188
Sibthorpe Pinchard, Elizabeth, *The Blind Child or Anecdotes of the Wyndham Family*, 180
sighted, 17, 19, 22, 57, 59, 61, 119, 202, 225, 227, 230, 233, 259, 271–72, 275, 279
sign language, 29–31, 34–37, 41

Singer Rowe, Elizabeth, 233
Singer, Peter, *Practical Ethics*, 16–21, 25, 27
Smart, Christopher, 184, 226
smell, 148, 176, 226–28, 232, 245, 274–75
Snellen chart, 40
soldiers, 24, 66–67, 73, 85–87, 89, 91, 94, 96
sound, 30, 218, 225, 229, 232–33, 241, 245, 275
specialism, 6–12, 69–70, 85, 94, 97, 104, 114–19, 125–28, 131–36, 143, 146, 154, 157, 165–72, 177–78, 182–83, 186–90, 194–95
spectacles, 59, 60
Spectator, 30, 34, 41, 56–68, 74
Spence, Joseph, 13, 239
spontaneous overflow, 250, 253, 254, 255, 256–58, 260, 262–63, 269, 272
St. Bartholomew's Hospital, 12, 73, 78, 86, 148, 177
St. Cecilia, 225–26
St. Edmunds-Bury, 13, 73, 199–205, 214–15, 221–23
Steele, Richard, 31, 68, 89
St. Matthew, Bethnal Green, 190
St. Thomas's Hospital, 12, 105, 106, 111, 135
styptic, 70, 91, 93–94
subscriber, 14, 180–81, 234–36, 239, 241, 249, 266, 271
Swift, Jonathan, 66–69, 80, 86, 105, 201, 212, 214–15; "Description of a City Shower," 201, 214–15; *Examiner*, 68, 212

taste, 235
Tatler, 31, 68–69, 74, 89, 214
taxation (parish), 188, 190–92, 200, 221–23
Taylor, John (writer and journal editor), 186
Taylor, John "Chevalier," 10, 11, 12, 15, 70, 115, 117, 128, 129–67, 168, 170, 172, 173; *An account of the mechanism of the eye*, 115, 132, 134–35, 142, 157–58, 171–72

Taylor, John, oculist of Hatton Garden, 6, 9, 10, 43–47, 57, 168–94
Taylor, William, 6, 10, 57, 178, 180–87
temptation, 230, 251
text-to-voice software, 19–20, 22
textbooks, 11–12, 65, 106
Tories, 31, 41, 68, 71, 212–13
touch, 6, 48–55, 61, 127, 165, 205, 231, 246

uniqueness, 4–5, 32–33, 35, 38, 41–42, 49–50, 275

Valentine's Day, 257–58, 263–65, 273–74
Variability, 4–5, 20–22, 28, 41, 277; capability, 4–5, 14; capacity, 4–5, 14; encounter, 5, 14, 34, 41, 58, 61, 70–71
Vincent, François-Andre, *Zeuxis Choosing as Models the Most Beautiful Girls of the Town of Croton*, 27–28

Wallis, John (deaf educator), 29–30
Walpole, Galfridus, 24, 38
Walpole, Robert, 113–34, 150
Ward, Joshua, 147–54; "Pill and Drop," 147, 149
Ware, James, 192
Whig, 31, 41, 68, 71–72, 77, 212–13
William III, 6, 67, 71, 80, 81–82
Williams, Raymond, 28–29, 32
work, 14, 19, 23, 26, 34–41, 44, 46, 65, 67, 72, 74, 79–81, 84–87, 92, 100, 110–11, 163, 189, 205, 207, 209, 221–23, 238, 239, 266, 268

York Buildings, 72
Young, Edward, 166–67, 235

Zwinger, Johann Rodolph, 137–38

Peculiar Bodies: Stories and Histories

Questioning the body as the historical subject of experiences "peculiar" to it, this series examines the myriad forms of the body—healthy, diseased, athletic, crippled, alluring, pious—across all disciplines, periods, and geographic contexts. The series embraces a range of historical, literary, and philosophical methodologies and theories around the idea of "the body."

CPSIA information can be obtained
at www.ICGtesting.com
Printed in the USA
LVHW091656031119
636193LV00002B/80/P